# Brain and Mind

Andreas Steck • Barbara Steck

# Brain and Mind

Subjective Experience
and Scientific Objectivity

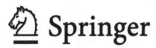
Springer

Andreas Steck
Professor of Neurology
University of Basel
Switzerland

Barbara Steck
Child and Adolescent Psychiatry and
  Psychotherapy
University of Basel
Switzerland

ISBN 978-3-319-37239-6      ISBN 978-3-319-21287-6 (eBook)
DOI 10.1007/978-3-319-21287-6

Springer Cham Heidelberg New York Dordrecht London
© Springer International Publishing Switzerland 2016
Softcover re-print of the Hardcover 1st edition 2016

Printed on acid-free paper

Springer International Publishing AG Switzerland is part of Springer Science+Business Media (www.springer.com)

# Foreword

I am not aware of any other book like this one. It represents a serious attempt to review the findings of contemporary neuroscience in broad brushstrokes—theoretical, empirical, and clinical—and to integrate them in a way that is both relevant and accessible to psychoanalytic psychotherapists (and other practitioners) working at the coalface of the mind–brain relationship.

By "coalface" I am referring to the *lived life* of the mind, and in particular to that aspect of it that we call mental suffering. The difficulties which bring people to psychotherapy are inevitably shaped partly by individual experiences and partly by biological universals—thus almost always by the interaction between these two. However, after the early works of Sigmund Freud which introduced such seminal concepts as libidinal drive and the Oedipus complex, and the like, psychoanalytic psychotherapists have by and large fallen woefully out of touch with developments in our understanding of the universal mechanisms that shape the mind—and therefore mental suffering.

This book seeks to redress this situation.

The authors are sensitive to the huge gulf that still separates the theoretical findings of the bench neuroscientist from the practical tasks facing the working psychotherapist, but they have sought to bridge the gap in the best possible way: via *clinical phenomena*. Also especially useful is their emphasis on development. The authors show how the new perspectives introduced by contemporary neuroscience provide practitioners with deeper understanding of the clinical and developmental problems they confront at the coalface.

I strongly recommend this book to every psychotherapist who acknowledges that there has been relevant progress in our knowledge of human biology since

Freud first published his *Three Essays on the Theory of Sexuality* more than a century ago. If you wish to acquaint yourself with this knowledge, I can think of no better place for you to start than with this book.

Mark Solms
President
South African Psychoanalytical Association

Chair of Neuropsychology
University of Cape Town and Groote Schuur Hospital
(Departments of Psychology and Neurology)
Groot Schuur
South Africa

# Preface

Our view of the human brain has been profoundly influenced by major developments in neuroscience. The goal of understanding the human brain always bears the inherent risk of biological or psychological reductionism. We present a perspective of the human mind in which personal history and subjective experiences are embedded in a framework that allows equal standing of the brain and the mind. To explain thoughts, feelings, and behavior, we have to be able to map mental representations in their full complexity. This mapping of brain structure and function is not new; today—due to the unprecedented development of technological innovations—links between physiological knowledge of the brain and features of the mind are conceivable. However, achieving a comprehensive theory of the mind and the brain is not yet within reach.

Jean-Pierre Changeux was one of the first neurobiologists to translate the basic facts of the neuronal structures and functions of the brain to the much broader scope of understanding mental functions. He advances the theory that the brain attains its adult and full pattern of connectivity by a process involving genetic and epigenetic factors. This model is at the base of our current understanding of brain plasticity— where remodeling on the one side and stabilization on the other are the two underlying functional aspects of the mind and brain throughout life—and at the root of neuronal and molecular mechanisms of learning and memory. Gerald Edelman presented a similar theory explaining the development and organization of higher brain functions based on an adaptive selection process of neuronal ontogenesis.

More recently, neuroscientists are taking advantage of the possibility to study and map large-scale neuronal networks investigating problems that were so far beyond the realm of neuroscience, such as the biological basis of consciousness. This theoretical approach—coupled with the incredible progress in neuroimaging— has revolutionized our way of considering the different stages of altered or diminished states of consciousness in clinical practice. While the centers, pathways, and neurotransmitters regulating alertness and awareness are well described and understood, fully translating what psychologists or philosophers call our conscious space or our lived mental experience in neuronal terms is still a formidable task.

The representational capacity of human memory grants us the many symbolic activities that characterize our mental lives and our many skills, including foremost language. Neuronal representations are not only widely distributed across brain regions but also depend on dynamic interactions between regions. Language—one of the most complex mental activities—is dependent on conceptual knowledge stored in vast regions of the brain, associated with sensory and motor control. Language and executive functions should not be separated but considered as part of a larger cognitive network. Language permits to communicate, exchange ideas, and establish contact with other persons. Language is related to conscious or unconscious content of the past, the present, or the future and contains shared realities and affects.

The brain does not function independently of the body, and this is especially true for emotions. There is an intense interest in understanding emotions and how they influence and affect our mental life. While the original definition of the limbic system and its boundaries laid down by James Papez and later by Paul McLean has been lately disputed, it is one of the most important parts of the brain controlling our emotions. Work on the limbic system remained for a long time in the hands of scientists studying animal behaviors like fear, aggression, and sexual arousal states. Psychiatry and neurology are increasingly looking at the role of the limbic system and its associated cortical and subcortical structures to understand behavioral and emotional disorders. Research on emotions boomed in the last two decades and has transcended the clinical and basic neuroscience fields. New models attempt to integrate neurobiological substrates to understand feelings and how we cope with fear and stress. Antonio Damasio has proposed that feedback from the body guides our behavior and eventually our decision-making abilities. Our reasoning and decision-making process is instinctive and influenced by our emotional evaluations. Rationality is always to some extent grounded in our bodies.

Jaak Panksepp, who has extensively studied neural mechanisms of emotions in animals, has joined forces with Mark Solms to lay the groundwork for a new discipline called neuropsychoanalysis. This scientific field is in fact not new, since it is what Sigmund Freud envisioned more than a century ago, when he proposed the basis of psychoanalytical theory. At this time however, neuroscience was in its infancy and could only provide limited answers to explain functional disorders of the nervous system. Neuropsychoanalysis seeks to connect psychoanalytical and neuroscientific perspectives of the mind and aims at advancing our understanding of scientific objectivity and subjective experience in mental life.

The results of infant research and the concepts of Anna Freud, Donald Winnicott, Wilfred Bion, Thomas Ogden, and many more greatly expanded the field of psychoanalytical interventions. The issue of childhood adversities in the development of mental disorder is a topic of considerable interest. Distress- and turmoil experiences of infants and young children have great impact on developmental structures and functions of the brain. Infant- and children's research show the importance of the quality of the early emotional relationship between infant and mother. Parents or primary caregivers' sensitive receptiveness to their infant and child's spontaneous expressions will shape his unique personality. Therefore, it is essential to focus attention on the child's inner world of desires and imagination, for which psychoanalytic understanding has greatly contributed. In child and adolescent psychiatry, it is fundamental to combine individual developmental changes, neurobiological endowment, unconscious mental life, interactive dialogues, subjective experience, and personal meaning. A child's desire for exchange with his primary significant caregivers motivates the creation of mental representations, which underlie his understanding of feelings, believing, and behaviors of other persons. The evolution of these processes reveals complex interactions between constitutionally determined capacities and environmental experiences; if these exchanges are impaired, disturbances of intrapsychic, interpersonal, and social relatedness ensue. Resilience research arose from an effort to better protect children, adolescents, and young adults of the impact of adverse life experiences. Critical life events find expression in sensations of pain, in coping- and grieving processes; they are always related to the subjective perception of an individual in the context of his biography.

Psychoanalytic psychotherapy is a treatment method intending to meet the needs of patients with mental health problems and patients with neurological or other somatic disorders. Psychoanalytic therapy tries to gain access to the subjective experience and personal meaning of a patient in his pain. Thanks to neuroscientific research, a lot has been learned about the important differences between various types of memories. Patients undergoing psychoanalytical treatment very often suffered traumatic experience in their personal history. The discovery of the different memory encodings has contributed to explain why some patients are unable to remember traumatic events; they were not explicitly encoded and therefore appear as affective memories in dreams, bodily sensations, and fantasies. The interpersonal exchange—a significant dialogue in a sustainable relationship—opens a window to the (un)conscious mental life of an individual. Especially for children suffering from developmental psychopathologies, the therapeutic aim—with respect to the anguish of the patient and his family—has to foster the child's developmental progression, helping him to experience a sense of coherence and personal continuity over time. The emergence of his self, his inner reality with feelings and fantasies, the frontier to his outer world, finally define a child's personal experience, his inner freedom, and creativity.

Neurologists, psychiatrists, psychotherapists, and psychologists are increasingly involved in neuroscientific research, creating very successful interdisciplinary fields such as affective neuroscience and neuropsychoanalysis. We are aware that there are huge gaps between neuroscience and psychotherapeutic disciplines with regard to their history and scope. But it is only the combination of clinical experiences with scientific facts that will help us better understand the brain–mind relationship. The authors' interest focuses on the complexity and interplay between neurobiological science, clinical manifestations, developmental aspects of disorders, and the individual's mind. Clinical vignettes are presented to illustrate our current understanding of the brain and mind couple as they demonstrate the complexity of a subject's mental functioning.

One major challenge dealing with various disciplines is the meaning of words and phrases that may carry different significance in interdisciplinary discussions.

There is no consistent universally agreed lexicon between disciplines. One way to escape these language formalisms is to avoid theoretical concepts that cannot be translated into every day terms. By leaving unnecessary complexities aside, this book attempts to bring a coherent picture of both the experimental and clinical neuroscientific fields. Our hope is to foster a dialogue between the different areas of the sciences of the mind and brain and to connect the interdisciplinary efforts that are needed to better help those who suffer from mental health- or neurological disorders.

Epalinges and Evolène, Switzerland                                          Andreas Steck

Barbara Steck

# Acknowledgments

We are especially grateful to friends and colleagues whose inspiration was central to the writing of this book. In particular we acknowledge the fruitful discussions with Dieter Bürgin. We are very thankful to Kewal Jain, member of the advisory board of Springer and Gregory Sutorius, senior editor Clinical Medicine at Springer New York for their personal commitment and support for this project. We are grateful to Mark Solms who has honored us with his foreword and we thank Antonio Damasio for his contribution and Dharmendra Modha for his comments.

We express our appreciation to Eric Bernardi for his professional drawing of the figures and to Hughes Cadas for helpful neuroanatomical advice. We thank the Springer Team for their careful attention to the production of the book and Melanie Price for language assistance.

Barbara Steck expresses her sincere gratitude to all patients who shared their personal experiences with her. Thanks to their confidence and responsiveness they allowed her to gain insight in their individual biographical history and their emotional life.

For simplification and readability we use mostly the male form. All names of the clinical vignettes have been changed.

# About the authors

Andreas Steck M.D. is Professor emeritus of Neurology and past Chair of the Department of Neurology, University Hospital, Basel, Switzerland. He is a fellow of the American Academy of Neurology and of the European Academy of Neurology.

Barbara Steck M.D. is a former Lecturer in Child and Adolescent Psychiatry and Psychotherapy at the University Hospital, Basel, Switzerland. She has a clinical background in Psychoanalysis and Family Therapy.

# Contents

**Part II**

**Part III**

**Part IV**

**Part X**

# Part I

# Chapter 1
# Consciousness

## The Problem of Consciousness

Historically, consciousness was defined by the English philosopher John Locke (1690, 1997) as "the perception of what passes in a man's own mind." The French philosopher René Descartes (1644, 1911) identified the mind with consciousness and, in his proposition of dualism, argued that the mind is independent from the body. René Descartes used the term "conscientia," which in modern terms means conscience or primarily moral conscience.[1] While for philosophers of mind the question of whether consciousness can be understood in a way that does not require a dualistic distinction between mental and physical entities remains an issue, the monist solution to the mind–brain problem, calling to an end of the division between mind and body, has come from the field of natural sciences, biology, and medicine.

For a long time, consciousness was a research topic avoided by most neuroscientists, because the experimental tools allowing exploration of a phenomenon that is classically defined in subjective terms were lacking. In the 1980s, an expanding community of neuroscientists began to address the question of consciousness giving rise to a stream of much acclaimed lay books[2] such as *Neuronal Man* by Jean-Pierre Changeux (1983), *The Remembered Present* by Gerald Edelman (1989), and *Descartes' Error* by Antonio Damasio (1995). In parallel, a considerable amount of

---

[1] John Locke (1632–1704) was interested in psychology and addressed topics such as the formation of self and consciousness. René Descartes (1596–1650) famously known for his statement "I think, therefore I am" shaped the philosophical discussion of the mind–body problem up to modern times.

[2] Jean-Pierre Changeux is a French neuroscientist who together with Dehaene is investigating the neuronal basis of cognitive functions. In his book *Neuronal Man* (*L'homme neuronal*), he proposes an elegant dialogue between the biological brain and the mind. Gerald Edelman is an American biologist (1929–2014) who turned late in his career to neuroscience. Influenced by his early work on the immune system, his model of the conscious brain is based on developmental selection. In a thoughtful book, *The Remembered Present,* he proposes an original biological theory of consciousnesses. Antonio Damasio is a neurologist who studies behavior, in particular emotions. In *Descartes' Error,* he calls for an end to the division between mind and body and contends that even our most rational decisions are rooted in emotions and feelings.

© Springer International Publishing Switzerland 2016
A. Steck, B. Steck, *Brain and Mind*, DOI 10.1007/978-3-319-21287-6_1

new experimental work on consciousness was and is being published by neuroscientists, psychologists, neurologists, and psychiatrists in specialized journals.

More recently, neurologists have begun to look at the problem of consciousness
by studying disorders of consciousness in patients with brain damage and disease
states leading to an altered level of consciousness, using brain-imaging techniques
such as functional magnetic resonance imaging (Owen 2008). With the development of the field of neuropsychoanalysis, the traditional matter of psychoanalysis,
such as the unconscious, implicit processing, the self, and free will, is being reana-
lyzed, and attempts are being made to integrate psychoanalytical concepts with
modern neuroscience (Solms and Turnbull 2002).

## Neurobiology of Consciousness

Among the brain's properties, the most fundamental is the generation of consciousness. Consciousness can be viewed as an emerging property of the brain and as such
is certainly one of the most complex biological phenomena.

The current conception that "consciousness is entirely caused by neurobiological processes and realized in brain structures" (Dehaene and Changeux 2004) is
widely shared by neuroscientists. Combining cognitive, neuroanatomical, neurophysiological, neuroimaging, and neurobiological methods, modern studies of consciousness describe its cognitive nature, its behavioral correlates, its possible
evolutionary origin, and its functional role. By taking into account the many levels
of organization on which the nervous system can be studied, from molecules to
synapses, from neurons to local circuits, and from large-scale networks to the hierarchy of mental representations they support, neuroscientific research avoided the
error to reduce consciousness to a low level of neural organization. While most
models attempt to identify the neuronal base of consciousness, a complete theory
will require new insights to explain how the neural events organize into larger-scale
active circuits, how the circuits themselves carry specific representations and forms
of information processing, and how these processes are ultimately associated with
conscious reports. Hence, a cognitive neuroscientific approach to consciousness
has to address both the architecture of mental representations and their neural
implementation (Dehaene and Changeux 2011). A theory of consciousness should
explain why some cognitive and cerebral representations are permanently or temporarily inaccessible to consciousness, the range of possible conscious contents,
how they map to specific cerebral circuits, and whether a generic neuronal mechanism underlies them all.

A satisfactory scientific theory of consciousness is still beyond reach. However,
different models relying on detailed biological, physiological, or clinical premises
have been proposed. The models of consciousness presented here are part of the
effort by neuroscientists to address an issue that until recently was considered
beyond the scope of neuroscientific research. Inherent to all the proposed models

is a degree of abstraction as well as a subjective experience, which might frustrate some readers. It is clear that at present, no single model of consciousness appears sufficient to account fully for the multidimensional properties of conscious experience, and although some of the models have gained prominence, none has been accepted as definitive. However, even without a general model of consciousness, our current understanding of how the brain works and how psychiatric or neurological disorders affect brain functions allows us to access and understand how we become conscious.

## Models of Consciousness

### *The Global Workspace Model*

Changeux and Dehaene have proposed a theoretical framework for the understanding of conscious phenomena: in this model, neuronal networks link through "bridging laws" molecular, neuronal, behavioral, and subjective representations into a coherent form (Dehaene et al. 1998; Dehaene and Naccache 2001). Their theory can be best explained by studying the issue of conscious access. When a piece of information becomes conscious, it is broadly available for multiple processes including action planning and voluntary redirection of attention and memory. This cognitive model emphasizes reportability as a key property of conscious representations, and a mental state is considered conscious when it is verbally reportable or internally accessible.

Yet we should not forget that our brain constantly works unconsciously. Automatic or unconscious cognitive processing is determined by multiple dedicated processors or modules (Baars 1988). Basically these modules are specialized neural circuits that process specific types of inputs. They include, for example, orientation-selective cortical columns in the visual system or the special purpose devices recognizing phonemes in sensory speech areas. These brain circuits are organized into functionally specialized unconsciously operating subsystems and form the basis of the so-called automated modularity of brain functioning.

A given process involving several mental operations can proceed unconsciously if a set of adequately interconnected modular systems is available to perform each of the required operations. For instance, a masked fearful face may cause unconscious emotional priming,[3] due to dedicated neural systems in the superior colliculus, pulvinar, and right amygdala associated with emotional valence to faces (Morris et al. 1998). Multiple unconscious operations can proceed in parallel so uncon-

---

[3] Priming is a term used by psychologists to characterize an implicit memory effect in which exposure to one stimulus affects the response to another stimulus.

scious processing is not limited to low-level or computationally simple operations. High-level processes may also operate unconsciously as long as they are associated with functional neural pathways established by evolution, laid down during development, or automatized by learning. For instance, motor skills used by athletes or musicians, word and sentence reading, and postural and balance control all require complex computations, yet there is considerable evidence that they can proceed automatically, nonconsciously, using specialized neural subsystems. This has been particularly well studied in musicians where experimental evidence (Zatorre et al. 1998; Schneider et al. 2002) provides strong links between specialized skills and particular brain structures.

On the other hand, the human brain must function clearly beyond automated modularity; otherwise we would be lost in a chaotic and uncontrolled state of mind. Our brain can flexibly and seemingly effortlessly recombine all these specialized tasks: once we are conscious of an item, such as a sentence we read in a book, we can readily perform a large variety of operations, including evaluation, memorization, and verbal report.

A modular view of the brain (Fodor 1983) is clearly not sufficient to account for the unified character of our conscious mental state. Baars (1988) proposed one of the first neurobiological models of consciousness that tries to fill this gap. Baars and Franklin (2007) described a "conscious access hypothesis" in a framework called "global workspace" (Fig. 1.1). This theory was conceived mainly from a cognitive psychological point of view and at first had little impact because the evidence was indirect and did not rely on anatomical or physiological bases. However, later developments in neuroimaging techniques broadly support his hypothesis.

The "Global Workspace" theory hypothesizes that a number of brain components constitute an integrative workspace that serves to reconcile the narrow momentary capacity of conscious contents by a widespread recruitment of unconscious brain functions, including long-term memory. Baars (1988), however, did not specify how the psychological construct of the conscious workspace was implemented in terms of neuronal networks. Different groups (Dehaene and Naccache 2001; Edelman and Tononi 2000; Edelman et al. 2011; Damasio 2010) have now integrated the theoretical framework into a neurobiological theory.

During decision making or discourse production, a subject brings to mind information conveyed from many different sources in a seemingly non-modular fashion. Furthermore, during the performance of a particularly difficult task, there is temporary automatic inhibition of some functions, allowing entry in a strategic or "controlled" mode of processing (Posner and Petersen 1990; Shallice et al. 2008). In order to establish a neurocomputational model of consciousness, it became clear that one had to postulate a distinct functional architecture, which goes beyond modularity and establishes flexible links among existing individual processors.

In recent years, the global workspace model has taken on an anatomical form (Dehaene and Changeux 2011). It emphasizes the role of groups of neurons with long-distance connections, particularly dense in prefrontal, cingulate, and parietal regions that are capable of interconnecting multiple specialized processors and broadcasting signals on a large scale in a spontaneous and sudden manner (Fig. 1.2).

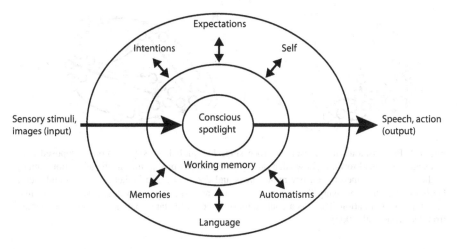

**Fig. 1.1** The global workspace. The global workspace theory of Baars consists of a cognitive architecture and is based on the principle that conscious brain events evoke widespread cortical activity. Conscious contents (conscious spotlight) need unconscious working specialized processors that operate in the backstage and compete with each other to gain access to the workspace (working memory) (Adapted from Baars and Franklin 2007)

These neurons form, what was referred to by Baars, as the "conscious spotlight" (Baars 1988; Baars and Franklin 2007, Fig. 1.1). This spotlight breaks the modularity of the nervous system and allows information reporting to and from multiple neural targets. It creates a global availability that is experienced as consciousness and results in reportability. The neuronal workspace hypothesis posits that the workspace neurons are reciprocally connected via long-distance axons to many, if not all, cortical processors permitting locally available information to be brought into consciousness. These neurons may be more densely accumulated in some areas than others. Anatomically, long-range cortico-cortical tangential and callosal connections originate mostly from the pyramidal cells of layers II and III of the cortex, which give or receive the so-called association efferents and afferents. These layers are thicker in the dorsolateral prefrontal and inferior parietal cortical structures (Goldman-Rakic 1988). The high concentration of neurons with long-distance axons in these areas may explain why they frequently appear coactivated in neuroimaging studies of conscious effortful processing. This model predicts that long-distance connections have been the target of recent evolutionary pressure in the course of hominization and are particularly well developed in our species.

The relative anatomical expansion of cortical areas rich in long-axon neurons, such as the prefrontal cortex, may have contributed to important changes in the functional properties of the workspace (Dehaene and Changeux 2004). Detailed anatomical studies of transcortical connectivity in the human brain revealed the presence of distant transcortical projections, which, for instance, directly link the right fusiform gyrus to multiple areas of the left hemisphere including Broca's and Wernicke's areas

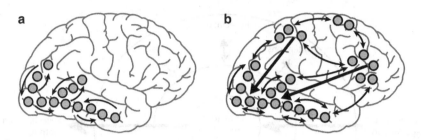

**Fig. 1.2** Preconscious and conscious processing. The global workspace model proposed here takes an anatomical form. It shows that during preconscious processing (**a**) the activation pattern of the brain is confined to sensory-motor areas and does not reach higher parieto-frontal areas. During conscious processing (**b**), the parieto-frontal areas become activated. *Long arrows* illustrate top-down attention. There is a continuum of in between states that are not shown (Adapted from Dehaene et al. 2006)

(Di Virgilio and Clarke 1997). The direct connection between the inferior temporal cortex and Wernicke's and Broca's areas is part of a large network linking higher-order visual and speech areas, including largely spread intrahemispheric and inter-hemispheric connections. One can speculate that these key components of the verbal reportability system are connected to many cortical areas given the overwhelming role of language in naming and understanding percepts and concepts.

While this model emphasizes cortico-cortical connectivity, it should be noted that corticothalamic columns are also important processing units in the brain. According to Llinás et al. (1998), the key aspect of neuronal organization, central to global functioning, is the rich thalamocortical interconnectivity and, particularly, the reciprocal nature of the thalamocortical neuronal loops. The interaction between specific and nonspecific thalamic loops suggests that rather than a gate into the brain, the thalamus represents a hub from which any site in the cortex can communicate with any other sites. Thus, long-distance connections between thalamic nuclei are contributing to the establishment of a coherent brain-scale state. Llinás et al. (1998) propose that consciousness is more a case of intrinsic brain activity than of external sensory drive. Llinas suggests that consciousness is an oneiric-like internal functional state, modulated—rather than generated—by the senses. To illustrate, he tells the example of how, in childhood, the sound of a curtain fluttering in the dark evokes very worrying images, corresponding to an oneiric perception. However, as soon as the lights go on, the worrying images go away, pointing to the modulatory role of the senses; in this case, the visual input changes the perception. The internal events we recognize as thinking, imagining, or remembering are, for the most part, related to intrinsic activity. This concept is in accordance with the fact that a very large percentage of the connectivity in the brain is recurrent and that much of its activity is related to intrinsic connectivity, not necessarily linked to the immediacy of sensory input. The thalamocortical theory of consciousness developed by Llinas, a founding father of modern brain science, has been further developed by Edelman and Tononi (2000) into what they call the dynamic core model.

## The Dynamic Core Model

The dynamic core model proposed by Edelman and Tononi (2000) and Tononi and Edelman (1998) emphasizes two basic properties of consciousness: conscious experience is integrated—each conscious scene is unified—and highly differentiated. At the same time and within a short period, we can experience a number of different conscious states. Neurobiological data indicate that neural processes associated with conscious experience are indeed highly integrated and highly differentiated. Changes in specific aspects of conscious experience correlate with changes in the activity of specific brain areas, whether the experience is driven by external stimuli, memory, or imagery and dreams. Conscious experience involves the activation or deactivation of widely distributed brain areas.

The transition between conscious controlled performance and unconscious automated performance is accompanied by a change in the degree to which neural activity is distributed within the brain. When tasks are novel, brain activation related to the task is widely distributed; when the task becomes automatic, activation is more localized. These observations suggest that when tasks are automatic and require little or no conscious control, the spread of signals influencing the performance of the task involves a more restricted and dedicated set of circuits which become "functionally insulated." This produces a gain in speed and precision but at the same time a loss in context sensitivity, accessibility, and flexibility, as Baars (1988) has suggested.

Tononi and Edelman (1998) propose that an underlying conscious experience does not extend to most of the brain but is restricted to varying subsets of neuronal groups. These neuronal groups constituting—on a time scale of hundreds of milliseconds—a unified neural process of high complexity are called the "dynamic core." By calling it the dynamic core, they mean to emphasize the function of integration (core) and the constantly changing activity pattern (dynamic). The dynamic core is a functional cluster: the participating neuronal groups are much more strongly interactive among themselves than with the rest of the brain. The dynamic core is tailored for high complexity: its global activity pattern must be selected within less than a second out of a very large repertoire. The dynamic core typically includes posterior corticothalamic regions involved in perceptual categorization, interacting with anterior regions involved in concept formation, value-related memory, and planning, although it is not necessarily restricted to the thalamocortical system. The term "dynamic core" deliberately does not refer to a unique invariant set of brain areas (such as the prefrontal or visual cortex), as the core may change in composition over time. The role of the functional interactions among distributed groups of neurons is more important than their local properties; the same group of neurons may at times be part of the dynamic core and underlie conscious experience, while at other times, they may be involved in unconscious processes. Since participation in the dynamic core depends on the rapidly shifting functional connectivity among groups of neurons rather than on anatomical proximity, the composition of the core can expand beyond anatomical limits and, in relation to particular conscious states, is expected to vary significantly. The dynamic core hypothesis avoids the idea that certain local intrinsic properties of neurons have, in some mysterious way, privileged correlation with consciousness. Instead, this hypothesis accounts for fundamental properties of conscious experience by linking them to global properties of particular neural processes. It emphasizes the fact that the dynamic core is a process since it is characterized in terms of time-varying neural interactions. It should not be viewed as a "thing" in a particular location or a specific structure in a given anatomical site.

An important characteristic of the dynamic core is fast integration of neural activity. The selection between different integrated states must be achieved within hundreds of milliseconds, thus reflecting the time course of conscious experience. While all these criteria are in line with our subjective perception of what consciousness is about, an essential prediction for the accuracy of the hypothesis is that in cognitive activities involving consciousness, there should be evidence of a large but distinct set of distributed neuronal groups that interact much more strongly among themselves than with the rest of the brain over fractions of a second. Various electrophysiological measurements support this hypothesis showing that when separate cortical areas contribute to a particular content of consciousness, they exhibit enhanced synchrony in the gamma frequency band[4] (Engel and Singer 2001). This specific change in neuronal synchrony provides the temporal binding and thus represents the neural correlate of conscious awareness (Canolty et al. 2006). These areas and patches of synchronous activity can be widely distributed across and within the cerebral hemispheres.

## *Epilogue*

All models describing the neural correlate of consciousness have in common the concept of a "global workspace," consisting of spatially dispersed, but interconnected neuronal groups in a widely distributed set of brain areas (Baars 1988; Edelman et al. 2011). Evidence also suggests that each separate area functions to process a distinctive feature of the overall conscious scene and that synchrony serves to "bind" these features together into an apparently seamless whole (Engel and Singer 2001). For example, it is possible to analyze the temporal distribution of neural activity generated in a subject's cortex using brain-imaging techniques, e.g., functional magnetic resonance imaging (fMRI) (Norman et al. 2006) or magnetoencephalography (MEG) (Srinivasan et al. 1999). From this information, we can deduce how mental states are represented in the brain; conscious perception of a visual stimulus is associated with significant increase in coherence between distant cortical neuronal populations measured by MEG recordings. These data suggest that during conscious perception, there is increased synchrony among distinct and distant neuronal groups.[5]

---

[4]Gamma waves are fast neural oscillations around 40 Hz. They are thought to be important in determining neuronal synchrony.

[5]New techniques such as optogenetics, so far limited to animal experimentation, offer both wide spatial coverage and high temporal resolution. They are helping to establish how mental representations map onto patterns of neural activity (Deisseroth 2014).

# Conscious Perception

In recent years, cognitive neuroscientists have begun to explore the means by which sensory information gains access to awareness. Conscious perception can be defined as the awareness of a sensory stimulus. To experimentally assess the introspective phenomena of conscious perception, a verbal report or account must be obtained. In this process, the working memory makes conscious events available and reportable. The current view is that conscious perception always reflects a memory process. Even the earliest stages in the sensory processing chain are not only concerned with intramodal sensory stimulation alone, but there is at the same time cross-modal activation of the sensory cortex. This takes place when the brain processes information relevant to the respective modality, independently of the sensory channel that triggered the representation of the content (Meyer et al. 2011). For example, we can see an image in the absence of the corresponding visual input when we deliberately recall a mental image or, incidentally, when we perceive a stimulus that activates a visual memory. In other words, there is more than just perception, and what really matters is the subject's perceptual experience.

Frontoparietal association cortices are crucial for information integration. Thus, information encoded in the workspace is available to many brain regions at once, including those responsible for motor behavior or verbal report. This global availability of information leads to what we subjectively experience as a conscious state (Dehaene and Changeux 2011). According to the models described above, top-down signals act as "generators of diversity," dynamically selecting the brain networks, that participate in a conscious state at any given moment. But there is more to it. A now widely shared hypothesis states that these top-down signals are "retroactivated" or reentered along the sensory pathways (Damasio 1989; Edelman and Tononi 2000). This implies that any sensory object we perceive automatically triggers the reexperience of associated images in the same, as well as other, modalities: seeing a red rose not only evokes the visual image, but may at the same time evoke any other associated sensory experience, for example, a smell. These images are stored in the association cortices. In a way, perception and memory recall are inseparable processes. To be consciously reexperienced, the images have to be reconverted to their explicit form: they are reconstructed from memory traces held in association cortices. The stream of consciousness is akin to a "remembered present" (Edelman 2001). In his book *The Remembered Present*, Edelman (1989) recapitulates the process involved in conscious experience as follows: the brain creates consciousness by recovering the past in the present, compares the past with the present, and restores the modified conception. The idea that perceptual images are not a direct reflection of the environment is well rooted in every day experiences. The perceptual field—unrolling continuously—constitutes a permanent conscious and unconscious in-depth experience of the world unfolding around us. Llinas and Paré suggest that consciousness is "an intrinsic property arising from the expression of existing dispositions of the brain to be active in certain ways" (Llinás and Paré 1991: p. 531).

Conscious perception is a process whereby the images we experience result from the association of signals that ascend and descend through mainly sensory systems.

In other words, conscious perception is the emerging product of sensory systems, just as motion is the product of signals descending through motor pathways.

## The Embodied Mind

An interesting contribution to the conceptualization of consciousness comes from an approach that considers how the body is represented in the brain. In this model, consciousness is "embodied" through the working of two distinct brain systems, the brain stem and the cortex (Solms and Panksepp 2012). Both systems are responsible for two different representations of our body. The brainstem, including the limbic system, performs functions associated with our internal body or milieu. This system is mostly implicated in the affective aspects of consciousness. This internal type of consciousness consists of emotional states rather than of cognitive objects of consciousness. In order to be turned into a conscious process, affective consciousness needs to be "externalized." This step requires the cortical mechanisms derived from the sensorimotor bodily representations. The internal body provides us only with a background consciousness. The experiencing subject—in order to truly perceive an object of consciousness—can "feel" this object only if it has been externalized, that is, presented by the classical senses in our cortical maps. The strong relationship between the two forms of consciousness relies on the functional integrity and interplay of the cortex and brain stem. This capacity to integrate clues across lines of information has been defined by psychologists as binding (Treisman 1999).[6] Only when binding is intact can objects be perceived by an experiencing subject. For example, seeing the yellow petals of a tulip is a visual experience of an object. This conscious experience is rarely limited to just seeing the color yellow, a kind of proto-object, as the visual experience will evoke the emotional and affective states at the same time. Thus, a perceptual visual event is recombined in a broader experience. Consciousness in essence is therefore as much affective as perceptual. Affects and emotions are not only interoceptive or subjective modalities but also intrinsic properties of the brain.

Current understanding of the encoding of neuronal networks suggests that there is a constant dialogue between afferent sensory information, reflecting surrounding events and outgoing pathways (Mesulam 2008). Consequently the brain can be viewed as a generator of predictions and interpretations. This inside–out brain activity denotes a clear volitional character. When we have a feeling it is often about something, demonstrating that affects may be directed toward an object. Here we add the important philosophical principle of the intentionality of consciousness. The phenomenological properties of a conscious experience should be understood as the result of informational processing within an intentional subject. Intentionality reflects the "directedness" of our mind in the process of thinking about something.

---

[6] The binding problem concerns how the unity of conscious perception originates from the combination of the activity of different neuronal populations. For example, how does the brain choose the correct sensory data to represent an object and not some illusory reconstruction of its features?

# Understanding the Human Brain by Studying Large-Scale Networks

At this point, we may ask what the real biological foundations of consciousness are. Can we really understand consciousness or even the more easily defined brain functions such as emotions, memory, and language? The human brain is by far the most complex organ with close to 100 billion neurons and an equal number of glial cells forming a wiring diagram of immense complexity. The challenge to understand the human brain is enormous. Since neuronal circuits operate in large ensembles, it does not make much sense to study a few neurons in a given region. Instead it will be through exploration of large neuronal networks that we will understand the "emerging" functions of a neuronal circuit. The rationale behind this principle is that—with each new level of complexity—a new property of the system will appear.

When we go from micro- to macrolevel, that is, when a system is growing in size, we deal with the properties of an ensemble and no longer individual components. This is best explained in the following example proposed by Erwin Schrödinger (1967), the discoverer of quantum physics: the sensation of color cannot be accounted for only by the light waves hitting the photoreceptors on the retina. To get a full feeling of the color sensation, we need to include all the nervous structures and processes starting in the retina and going along the visual pathways to the occipital cortex and association cortical areas.[7]

For an "emergent" level analysis of brain circuits, we need to record and image every spike and action potential from every neuron and synapse within a circuit; this is not yet possible. Today we can only record single cell activity of a few neurons at a time. Imaging techniques like fMRI and MEG can map whole brain activity patterns, but are unable to record a single cell or specific synaptic activity. Furthermore, the temporal resolution is far too slow to detect the rapid neuronal firing activity.

There are currently new techniques being developed to study large-scale brain network functions. Neuroscientists in both the United States and Europe (Alivisatos et al. 2012; Kandel et al. 2013) have called for an international effort aimed at mapping brain functions and reconstructing the full recording of neuronal activity across complete networks. This brain mapping will directly address the "emergent" level of functions, shedding light on our understanding of higher brain functioning. Neurobiologists believe that the study of so-called large brain networks will bring answers to cognitive and affective dysfunctions in neurological and psychiatric disorders (Menon 2011). These networks reflect functional connectivity between discrete regions of the brain and thus provide us with a window to study structure–function relationships. Among these large-scale networks, the following should be of particular interest to study.

---

[7] Philosophy often refers to the emergence of subjective conscious experience by using the term qualia. Damasio (2010) suggests correctly that while the qualia issue is traditionally regarded as a problem of consciousness, it should be more appropriately considered as a concept applied to the problem of mind. All conscious experiences or mental processes are accompanied by feelings and qualia refer to this subjective experience.

The default mode network (DMN) comprises the posterior cingulate cortex, the medial prefrontal cortex, the medial temporal lobe, and the angular gyrus (Fig. 1.3a). This network forms an integrated system for internally focused attention and is the mode that we use for our inner mental conversations. We actually spend much more time in this mode than in any other. It is typically deactivated during stimulus-driven cognitive processes, but is particularly active during episodic memory retrieval. Reduced functional connectivity in the DMN occurs in patients with neurodegenerative disorders such as Alzheimer's disease, as well as in subjects with genetic risk factors for Alzheimer's disease (Brown et al. 2011). We shall come back to the properties of the DMN in clinical view of consciousness.

The cognitive control network (CCN) or central executive network (CEN) is the brain network responsible for high-level cognitive functions such as planning, decision making, and the control of attention and working memory. It is a frontoparietal system (Fig. 1.3b). The CEN and DMN are thought to be alternatively active: self-reflection ceases when we are actively performing a task and conversely the CEN is turned off in self-reflection.

The affective network, another intensively studied network, involves the limbic system and anterior cingulate cortex. It is called the salience network (SN) and is involved in detecting and integrating relevant interoceptive, autonomic, and emotional information (Seeley et al. 2007). It is a kind of somatic marker network because it generates the somatic sensation that accompanies emotions. Extensive data exist describing alteration of this network in depression and anxiety resulting in decreased ability to focus on cognitive tasks, excessive rumination, and emotional and visceral dysregulations (Stein et al. 2007).[8]

These networks can be dysregulated and the connections between them altered in neurological or psychiatric disorders (Sheline et al. 2010). They are developmentally regulated (Supekar et al. 2010) and their development can be affected and compromised by early life traumatic experiences resulting in maladaptive changes. This is in line with evidence that early life stressors are of importance in the predisposition for mental disorders.

Classical brain lesion studies have been instrumental in uncovering essential aspects of major neurological disorders following brain damage. Major advances in our understanding of disorders of consciousness, memory, emotion, and language would not have been possible without the study of patients suffering from discrete and specific brain lesions. Conversely, brain lesion studies will not further the understanding of psychiatric disorders such as depression and schizophrenia, which will have to await the knowledge of how alterations in large neuronal networks impact not only information processing but mental functioning. In future, functional

---

[8] Aberrant intrinsic organization and interconnectivity of the SN, CEN, and DMN are thought to play a role in many psychiatric and neurological disorders. For example, a functional deficit in the insular–cingulate SN gives rise to aberrant engagement of the frontoparietal CEN, compromising cognition and goal-relevant adaptive behavior. For a more detailed discussion of the role of large-scale brain networks in psychopathology, see Menon (2011).

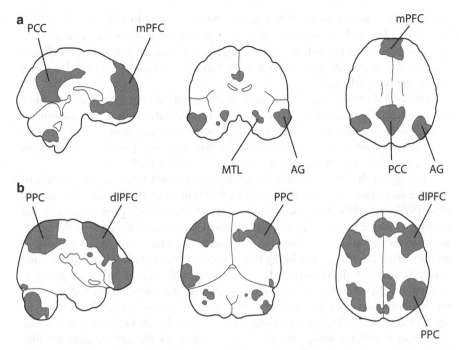

**Fig. 1.3** The major neurocognitive networks. (**a**) The default mode network (DMN) is a network which includes the posterior cingulate cortex (PCC), the medial prefrontal cortex (mPFC), the medial temporal lobe (MTL), and the angular gyrus (AG). (**b**) The central executive network (CEN) is a frontoparietal system anchored in the dorsolateral prefrontal cortex (dl PFC) and the posterior parietal cortex (PPC) (Adapted from Menon 2011)

mapping analyses will also be a tool to understand brain networks defining higher-order consciousness in humans.

# Challenges

The relationship between the structure of the nervous system and its function is still poorly understood. This is the main reason why a unified model of consciousness remains a challenge. Lichtman and Denk (2011) review the challenges of imaging brain circuits and points to some of the technical difficulties we are confronted with when trying to bridge the structure–function divide. A major problem concerns the immense structural and functional diversity of cell types in the brain: neuronal cellular architecture is extremely variable from one region to the other.

A second unique feature of the nervous system is that structural connectivity may ultimately determine function, but does not constitute a map of functions. The nervous system depends on rapid reversals of membrane potentials, called action potentials, to transmit signals between one part of a neuron to a distant part as well as smaller, slower changes in membrane potentials at sites of synaptic contact (i.e., synaptic potentials) to mediate the exchange of information between one cell and the next. Action potentials typically last a few milliseconds, which means that direct measuring is a challenge.

A third challenge is the fact that the brain is organized over a range of six orders of magnitude, from the macroscopic level at the centimeter scale to the micrometer level of synaptic connection. MRI provides a view of the macroscopic level, whereas an electron microscope is needed to visualize synapses. New powerful technologies will be required to get the complete "wiring diagram" of the brain.

The biggest challenge remains the ability to record activity of large numbers of neurons in a circuit and to understand its functions. Positron emission tomography (PET) and MRI detect activation of broad regions but cannot measure the activity of single neurons. To analyze the most interesting functions of the brain, such as perception or consciousness, we should first know what levels of cellular activity produces them. It is likely to be in the range of millions of neurons and similarly analysis of the same order of magnitude of neurons will be required to understand dysfunctions at the root of psychiatric disorders. At present, one can record individual cells in relatively small regions of the brain. Given the very short time scale at which neurons fire, milliseconds, the challenge of constructing an activity map is immense. One also has to be sure that the method does not alter brain activity. "Brain mapping" is likely to be established first in animal models. A human brain activity map remains a long way into the future for technical and possibly ethical reasons.

MRI has a spatial resolution of about one millimeter for structural analysis or functional imaging. This resolution corresponds to about 80,000 neurons and 4.5 million synapses which is way above the cellular scale, but provides information at the level of brain areas such as subcortical nuclei or gyri. The integration of information at the level of cortical layers, columns, or microcircuits will require new ultrahigh-resolution techniques in association with computational science and next-generation neuro-technologies (Insel et al. 2013; Hill et al. 2012). These techniques will be required to study local connectivity—the smallest functional unit of the brain may contain 80–100 neurons—and understand what happens in diseases when networks fail (Stam and van Straaten 2012).

It is not known how many neurons and synapses need to be activated to construct a synthetic neural model of consciousness. If it is necessary to stimulate a workspace containing millions of neurons and billions of synapses, modeling may be very difficult because of limits on processing speed and active memory capacity. But so far, it appears that a much smaller number of stimulated neurons and synapses might prove sufficient to give rise to a particular mental property such as an image or a thought.

In order to describe complex mental images or behaviors that are inscribed in large-scale neuronal networks, neuroscientists are constructing increasingly sophisticated computational models (Eliasmith et al. 2012; Kandel et al. 2013). The idea to use computational power to simulate the activity of the human brain is hardly new. Even in the early days of computers in the 1940s, they were referred to as electronic brains and as they become more capable of performing increasingly complex tasks, we now speak of artificial intelligence.

To build faster computers with increasing memory, technological engineering is the real guide. Computational power is now reaching sufficient levels, to investigate cortical circuits such as neocortical columns, and as computing capacities are developed, simulation of large-scale brain networks will become possible.

The current trend in computer development reveals however an increasing divergence in terms of operating frequency and energy demand in comparison to the brain (Fig. 1.4). A major problem with supercomputers simulating brain function is the enormous power required, in the range of gigawatts. They are also not very efficient at pattern recognition, for example, face and voice identifications, situations where the human brain performs infinitely better. Therefore, researchers are now trying to build biologically derived computer models that capture aspects of the neuroanatomy and neurophysiology in the brain to assimilate organizational principles that underlie basic cognitive functions. In order to build such artificial brains, neuromorphic chips have been designed that simulate the interconnectivity of the brain (Merolla et al. 2014).

If we compare the energy needed to generate one synaptic event between a supercomputer and the human brain, we become aware of the incredible contrast between the artificial and the human situation. "It is estimated that one synaptic event in a large computer consumes the energy of a few micro joules, while in a neuromorphic computer it comes down to a few pico joules. This must be put in perspective with the brain that needs a few femto joules per synaptic event. It is

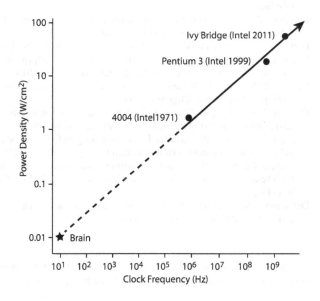

**Fig. 1.4** The current trend in computer development is leading away from the brain's operating point in terms of power density and clock frequency (Adapted from Merolla et al. 2014)

obvious that neurons and synapses in the brain have significantly more biophysical and biochemical richness than what is possible to capture today in silicon."[9]

We are far away to understand the "grand design" at the root of the computational ability of our brain. Researchers believe that combining advances in neuroscience and computation science will help us unravel higher cognitive brain functions. Starting from individual neurons and going to large-scale neuronal networks, we should learn how to test the role of defined neuronal elements in behavior. These developments are currently taking place in many research laboratories worldwide and are supported by recent political initiatives both in Europe and the United States. We may expect from these big initiatives fundamental discoveries of normal brain functioning and foremost a better understanding of neurological and psychiatric disorders.

# References

Alivisatos AP, Chun M, Church GM, Greenspan RJ, Roukes ML, Yuste R. The brain activity map project and the challenge of functional connectomics. Neuron. 2012;74(6):970–4. doi:10.1016/j.neuron.2012.06.006.

Baars BJ. A cognitive theory of consciousness. Cambridge: Cambridge University Press; 1988.

Baars BJ, Franklin S. An architectural model of conscious and unconscious brain functions: Global Workspace Theory and IDA. Neural Netw. 2007;20(9):955–61.

Brown JA, Terashima KH, Burggren AC, Ercoli LM, Miller KJ, Small GW, et al. Brain network local interconnectivity loss in aging APOE-4 allele carriers. Proc Natl Acad Sci U S A. 2011;108(51):20760–5. doi:10.1073/pnas.1109038108.

Canolty RT, Edwards E, Dalal SS, Soltani M, Nagarajan SS, Kirsch HE, et al. High gamma power is phase-locked to theta oscillations in human neocortex. Science. 2006;313(5793):1626–8.

Changeux, Jean-Pierre. L'Homme neuronal. Fayard Paris 1983 (1985 Neuronal man: the biology of mind).

Damasio AR. Time-locked multiregional retroactivation: a systems-level proposal for the neural substrates of recall and recognition. Cognition. 1989;33(1-2):25–62.

Damasio A. Self comes to Mind. New York: Vintage Books; 2010. ISBN 978-0-307-47495-7.

Dehaene S, Changeux JP. Experimental and theoretical approaches to conscious processing. Neuron. 2011;70(2):200–27. doi:10.1016/j.neuron.2011.03.018.

Dehaene S, Naccache L. Towards a cognitive neuroscience of consciousness: basic evidence and a workspace framework. Cognition. 2001;79(1-2):1–37.

Dehaene S, Kerszberg M, Changeux JP. A neuronal model of a global workspace in effortful cognitive tasks. Proc Natl Acad Sci U S A. 1998;95(24):14529–34.

Dehaene S, Changeux JP, Naccache L, Sackur J, Sergent C. Conscious, preconscious, and subliminal processing: a testable taxonomy. Trends Cogn Sci. 2006;10(5):204–11.

Dehaene S, Changeux JP. Neural mechanism for access to consciousness. In: Gazzaniga MS, editor. The cognitive neurosciences, Consciousness, vol. X. IIIth ed. Cambridge: MIT Press; 2004. p. 1145–58.

Deisseroth K. Circuit dynamics of adaptive and maladaptive behaviour. Nature. 2014;505(7483):309–17. doi:10.1038/nature12982.

---

[9] (D. S. Modha, IBM Research, Almaden, San Jose, CA, USA, personal communication). The joule is a unit of energy. A micro joule is $10^{-3}$ J, a pico joule is $10^{-12}$ J, and a femto joule is $10^{-15}$ J.

Descartes R. The Principles of Philosophy. Translated by E. Haldane and G. Ross. Cambridge: Cambridge University Press; 1644/1911.

Di Virgilio G, Clarke S. Direct interhemispheric visual input to human speech areas. Hum Brain Mapp. 1997;5(5):347–54. doi:10.1002/(SICI)1097-0193(1997)5:5<347::AID-HBM3>3.0.CO;2-3.

Edelman GM. The remembered present: a biological theory of consciousness. New York: Basic Books; 1989. ISBN 9780465069101.

Edelman G. Consciousness: the remembered present. Ann N Y Acad Sci. 2001;929:111–22. Review.

Edelman GM, Tononi G. A universe of consciousness. New York: Basic Books; 2000. ISBN 978-0-465-01377-7.

Edelman GM, Gally JA, Baars BJ. Biology of consciousness. Front Psychol. 2011;2:4. doi:10.3389/fpsyg.2011.00004. eCollection 2011.

Eliasmith C, Stewart TC, Choo X, Bekolay T, DeWolf T, Tang Y, et al. A large-scale model of the functioning brain. Science. 2012;338(6111):1202–5. doi:10.1126/science.1225266.

Engel AK, Singer W. Temporal binding and the neural correlates of sensory awareness. Trends Cogn Sci. 2001;5(1):16–25.

Fodor JA. The modularity of mind. Cambridge: MIT Press; 1983.

Goldman-Rakic PS. Topography of cognition: parallel distributed networks in primate association cortex. Annu Rev Neurosci. 1988;11:137–56.

Hill SL, Wang Y, Riachi I, Schürmann F, Markram H. Statistical connectivity provides a sufficient foundation for specific functional connectivity in neocortical neural microcircuits. Proc Natl Acad Sci U S A. 2012;109(42):E2885–94. doi:10.1073/pnas.1202128109.

Insel TR, Landis SC, Collins FS. Research priorities. The NIH BRAIN Initiative. Science. 2013;340(6133):687–8. doi:10.1126/science.1239276.

Kandel ER, Markram H, Matthews PM, Yuste R, Koch C. Neuroscience thinks big (and collaboratively). Nat Rev Neurosci. 2013;14(9):659–64. doi:10.1038/nrn3578.

Lichtman JW, Denk W. The big and the small: challenges of imaging the brain's circuits. Science. 2011;334(6056):618–23. doi:10.1126/science.1209168.

Llinás RR, Paré D. Of dreaming and wakefulness. Neuroscience. 1991;44(3):521–35. Review.

Llinás R, Ribary U, Contreras D, Pedroarena C. The neuronal basis for consciousness. Philos Trans R Soc Lond B Biol Sci. 1998;353(1377):1841–9. Review.

Locke J, Woolhouse R, editors. An Essay Concerning Human Understanding. New York: Penguin; 1997.

Menon V. Large-scale brain networks and psychopathology: a unifying triple network model. Trends Cogn Sci. 2011;15(10):483–506. doi:10.1016/j.tics.2011.08.003.

Merolla PA, Arthur JV, Alvarez-Icaza R, Cassidy AS, Sawada J, Akopyan F, et al. Artificial brains. A million spiking-neuron integrated circuit with a scalable communication network and interface. Science. 2014;345(6197):668–73. doi:10.1126/science.1254642.

Mesulam M. Representation, inference, and transcendent encoding in neurocognitive networks of the human brain. Ann Neurol. 2008;64(4):367–78. doi:10.1002/ana.21534. Review.

Meyer K, Kaplan JT, Essex R, Damasio H, Damasio A. Seeing touch is correlated with content-specific activity in primary somatosensory cortex. Cereb Cortex. 2011;21(9):2113–21. doi:10.1093/cercor/bhq289.

Morris JS, Ohman A, Dolan RJ. Conscious and unconscious emotional learning in the human amygdala. Nature. 1998;393(6684):467–70.

Norman KA, Polyn SM, Detre GJ, Haxby JV. Beyond mind-reading: multi-voxel pattern analysis of fMRI data. Trends Cogn Sci. 2006;10(9):424–30.

Owen AM. Disorders of consciousness. Ann N Y Acad Sci. 2008;1124:225–38. doi:10.1196/annals.1440.013. Review.

Posner MI, Petersen SE. The attention system of the human brain. Annu Rev Neurosci. 1990;13:25–42. Review.

Schneider P, Scherg M, Dosch HG, Specht HJ, Gutschalk A, Rupp A. Morphology of Heschl's gyrus reflects enhanced activation in the auditory cortex of musicians. Nat Neurosci. 2002;5(7):688–94.

Schrödinger E. What is life? Cambridge University Press. 1967.

Seeley WW, Menon V, Schatzberg AF, Keller J, Glover GH, Kenna H, et al. Dissociable intrinsic connectivity networks for salience processing and executive control. J Neurosci. 2007;27(9):2349–56.

Shallice T, Stuss DT, Alexander MP, Picton TW, Derkzen D. The multiple dimensions of sustained attention. Cortex. 2008;44(7):794–805. doi:10.1016/j.cortex.2007.04.002.

Sheline YI, Price JL, Yan Z, Mintun MA. Resting-state functional MRI in depression unmasks increased connectivity between networks via the dorsal nexus. Proc Natl Acad Sci U S A. 2010;107(24):11020–5. doi:10.1073/pnas.1000446107.

Solms M, Panksepp J. The "id" knows more than the "ego" admits: neuropsychoanalytic and primal consciousness perspectives on the interface between affective and cognitive neuroscience. Brain Sci. 2012;2(2):147–75. doi:10.3390/brainsci2020147.

Solms M, Turnbull O. The Brain and the Inner World. New York: Other Press; 2002.

Srinivasan R, Russell DP, Edelman GM, Tononi G. Increased synchronization of neuromagnetic responses during conscious perception. J Neurosci. 1999;19(13):5435–48.

Stam CJ, van Straaten EC. The organization of physiological brain networks. Clin Neurophysiol. 2012;123(6):1067–87. doi:10.1016/j.clinph.2012.01.011.

Stein MB, Simmons AN, Feinstein JS, Paulus MP. Increased amygdala and insula activation during emotion processing in anxiety-prone subjects. Am J Psychiatry. 2007;164(2):318–27.

Supekar K, Uddin LQ, Prater K, Amin H, Greicius MD, Menon V. Development of functional and structural connectivity within the default mode network in young children. Neuroimage. 2010;52(1):290–301. doi:10.1016/j.neuroimage.2010.04.009.

Tononi G, Edelman GM. Consciousness and complexity. Science. 1998;282(5395):1846–51.

Treisman A. Solutions to the binding problem: progress through controversy and convergence. Neuron. 1999;24(1):105–10. 1.

Zatorre RJ, Perry DW, Beckett CA, Westbury CF, Evans AC. Functional anatomy of musical processing in listeners with absolute pitch and relative pitch. Proc Natl Acad Sci U S A. 1998;95(6):3172–7.

# Chapter 2
# Clinical View of Consciousness

## Introduction

A definition of consciousness should include an implicit philosophical dimension: that is, consciousness is self-reflective and passive but also intentional and somehow timeless. Consciousness is about what might be described as awareness of inner states or—as Solms puts it—a kind of internal sensory modality that perceives the processes occurring within us (Solms and Turnbull 2002). During sleep, consciousness fades in and out on a regular basis. Consciousness is a given property of the mind and depends very much on the way our brain is functioning.

Obviously consciousness evolves with brain states, and as the brain is in a constant state of change, fluctuating between continuums of wakefulness–drowsiness–sleep cycles, one has to account for the many dimensions that consciousness takes. Consciousness in the waking state is obviously different from consciousness in sleep where in the various stages of sleep, mentation occurs in the form of dreams. We also have to consider the very many altered states of consciousness that have been described by neurologists (Table 1.1, Vaitl et al. 2005). They are part of a large behavioral repertoire of both physiological and pathological states of consciousness, of which we start to better understand the neural correlates.

Consciousness in neurological terms has two dimensions: wakefulness and awareness (Fig. 2.1). Wakefulness is a quantitative aspect of consciousness and can be divided in categories such as alert, somnolent, stuporous, or comatose. Wakefulness is critically determined by subcortical arousal systems. As we fall asleep, the level of wakefulness decreases and as a consequence, awareness of the environment is diminished. Awareness corresponds to a qualitative dimension of consciousness and can be equated to the "content" of consciousness.

Neurologists are concerned with issues such as the level or state of consciousness and the different conditions associated with impaired awareness. Psychiatrists are more interested in the content of consciousness. Since Freud, the study of the unconscious has been at the forefront of psychoanalytical research and practice. Modern neuroscience is bringing insight into the functioning of the brain and offers some explanation for the different aspects of consciousness. We now know that the conscious dimension of brain activity is a very limited part of the mind and of our mental life. Functional

© Springer International Publishing Switzerland 2016
A. Steck, B. Steck, *Brain and Mind*, DOI 10.1007/978-3-319-21287-6_2

neuroimaging and large-scale brain activity mapping are changing our understanding of patients with coma, brain damage, and related states and opening new avenues for the study of sleep, dreams, and neuropsychiatric disorders (Insel et al. 2013).

## The Pathophysiology of Reduced Consciousness

The two physiological components of conscious behavior, namely, arousal (vigilance) and content of consciousness (presence of mind), may be affected differently in brain pathophysiology, depending on the type and distribution of the underlying brain disease. Disturbance of arousal primarily affects wakefulness and awareness and leads to obtundation (a reduced level of alertness or consciousness), stupor, and coma. This aspect of consciousness is normally described in quantitative terms. The Glasgow Coma Scale,[1] which was designed to evaluate altered levels of consciousness after head trauma, is widely used in clinical practice. States of reduced arousal are caused by lesions of the ascending reticular activating system (ARAS).[2] This arousal system is anatomically represented by a number of structures in the rostral brain stem tegmentum and the diencephalon and their projections to the cerebral cortex. It contains a complex network of neurons projecting from multiple brain-stem nuclei to the cortex via thalamic and extra thalamic pathways. Principal among these are acetylcholine-producing neurons of the peribrachial nuclei, made up of the pedunculopontine tegmental and lateral dorsal tegmental nuclei. This group of neurons projects rostrally in two major pathways: (1) a dorsal pathway that synapses with the midline and nonspecific thalamic nuclei and sends a glutaminergic

| Table 1.1 Altered states of consciousness | |
|---|---|
| *Spontaneously occurring* |
| Daydreaming |
| Drowsiness, hypnagogic states |
| Sleep, dreaming |
| *Psychologically induced* |
| Rhythm-induced trance (drumming and dancing) |
| Relaxation, meditation |
| Hypnosis |
| *Disease induced* |
| Psychiatric disorders, psychosis, depression |
| Neurological disorders, coma, vegetative state, epilepsy |
| *Toxic or pharmacologically induced* |

*Source*: Adapted from Vaitl et al. (2005)

---

[1] The Glasgow Coma Scale (GCS) is a clinical score to assess the level of consciousness in a patient. The GCS was originally described by two physicians from the University of Glasgow.

[2] The discovery of the ARAS by Giuseppe Moruzzi and Horace Magoun dates back to 1949. They showed that stimulation of the brain stem reticular formation evoked an arousal reaction (Moruzzi and Magoun 1949).

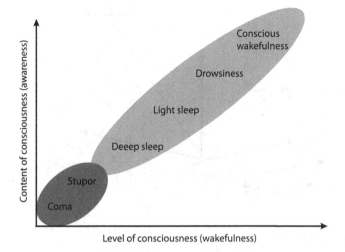

**Fig. 2.1** The two dimensions of consciousness: wakefulness and awareness (Adapted from Laureys 2005b)

projection to large areas of the cerebral cortex and (2) a ventral pathway from the rostral brain stem tegmentum that reaches the basal forebrain, especially the posterior hypothalamus, where axon terminals act on neurons that synthesize histamine, hypocretin, and other neurotransmitters (Young 2009) (Fig. 2.2). The connections to the hypothalamus are important for the regulation of the circadian sleep–wake cycle; the thalamus plays a key role in modulating the interactions between brainstem arousal networks and cortical awareness networks.

When consciousness fades, cognitive and mnestic functions are degraded and the contents of consciousness become fragmented and disordered; depending on the extent of the disturbance, confusion, lethargy, and finally a vegetative state ensue. Disorders of consciousness result from either toxic-metabolic or extensive structural disorders of the cerebral cortex. The limbic system and mesial frontal areas play a dominant role in shaping conscious behavior. Reduced functioning of large areas of both hemispheres also results in a diminished arousal state. Consciousness fades and eventually vanishes when anesthetics cause functional disconnection and interrupt cortical neuronal communication. Anesthesia has common behavioral and electrophysiological characteristics with sleep. However, recent literature suggests that the transition process between anesthesia-induced alteration of consciousness and the shift from wake state to sleep state is not driven by the same sequence of events. Anesthesia primarily affects the cortex with subsequent repercussions on the activity of subcortical networks, while sleep originates in subcortical structures[3] with subsequent repercussions on thalamocortical interactions and cortical activity (Bonhomme et al. 2011).

---

[3] The reversible unconsciousness of sleep relates to dynamic inhibition of the neurotransmitter systems involved in arousal. Sleep centers are mainly in the preoptic region of the hypothalamus and use γ-amino butyric acid (GABA), an inhibitory neurotransmitter. Adenosine, a neuromodulator, also provides feedback inhibition of the arousal system. For review, see Young (2009).

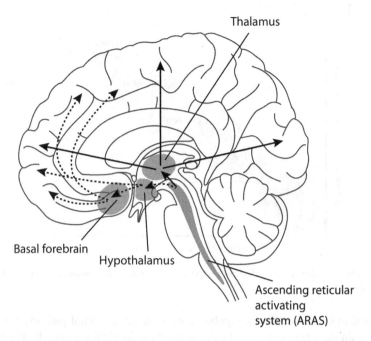

**Fig. 2.2** The ascending reticular activating system (ARAS). The nuclei and pathways of the dorsal and ventral components of the ARAS originate in the cholinergic cells of the reticular formation. The dorsal pathway (*bold arrows*) activates the cerebral cortex via the thalamus. The ventral pathway (*dotted arrows*) projects to the hypothalamus and basal forebrain, which in turn projects to the cortex (Adapted from Reinoso-Suarez 2005 and Brown et al. 2012)

## The Construction of the Conscious Brain

The neurologist Damasio (2010) proposed a theory of consciousness based on an evolutionary perspective and clinical behavioral practice. He approaches the problem of consciousness by referring to a neurobiological theory of emotions and feelings rooted in the body. Rewards and emotions are viewed as part of the bio-regulatory machinery. Subjective feelings of pleasure and resulting positive emotions represent key functions of rewards (Schultz 2013). When a subject is confronted with a significant emotional challenge, he experiences a very profound change in the state of his body, of the internal milieu. Damasio (2010) suggested a framework in which representations of the internal milieu, the viscera, the muscles, and the skin start in a very fragmentary way at the level of the spinal cord and continue progressively to the brainstem, hypothalamus, and beyond toward the cortex and to more and more organized maps. William James[4] already stated that emotions happen in the body and profoundly change the state of the body. While the role of the body was neglected in emotion studies during the first part of the twentieth century, authors like Panksepp (2001), LeDoux (2000), and Damasio (1999) are now emphasizing the link between body and emotions.

When asking the question if emotions are necessarily conscious, Damasio answers that in evolution, emotions arose in primitive organisms long before consciousness emerged. Emotions existed to benefit survival. When a threatened octopus responds by ink reaction, we can postulate that there is fear emotion. But this simple creature is unlikely to have a representation of its own organism or self. In humans, the self serves as the basis from which brain mechanisms will lead to consciousness, allowing, among other things, to develop feelings. In his book *The Feelings of What Happens,* Damasio (1999) makes the point that consciousness appears at a pivoting point between emotion and feeling. He states that emotions are basically unconscious, whereas feelings are conscious. Consciousness is an important evolutionary trait that allows us to "feel" our emotions.

Consciousness is not restricted to humans. The idea that we have consciousness because we have language is profoundly wrong. The story goes the other way: we have language because we have consciousness. In humans, consciousness does take a growing magnitude because of language and because of an enormous extension of memory capacity, for both the past and "the future". What I call memory of the future is this: unlike most creatures, humans are deeply involved with planning. This is happening continuously and we are also continuously memorizing our plans. So we have, at any given time, not only a memory of our past—highly organized—but also a memory for our anticipated future. This is a big difference relative to other animals that are capable of many smart things but not long term planning. So when you add our memory and our planning to language, you achieve a dimension of consciousness that is really extraordinary.

I am firmly convinced that we will find consciousness all the way down—it's not a primate property—birds have it and I would be surprised if reptiles and fish hadn't.

The critical development for consciousness is that not only can one build a representation of oneself which, at the core, means a representation of one's internal state, but one can also build a representation of one's internal state being changed by something else. In order to achieve that, one needs a remarkable layering in the brain, so that we have structures that literally look at other structures. By the way, I am not certain—and that is out of sheer ignorance—that a fruit fly cannot do this; her brain may have what is necessary to do this. But I believe that what does happen with us is that we can represent the internal milieu—in structures from paralimbic and limbic areas to the hypothalamus. Within these areas we can create a pretty vivid representation of the internal milieu and the state of the viscera.

Coming back to insects, bees for example, there is evidence that they can build and use maps of their environment. But there is so far no evidence that the same is possible for maps of the internal milieu. This relates to the notion of self. The "protoself" is the representation of the internal milieu, for example, of the viscera. It's really a cognition of the interior. We have several adaptive behaviors that are built on the cognition of the exterior, but may

---

[4] William James (1842–1910) is an American psychologist whose writings on emotions have inspired contemporary neuroscientists such as Damasio and LeDoux.

be that once we can understand more about the cognition of the interior and about the sorts of maps involved, we can better understand the origin of the mind. (Excerpt from Damasio's viewpoint at a round table discussion "Exploring the minded brain," Basel 1998, by permission of the author.)

## The Hierarchy of Consciousness

When one is awake and alert and not actively engaged in a particular cognitive task, a neural network comprising the lateral parietal, ventromedial prefrontal, middorso-lateral prefrontal, and anterior temporal cortices exhibits a remarkably high metabolic activity with multiple hot spots in these regions (Cavanna and Trimble 2006). This baseline state of neural activity is necessary to assume a continuous representation of the self. This mode of function of the brain has been called the default mode.[5] It subserves conceptual information processing as opposed to perceptual processing; it is essentially involved in the processing of endogenous signals such as representations of information in the form of mental images or spontaneous thoughts. This all happens in the context of general body awareness, upon which extended consciousness is constructed.

Consciousness exists in a hierarchy of stages, each building upon (and dependent on) its predecessor(s). According to Damasio (1999), core consciousness arises when the brain generates a representation of the relationship between the organism (the self) and an environmental stimulus. The state preceding core consciousness is the protoself, a nonconscious collection of representations of the multiple dimensions of the current state of the organism. The state following core consciousness is extended consciousness, the capacity to be aware of a large collection of entities and events and the ability to generate a sense of individual perspective or ownership.

When we consider these hierarchy definitions, there is an obvious similarity with Daniel Stern's description of the development of the sense of self where "the emergent self" that Stern evokes is conceptualized by Damasio as the "protoself." Stern, a psychoanalyst who specialized in infant development, proposes that the self is

---

[5] An unexpected finding that dates back to the introduction of fMRI in the early 1990s is the discovery of the brain default mode network (DMN) (Buckner 2012). The network is a set of brain regions that are tightly correlated and activated when an individual lies at rest in an imaging machine (fMRI). It contains parts of the medial and ventral temporal lobe, parietal cortex, medial prefrontal cortex, and cingulate cortex. This default brain network observed in fMRI corresponds to a state in which subjects are not accomplishing a task but are left in an idle state where they can dream or think about anything they like. This freewheeling mental activity involves a large portion of our brain, concerned with self-awareness, consciousness, and planning behavior. The DMN is also described in the previous chapter.

layered and that an infant will successively develop an increasingly interpersonal sophisticated sense of self. He distinguished four main senses of self (Stern 1985):

- The sense of an emergent self, which forms from birth to age 2 months.
- The sense of a core self, which forms between the ages of 2 and 6 months.
- The sense of a subjective self, which forms between 7 and 15 months.
- Afterward—as development proceeds—a sense of a verbal self with the ability to tell a narrative about one's own experience and thus referring verbally to the world will emerge.

It is interesting to note that Stern's phases of the development of the sense of self map neatly into Damasio's (1999) neuropsychological descriptions: the protoself, core consciousness, and extended consciousness. Where the emergent self that Stern describes is conceptualized by Damasio as the protoself, Stern's core self is the product of core consciousness. This brings an interesting parallel between the neural self and the psychoanalytical theories of self, which—as Freud himself believed—are rooted in biology.

Damasio's work on the embodied mind (1999, 2010),[6] where the traditional sharp separation between body and mind is no longer maintained, is helpful for understanding the nature of "primary consciousness" in infancy. Basically all mental acts (perception, feeling, cognition, remembering) are accompanied by input from the body. This input is what Damasio calls "background feelings" and what Stern (2010) calls "vitality affects." As we are involved in a constant flow of mental activity, our body is never doing nothing. The bodily signals, even if they are in the background, are in the words of Stern (1985), "the continuous music of being alive" (Introduction p. XVIII).

## When Consciousness Fades

### *Anesthesia*

The introduction of anesthesia into clinical medicine led to a revolution in the nineteenth century, allowing patients to undergo surgery and other procedures without the distress and pain they would otherwise experience. In a famous demonstration "Insensibility during surgical operations produced by inhalation," the Bostonian surgeon Bigelow reported in 1846 the first use of ether as an anesthetic. Anesthesia causes lack of awareness and according to Bigelow "during the operation the patient muttered, as in a semi-conscious state" (1846: p. 309); it was clear to the physicians involved that consciousness was impaired. Since then, research on how anesthetics bring unconsciousness has provided critical insights into the science of

---

[6] The term embodied mind, as seen previously, has been taken up by many neuroscientists and refers to how mind and body depend on each other.

consciousness. The advent of cellular electrophysiology and molecular biology techniques demonstrated that proteins, namely, receptors and ion channels on neurons, were the most likely targets for the anesthetic effect (Alkire et al. 2008). Anesthetics are thought to work by interacting with ion channels, mostly K+ channels and receptors such as γ-aminobutyric acid (GABA), N-methyl-D-aspartate (NMDA), glycine, serotonin, α-amino-3-hydroxy-5-methyl-4-isoxazolepropionic acid (AMPA), and acetylcholine (ACh), which regulate membrane potentials and synaptic transmission in key regions of the brain and spinal cord. The ion channel targets are differentially sensitive to the various anesthetic agents producing diverse effects (Kopp Lugli et al. 2009). Basically anesthetics inactivate neurons by impairing their ability to fire either by increasing inhibition or decreasing excitation, thus altering neuronal activity. This is reflected by changes in EEG activity: there is a transition from the low-voltage, high-frequency pattern of wakefulness (known as activated EEG) to the slow-wave EEG of deep sleep and finally to an EEG burst-suppression pattern characteristic of severely reduced brain activity as observed in anesthesia (Fig. 2.3). As anesthetic doses increase, the downstate becomes progressively longer and eventually a flat EEG will appear, signaling cessation of the brain's electrical activity. This is one of the criteria for brain death (Wijdicks 2001). It is assumed that at some level of anesthesia between behavioral unresponsiveness and the induction of a depressed slow EEG, consciousness fades.

It is generally accepted that for consciousness to exist, our brain must be capable of integrating information (Tononi 2004). Consciousness is lost when this is no longer possible, as in anesthesia, when there is a breakdown of connectivity and thus of integration of information. The level of brain consciousness is directly related to the repertoire of all the different bits of information that can be discriminated and integrated. The integration or binding factor is the functional cluster or dynamic core that we described in the previous chapter. In anatomical terms, this functional cluster corresponds to the thalamocortical complex, the assumed target for anesthesia. This thalamocortical complex[7] is a unique structure allowing functional integration of specialized cortical areas (Fig. 2.4) and behaves as an entity endowed with a large number of discriminable states. By contrast, other parts of the brain made up of small, quasi-independent modules, such as the cerebellum and the basal ganglia that are implicated in motor control, are not sufficiently integrated and so contribute less to conscious experience. Accordingly, they can suffer lesion without loss of consciousness (Tononi 2004).

Consciousness is not an all-or-none property, but consists of specific states that increase in proportion to the system's repertoire. The shrinking or dimming of consciousness during sedation is consistent with this idea. On the other hand, the abrupt loss of consciousness at a critical concentration of anesthetics suggests that the integrated repertoire of neural states can suddenly collapse (Vyazovskiy et al. 2008).

---

[7] The rich thalamocortical interconnectivity is central to the activity generating consciousness. As discussed previously, all models of consciousness refer to this system.

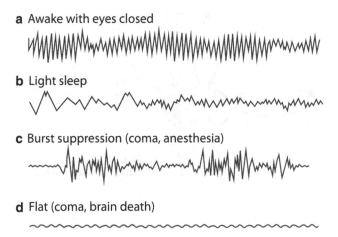

**a** Awake with eyes closed

**b** Light sleep

**c** Burst suppression (coma, anesthesia)

**d** Flat (coma, brain death)

**Fig. 2.3** Electroencephalographic (EEG) patterns. EEG activity during awake state, sleep, coma, and brain death. The burst-suppression pattern is observed in coma and anesthesia (Adapted from Brown et al. 2010)

## *Minimally Conscious State*

In the 1970s, neurologists described a chronic vegetative state or coma vigil, a condition in which patients recovering from a coma could open their eyes (spontaneously or after stimulation), but remained without communication or behavioral signs of consciousness. It was and still is standard procedure to use behavioral scales to assess a patient's unconscious state based on the absence of motor responsiveness. For example, if a patient opens his eyes and makes rowing eye movements but fails to engage in activity of intentional eye movements, the patient is clinically considered as being unconscious.

Over the last decade, as neurologists started using new methods of assessment of the level of cognitive functioning, especially functional MRI (fMRI), the term unresponsive wakefulness syndrome or minimally conscious state was introduced to describe a group of patients who previously would have been considered to be in a vegetative state by classical clinical assessment (Bruno et al. 2011). In these patients, fMRI reveals an unexpected capacity for voluntary mental imagery, as the following example demonstrates.

Owen (Owen et al. 2006) used fMRI to study a patient who appeared to be in a vegetative state. The patient was a young lady who, after sustaining a severe traumatic brain injury, remained unresponsive and was diagnosed with a chronic vegetative state. She was asked to perform two mental imagery tasks—imagining playing tennis and walking through the rooms of her house—tasks associated with differential activation of a number of distinct cortical brain regions. Surprisingly the resulting brain response patterns in the patient were comparable with those observed in healthy, awake controls performing the same mental imagery tasks. These functional

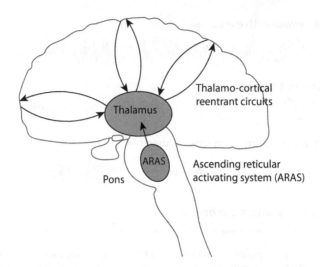

**Fig. 2.4** Consciousness and the thalamocortical system. Consciousness depends on the activation of the thalamus—by the ascending reticular activating system (ARAS)—and on the thalamocortical reentrant circuits. Conscious experience requires rapid bidirectional interactions among distributed neuronal populations

neuroimaging studies offer the possibility to directly measure brain activity in severely brain-damaged patients at rest and during external activation. The technique allows the visualization of neural motor-independent commands, such as the presence of voluntary mental imagery. Owen and Cruse thus conclude that the patient was responding to verbal commands and therefore retained a level of awareness not apparent by her behavior (Cruse and Owen 2010).

The important question is whether the evidence of brain activation by fMRI in patients with disorders of consciousness (Laureys et al. 2002; Boly 2011; Owen 2013) indicates conscious awareness or not. Could it be that these patients retain discreet islands of subconscious cognitive functions which persist in the absence of their awareness? There are many studies in healthy volunteers, from implicit learning to speech perception during anesthesia (Davis et al. 2007; Owen 2013), demonstrating that many aspects of human cognition can go on in the absence of awareness. It could be argued that these patients do not have a conscious experience associated with stimuli or task processing. On the other hand, since there are many definitions of consciousness or self-consciousness, the question whether these patients are conscious or not remains open. If we accept that consciousness is based on intentional behavior, it would be appropriate to use a method to determine if a subject is consciously aware by testing ability to communicate through a recognized behavioral response. This definition may however be too restrictive if one contends that conscious awareness remains even if the ability to communicate is lost.

The debate also revolves around the issue of whether the cortical activity measured by fMRI is sufficient to indicate conscious awareness. From a neurobiological view point, one can assert that activation of cortical regions in patients with disorders of consciousness may be considered as a neural marker of consciousness. Depending on the regions that are activated, such as the parietal lobe contributing to speech or movement recognition, or the amygdala, implying emotional response, fMRI studies provide us with reliable neural responses in individual patients, showing us a picture of their remaining brain function. What we observe both clinically and experimentally in patients in the minimally conscious state is a kind of impaired and severely diminished core consciousness. Consciousness in a normal awake person is unified, that is, we have a single state of consciousness. The unity of consciousness breaks down in the context of neurological or psychiatric disorders. For some authors like Bayne (2011), talking about levels of consciousness is misleading because it implies that there are states of consciousness that can be arranged in a hierarchical mode. He proposes to view diminished states of consciousness as "background states." Examples of background states include drowsiness, the REM dream state, the minimal conscious state, epileptic seizures, or hallucinatory states to name a few. Subjects or patients in these altered states of consciousness are not able to feel the full quality and all impressions that consciousness provides in the state of normal wakefulness.

In this respect, it is interesting to look at the default mode network (DMN). This network contains some of the most metabolically active regions of the human brain at rest and has been proposed to play a key role in maintaining a state of readiness of internal representations (Schiff 2012).[8] Specific structural impairments of the DMN in patients with disorders of consciousness can help categorize subjects with minimally conscious state and be correlated with clinical outcome (Fernández-Espejo et al. 2012). The integrity of thalamocortical connections, especially the connections between the thalamus and the posterior cingulate gyrus, is essential for the presence of reflective behavior in patients with impaired consciousness.

To summarize, there are two different supporting networks for awareness (Demertzi et al. 2013). One component consists mainly of the lateral parts of the prefrontal and posterior parietal cortex and is responsible for external awareness. This is awareness of what we perceive through our senses (seeing, feeling, hearing, smelling, and tasting). The second component comprises medial brain structures such as the medial prefrontal cortex, thalamus, and anterior and posterior cingulate cortex and is involved in internal awareness, that is, self-mentation. The intrinsic network corresponds to the DMN, while the extrinsic system corresponds to the cognitive control network (CCN), the brain network that is active during goal directed behavior. The global "workspace" of Dehaene and Changeux (2011) and the "dynamic core" of Edelman and Tononi (2000) encompass these two systems. Any disruption, either within or between these systems, will result in an altered state

---

[8] As seen previously, the DMN is composed of thalamocortical connections that include the medial prefrontal cortex, the posterior cingulate cortex, and the temporoparietal region.

of consciousness. For example, in hypnosis where people report a sense of dissociation from the environment, there is a reduction in the functional connectivity of the external awareness system (Demertzi et al. 2013). The study of how the two systems support the dynamic functioning of consciousness is helping us to understand how conscious mentation functions in both health and disease.

## Altered Consciousness in Neurological Disorders

Several neurological disorders lead to altered consciousness. We have discussed new studies that help us to better understand the most extreme states of impaired consciousness—persistent vegetative state and anesthesia—where core consciousness and extended consciousness are profoundly affected. Let us now look at clinical examples of patients with neurological disorders affecting or impairing consciousness.

### *Disconnection and Neglect*

Neurological data indicate that integration of distributed neuronal populations through specific interactions is required for conscious experience. Patients with disconnection syndromes, in which one or more brain areas are anatomically or functionally disconnected from the rest of the brain, display a number of neurological symptoms depending on which pathway is affected. Damage to a region or disconnection of one or more regions will disrupt or alter the corresponding functions. Already in the nineteenth century, Carl Wernicke showed that a form of aphasia results from disconnection of the sensory speech and motor speech areas. This type of aphasia is called conduction aphasia (Benson et al. 1973). This disorder is characterized by fluent speech but impaired repetition of words or phrases with difficulty in naming.

The corpus callosum[9] is recognized as the principal information transfer pathway between brain regions and is consequently an important site of disconnecting lesions. Although the corpus callosum is a single anatomical structure, it represents the discrete interconnection of a number of specific cortical centers. Patients who have had brain tumors, brain infarction, or surgical resection for uncontrollable seizure disorders primarily provided the knowledge about the neuropsychology of interhemispheric disconnection. One of the most surprising results is that—in ordinary social situations—these patients are indistinguishable from normal people except for some memory problems. This suggests that the corpus callosum and specifically the connections between both cerebral hemispheres may not play an essential role in the formation of consciousness, but that the wiring between both sides of the brain is important for specialized conscious tasks. Appropriate testing methods sensitive to

---

[9] The corpus callosum is a thick band of nerve fibers connecting the two hemispheres.

lateralization of function that is hemispheric specialization[10] are indeed needed to expose neuropsychological deficits resulting from lack of interhemispheric transfer.

The hemispheric specialization typical of human subjects results in unique neuropsychological syndromes (Gazzaniga 1995). A classic example of a disconnection syndrome is the inability of right-handers to name or describe an object in the left hand even when it is being appropriately manipulated because the afferent sensory information of the left hand is projected onto the right hemisphere and cannot be transferred to the speech area on the left side of the brain. Such a situation is reported in detail by Geschwind and Kaplan (1998). The patient, suffering from a brain tumor that affected the corpus callosum, could not write (spontaneously or to dictation) with his left hand but succeeded easily with the right hand. Tactile object naming (stereognosis) was performed normally with the right hand but not with the left; the patient failed to name objects placed in the left hand (if hidden from view). His right hand followed commands flawlessly, but he made many errors with the left. This case study shows that callosal disconnection does not lead to generalized impairment in consciousness but to well-defined and focal neuropsychological deficits. Whether psychiatric dissociation syndromes and conversion disorders may originate from a similar alteration of interactions between specific brain regions—although in these cases the nature of the disconnection would be functional rather than lesional—is a debated subject.

Along these lines, a look at hypnotic states is of interest. Hypnosis is a procedure which can induce alterations in perception or memory in the subject: for example, in hypnotic analgesia, the subject fails to show discomfort to a normally painful stimulus. This state of analgesia can be interpreted as a disconnection or failure to process painful stimuli in the brain. As seen previously, the hypnotic state is characterized by reduction in functional connectivity in the external awareness system. This disconnection leads to impaired processing of exterior phenomenal awareness, resulting in decreased pain perception.

Attention is considered as a prerequisite of consciousness, as exemplified by our failure to consciously perceive an event when our attention is not or otherwise engaged: so-called inattentional blindness (Mack and Rock 1998). Brain-lesion patients suffering from hemineglect provide a striking illustration of the role of attentional factors in consciousness (Driver and Vuilleumier 2001). Hemineglect results from unilateral brain damage affecting the parietal region, which is involved in the orientation of attention to space and objects to the other side of the body. Neglect patients fail to attend to stimuli located in the contra-lesion space, e.g., on the left following a right-sided lesion. The focus of attention seems permanently biased toward the right half of space, and patients behave as if the left half is unavailable to conscious process. Thus, neglect involves a dramatic loss of awareness. These few examples show that, while we normally enjoy the full range of perceptual awareness, this faculty is markedly limited in patients with disconnection or neglect syndromes.

---

[10] The left hemisphere is specialized for language and speech, while the right hemisphere is involved in such tasks as attention regulation and facial recognition.

## *Epilepsy*

Epilepsy is a condition recognized since the beginning of recorded history. Originally it was thought to have a divine or spiritual origin. Hippocrates (460–377 BC) rejected the idea that "Epilepsy was a sacred disease[11] caused by evil spirits" and not believing in superstitions, declaring epilepsy as a disease of the brain. Before him, Punarvasu Ātreya described epilepsy as loss of consciousness (Eadie and Bladin 2001). Normally the brain functions as a complex anatomical and functional network. Epilepsy is characterized by the unexpected emergence of an abnormal brain dynamic state with excessive neuronal firing and synchronization of neural networks. In the healthy brain, there is a subtle interplay in rapid formation and disappearance of functional connections between different brain regions. In epilepsy, this fragile "binding" is disturbed either by excessive connectivity or disconnection (Stam and van Straaten 2012). The breakdown of the normal modular brain structure and of its intrinsic "fragile binding" results in many symptoms, ranging from abnormal sensations to attention deficits and altered consciousness. Much of the progress in comprehension of brain functions is related to a better understanding of local activation of functional brain units. It is obvious, and the study of epilepsy demonstrates very clearly that sudden and out of context activation of functional brain units will perturb functional brain connectivity. Any movement away from the optimal hierarchical modularity of the brain network results in the dazzling variety of symptoms seen in epilepsy, but also in other paroxysmal disorders such as migraine. It is becoming increasingly clear that regulated auto organizing activity in vast populations of neurons is a prerequisite for normal brain functioning.

Epileptic attacks can take many different forms. There may be transient loss of consciousness as seen in generalized seizures or absence seizures. In partial seizures, the symptoms may be very varied depending on the localization of the epileptic discharge. There may be motor symptoms such as limb movements and sensory symptoms with abnormalities of vision, sound, smell, or other sensations, as well as psychic alterations such as feelings of joy or fear, senses of false familiarity, or unusual thoughts. Partial seizures may be confined to the epileptic focus or may spread to others areas of the brain, leading to a generalized attack.

Some patients live very strange experiences during a seizure. A patient who was suffering from temporal lobe epilepsy with olfactory symptoms reported strange feelings of what could be called a dissociation of consciousness (Efron 1956). "I can be perfectly well, when suddenly I feel snatched away. I seem to feel as if I am in two places at once, but in neither place at all. All this time I feel that I am remote." (p. 270). This kind of very particular experience with dissociation of consciousness is akin to hallucinatory experiences and can be considered as a state of "fragmented" consciousness.

---

[11] Sacer, from Latin, means not only "holy," "consecrated," but also "wicked," "horrible."

Oliver Sacks has devoted an entire book to hallucinations.[12] Hallucinations, taken as sensations arising out of context, for example, seeing things or hearing voices that are not actually real, not only belong to the domains of neurology or psychiatry but are commonly encountered in situations such as extreme sensory deprivation and intoxication, especially with the use of hallucinogenic drugs, leading to a large range of altered states of consciousness with a variety of perceptual distortions.

Compared to the study of epilepsy, few other neurological conditions have given us so many insights into the working and organization of the nervous system. Wilder Penfield[13] took up the challenge to record the human cortex in the awake, epileptic patient and was able to locate sensory and movement areas. By stimulating these specific sensory and motor areas in a given patient, he found the exact cortical map corresponding to his specific type of symptoms. The removal of this particular area or the epileptic focus led—in the cases where it could be safely performed—to the cessation of the seizures.

The study of epileptic seizures also has the potential to contribute a great deal to our understanding of consciousness. Absence seizures are classically described as an abrupt and sudden onset of impairment of consciousness, interruption of ongoing activities, a blank stare, and possibly a brief upward rotation of the eyes. If the patient is speaking, speech is slowed or interrupted; if walking, he or she stands transfixed; if eating, food intake is stopped. Usually the patient is unresponsive when spoken to. The attack lasts from a few seconds to a few minutes and disappears as rapidly as it starts.

The assumption that patients undergoing an absence seizure are no longer conscious is increasingly disputed (Bayne 2011). Whether these patients are conscious depends on how we define consciousness. If reportability is a necessary condition, then patients experiencing absence epilepsy cannot be considered conscious. This restricted definition would prevent us from ascribing consciousness to animals, infants, and many cognitively impaired patients. Bayne suggests a more broad approach that takes into account the evidence of voluntary mental imagery. We have previously seen that mental imagery production in patients with minimally conscious state is taken as an indicator of consciousness (Owen et al 2006).

Such a volition-based approach to consciousness would suggest that many absence seizures patients are conscious, albeit in a diminished manner. This is illustrated by the case of a 9-year-old boy reported by Gloor (1986, cited in Bayne 2011: p. 50): "He had a vacant look on his face. I asked him to close his eyes, but he did not comply even though the command was repeated. I then said Ricky can you hear me? To which he replied promptly by saying yes. After the attack, questioning revealed that he remembered that I had asked him to close his eyes." It seems that the capacity to perform single motor tasks on command is more likely to be disrupted

---

[12] Oliver Sacks (1933–2015) was a British-American neurologist who has written extensively about his experience with neurological patients. In his book *Hallucinations (2012)*, he recounts hallucination narratives.

[13] Wilder Penfield (1891–1976) was a Canadian neurosurgeon and neurophysiologist who worked at the Montreal Neurological Institute.

than the capacity to encode items in short-term memory. Clinicians have known for a long time that there is substantial variability in the degree of impaired consciousness from one patient to another and that absence seizures can affect some cognitive tasks while sparing others.

Loss of consciousness is not an all-or-nothing phenomenon (Laureys 2005a). Selective loss of consciousness and the resulting cognitive impairment described in these clinical examples teaches us that the content of any conscious state is—in pathological conditions—no longer under global control such as by the "global workspace," in the model proposed by Dehaene and Changeux (2011) and Edelman and Tononi (2000). The content of consciousness can indeed be extremely fragmented.

The notion that consciousness is fragmented is particularly apparent from the observation of patients with temporal lobe epilepsy. In this type of seizure, patients can experience feelings of depersonalization together with multiple fragmentized sensory states, such as visual or auditory hallucinations. These psychic phenomena, called aura, usually precede an observable seizure and can take the form of cognitive automatisms such as derealization or depersonalization; affective automatisms such as attacks of terror, pain, sadness, and joy; or perceptive hallucinatory like phenomena (Alvarez-Silva et al. 2006).

Depending on how the "personality fragments" are related, or if they fail to relate, we can argue that during a temporal lobe seizure, consciousness is not unified. It is as if the abnormal electrical activity taking place would "unbind" the functional connectivity of the brain. These clinical examples can be taken as evidence for a phenomenal fragmentation of consciousness, and this is a view shared by neurologists and neuroscientists. While mainstream empirical and philosophical findings hold that consciousness is unified, we should consider the possibility that the contents of consciousness no longer occur in a single phenomenal state in a patient undergoing a seizure (Bayne 2011).

Most current neurobiological models of consciousness propose some form of centralized consciousness module or workspace and are therefore best understood in holistic terms. These systems allow a subject to be conscious and ensure that his conscious state will be unified. However, as long as the general enabling mechanism involved in mediating the transition from unconscious to conscious is not clearly understood, the debate about the degree to which consciousness is unified will continue, especially in view of clinical examples showing that breakdown of consciousness is common.

## Narcolepsy

Narcolepsy is a chronic neurological disorder that combines the unique association of sleep attacks and episodes of muscle weakness, triggered by excitement. In 1880 the French neurologist Jean-Baptiste Gélineau (1880) reported the case of a wine merchant who had episodes of a sudden loss of muscle tone so that he would fall to the ground while remaining conscious.[14] These episodes of sudden muscle atonia, triggered by strong emotions, laughter being the most common, are called cataplexy. The other major symptom in this affection is excessive daytime sleepiness: patients fall asleep during the day with sometimes up to more than hundred episodes, lasting from a few seconds through several minutes of micro-sleep attacks. While we normally have a well-ordered sleep–wake cycle with sleep occurring mostly at night, patients with narcolepsy suffer from irresistible sleep attacks, feeling a strong urge to sleep, often against a background of extreme drowsiness. These "in between states" with repeated sleep attacks occur while the patient is at school or work, compromising normal daily activities. Driving a car is very dangerous for patients with narcolepsy.

The symptoms of narcolepsy may be understood as a consequence of loss of control of the normal boundaries between sleep and wake states. Sleep attacks, sleep paralysis, and hallucinations represent "in between states," with intrusion of elements of rapid eye movement (REM) sleep into the wakeful state. Cataplexy is due to the activation of glycinergic and gabaergic neurons in the reticular formation, which project onto spinal motoneurons resulting in their hyperpolarization and leading to muscle atonia (Luppi et al. 2011). Unchecked excitation from the amygdala during an emotional state is at the origin of this activation. In other words, the physiological mechanism leading to muscle atonia during REM sleep is accidentally activated in narcolepsy due to regulatory failure by the wake-promoting system. Discovery of these mechanisms came from genetic studies in dogs suffering from narcolepsy (Lin et al. 1999).

As a young researcher, Mignot (Lin et al. 1999) worked with dogs suffering from narcolepsy, in the sleep laboratory of William C. Dement, one of the scientists who discovered REM sleep. Narcolepsy was known to occur in animals and had been particularly studied in Labrador retrievers where it follows a genetic trait. The gene responsible, discovered by Mignot (1999), turned out to be the receptor for a family of peptides called hypocretins. Hypocretins are hypothalamic neuropeptides that play a key role in the regulation of wake-promoting systems. Loss of hypocretin leads to a "fragilization" of wakefulness that causes an inability to remain awake for extended periods (Bourgin et al. 2008). Hypofunction of the hypocretin system in the central nervous system leads to interference in other chemical systems of sleep regulation (Fig. 2.5), especially the locus coeruleus, a principal site for the production of norepinephrine. Hypocretin deficiency results in low levels of norepinephrine, a catecholamine playing a crucial role in alertness and arousal.

Narcolepsy patients have no hypocretin in their spinal fluid, indicating loss of brain hypocretin. But what causes this initial loss? Contrary to a genetic disease in dogs, human narcolepsy is a sporadic condition. The specific loss of hypocretin-producing neurons in narcoleptic patients results from an autoimmune attack on the hypocretin-secreting cells in a process called molecular mimicry. The mechanistic

---

[14] Narcolepsy is a rare disease affecting one in 2000 persons. The condition is described here because it offers a unique insight in the neurobiological mechanisms of regulation of sleep–wake cycles. Recent advances in the causes of narcolepsy may be relevant for a better understanding of other neurological and psychiatric disorders.

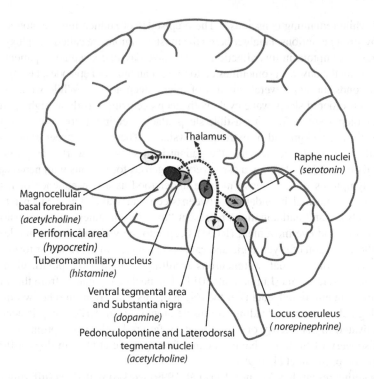

**Fig. 2.5** Hypocretin projections in the brainstem. Hypocretin neuronal projections (black, dotted lines) are present throughout the brainstem and make contact with a variety of brain stem nuclei involved in cholinergic, histaminergic, dopaminergic, serotonergic, and noradrenergic activities. Hypoactivity of hypocretin function leads to narcolepsy. Recent studies point also to a role of hypocretin hypofunction in anxiety disorders and depression (Johnson et al. 2012) (Adapted from Silber and Rye 2001)

explanation proposed is the activation of the immune system by a virus carrying a molecular structure similar to epitopes found in hypocretin-secreting cells (De la Herrán-Arita et al. 2013). Hypocretin-producing cells are destroyed by this autoimmune reaction resulting in narcolepsy. Currently, replacement therapies acting on the hypocretin system are available, while new treatment options using immunomodulation are under development (De la Herrán-Arita and García-García 2013).

Generally multiple factors contribute to the development of an autoimmune disease; in narcolepsy a combination of genetic susceptibility of the immune system and a viral or bacterial winter-related infection seem to be the main culprits (Mahlios et al. 2013). An interesting parallel can be drawn with encephalitis lethargica, described by von Economo in the 1930s.[15] Encephalitis lethargica appeared during the successive waves of influenza pneumonia that started in 1918 and peaked in the 1920s (Ravenholt and Foege 1982). It was characterized by a hypersomnolence associated with psychotic symptoms and a movement disorder presenting features of Parkinson's disease. These patients had midbrain lesions, including the posterior hypothalamus, hence affecting

---

[15] Constantin von Economo (1876–1931) was an Austrian psychiatrist and neurologist.

hypocretin-secreting neurons. Although narcolepsy and the encephalitis lethargica described by von Economo are distinct diseases, they share a sleep disorder. Both disorders are triggered by upper airway infections such as influenza. It is speculated that other neuropsychiatric conditions, such as movement disorders in children, result from similar autoimmune mechanisms following an infection.[16]

## Alzheimer's Disease

Alzheimer's disease,[17] the major cause of cognitive impairment in the elderly, is characterized prominently by memory loss, insidiously robbing patients of the ability to remember, to reason, and to make informed judgments. As the disease progresses, profound degradation of consciousness occurs. The extended consciousness, which holds autobiographical memories allowing us to be aware of an almost unlimited amount of images and events, is affected. We witness in these patients a slow mental decline characterized by impaired intellectual agility, reducing the subject's individual perspectives. This is characterized by personality changes and deficits in social cognition. The alterations also touch the capacity to evaluate personal emotional relevance of everyday information, to maintain and access common social knowledge, to process higher-order items about beliefs and intentions, and to generate and select behavioral responses (Shany-Ur and Rankin 2011).

There are no such terrible losses than those of our emotional and intellectual identity. As the disease progresses, the core consciousness or self-consciousness is affected, and the patient's sense of self is impaired. In a sense, the central deficit in Alzheimer's disease is impaired self-consciousness (Gil et al. 2001). But alteration of self-consciousness is heterogeneous and partial, so that it cannot be said that patients are unaware of existing or, more generally, that reflexive consciousness no longer remains.

The self-awareness deficit most commonly observed is anosognosia. This diminished awareness to know or recognize one's own illness has been used synonymously with loss of insight. Anosognosia is a term that was originally used to refer to a reduced awareness of hemiplegia in stroke patients and is observed in patients with a parietal lesion. As noted before, the parietal lobe, mostly on the right side, has important functions in updating sensory-body representations. The term anosognosia is now applied to reduced awareness of any symptoms (Mendez and Shapira 2011).

Patients diagnosed with dementia of the Alzheimer's type typically display a lack of awareness of their deficits and insist that nothing is wrong with them. The degree of anosognosia is correlated with the severity of dementia, but also with the

---

[16] For example, several pediatric movement disorders have been linked to autoimmune derangements triggered by viral or bacterial infections, though the link remains controversial (Wolf and Singer 2008). There is also evidence supporting a role for an immune dysregulation in the development of psychosis spectrum disorders.

[17] Alzheimer's disease (AD) is the most common neurodegenerative disorder of the brain. The etiology of AD is still not well understood. For a discussion of the many factors, including genetic susceptibility traits responsible for this condition, the reader is referred to publications in specialized journals.

severity of involvement of frontal functions (Starkstein et al. 1996). Anosognosia in Alzheimer's disease is also the result of the inability to update information about the self, due to memory impairment, leading to a "petrified self," frozen in time (Mograbi et al. 2009). One of the main features of consciousness is the capacity to integrate the many different sensory inputs, cognitions, and emotions in one single unified scene. The diffuse brain damage in Alzheimer's disease, resulting in impaired information transfer, leaves the patient with a limited and less flexible self-knowledge. The patient tries to elaborate his accomplishments and his abilities in his remote past, in older memories, leading to an outdated sense of self. In addition, due to the anterograde memory problems, experience of current tasks is poorly integrated. Thus, memory impairment in Alzheimer results in incoherence in the structure of the self and in broader terms, an altered consciousness (Mograbi et al. 2009).

# References

Alkire MT, Hudetz AG, Tononi G (2008) Consciousness and anesthesia. Science 322(5903): 876–80. doi:10.1126/science.1149213, Review

Alvarez-Silva S, Alvarez-Silva I, Alvarez-Rodriguez J, Perez-Echeverria MJ, Campayo-Martinez A, Rodriguez-Fernandez FL (2006) Epileptic consciousness: concept and meaning of aura. Epilepsy Behav 8(3):527–33

Bayne T (2011) The presence of consciousness in absence seizures. Behav Neurol 24(1):47–53. doi:10.3233/BEN-2011-0318

Benson DF, Sheremata WA, Bouchard R, Segarra JM, Price D, Geschwind N (1973) Conduction aphasia. A clinicopathological study. Arch Neurol 28(5):339–46

Bigelow HJ (1846) Insensibility during surgical operations produced by inhalation. The Boston medical and surgical journal XXXV(16):309–316

Boly M (2011) Measuring the fading consciousness in the human brain. Curr Opin Neurol 24(4):394–400. doi:10.1097/WCO.0b013e328347da94, Review

Bonhomme V, Boveroux P, Vanhaudenhuyse A, Hans P, Brichant JF, Jaquet O et al (2011) Linking sleep and general anesthesia mechanisms: this is no walkover. Acta Anaesthesiol Belg 62(3):161–71

Bourgin P, Zeitzer JM, Mignot E (2008) CSF hypocretin-1 assessment in sleep and neurological disorders. Lancet Neurol 7(7):649–62. doi:10.1016/S1474-4422(08)70140-6

Brown EN, Lydic R, Schiff ND (2010) General anesthesia, sleep, and coma. N Engl J Med 363(27):2638–50. doi:10.1056/NEJMra0808281

Brown RE, Basheer R, McKenna JT, Strecker RE, McCarley RW (2012) Control of sleep and wakefulness. Physiol Rev 92(3):1087–187. doi:10.1152/physrev.00032.2011, Review

Bruno MA, Vanhaudenhuyse A, Thibaut A, Moonen G, Laureys S (2011) From unresponsive wakefulness to minimally conscious PLUS and functional locked-in syndromes: recent advances in our understanding of disorders of consciousness. J Neurol 258(7):1373–84. doi:10.1007/s00415-011-6114-x

Buckner RL (2012) The serendipitous discovery of the brain's default network. Neuroimage 62(2):1137–45. doi:10.1016/j.neuroimage.2011.10.035

Cavanna AE, Trimble MR (2006) The precuneus: a review of its functional anatomy and behavioural correlates. Brain 129(Pt 3):564–83

Cruse D, Owen AM (2010) Consciousness revealed: new insights into the vegetative and minimally conscious states. Curr Opin Neurol 23(6):656–60. doi:10.1097/WCO.0b013e32833fd4e7

Damasio A (1999) The feeling of what happens. Harcourt Brace, New York. ISBN 0-439-0073-0

Damasio A (2010) Self comes to Mind. Vintage Books, New York. ISBN 978-0-307-47495-7

Davis MH, Coleman MR, Absalom AR, Rodd JM, Johnsrude IS, Matta BF et al (2007) Dissociating speech perception and comprehension at reduced levels of awareness. Proc Natl Acad Sci U S A 104(41):16032–7

Dehaene S, Changeux JP (2011) Experimental and theoretical approaches to conscious processing. Neuron 70(2):200–27. doi:10.1016/j.neuron.2011.03.018

De la Herrán-Arita AK, García-García F (2013) Current and emerging options for the drug treatment of narcolepsy. Drugs 73(16):1771–81, Review

De la Herrán-Arita AK, Kornum BR, Mahlios J, Jiang W, Lin L, Hou T et al (2013) CD4+ T cell autoimmunity to hypocretin/orexin and cross-reactivity to a 2009 H1N1 influenza A epitope in narcolepsy. Sci Transl Med 5(216):216ra176. doi:10.1126/scitranslmed.3007762

Demertzi A, Vanhaudenhuyse A, Brédart S, Heine L, di Perri C, Laureys S (2013) Looking for the self in pathological unconsciousness. Front Hum Neurosci 7:538. doi:10.3389/fnhum.2013.00538, Review

Driver J, Vuilleumier P (2001) Perceptual awareness and its loss in unilateral neglect and extinction. Cognition 79(1-2):39–88, Review

Eadie MJ, Bladin PF (2001) A disease once sacred: a history of the medical understanding of epilepsy. John Libbey Eurotext, Montrouge. ISBN 978-0-86196-607-3

Edelman GM, Tononi G (2000) A universe of consciousness. Basic Books, New York. ISBN 978-0-465-01377-7

Efron R (1956) The effect of olfactory stimuli in arresting uncinate fits. Brain 79(2):267–81

Fernández-Espejo D, Soddu A, Cruse D, Palacios EM, Junque C, Vanhaudenhuyse A et al (2012) A role for the default mode network in the bases of disorders of consciousness. Ann Neurol 72(3):335–43. doi:10.1002/ana.23635

Gazzaniga MS (1995) Principles of human brain organization derived from split-brain studies. Neuron 14(2):217–28, Review

Gélineau JB (1880) De la narcolepsie. Gazette des Hôpitaux 53:626–628

Geschwind N, Kaplan E (1998) A human cerebral deconnection syndrome: a preliminary report. 1962. Neurology 50(5):675–685

Gil R, Arroyo-Anllo EM, Ingrand P, Gil M, Neau JP, Ornon C et al (2001) Self-consciousness and Alzheimer's disease. Acta Neurol Scand 104(5):296–300

Gloor P (1986) Consciousness as a neurological concept in epileptology: a critical review. Epilepsia 27(Suppl 2):S14–26

Insel TR, Landis SC, Collins FS (2013) Research priorities. The NIH BRAIN Initiative Science 340(6133):687–8. doi:10.1126/science.1239276

Johnson PL, Molosh A, Fitz SD, Truitt WA, Shekhar A (2012) Orexin, stress, and anxiety/panic states. Prog Brain Res 198:133–61. doi:10.1016/B978-0-444-59489-1.00009-4, Review

Kopp Lugli A, Yost CS, Kindler CH (2009) Anaesthetic mechanisms: update on the challenge of unravelling the mystery of anaesthesia. Eur J Anaesthesiol 26(10):807–20. doi:10.1097/EJA.0b013e32832d6b0f

Laureys S, Faymonville ME, Peigneux P, Damas P, Lambermont B, Del Fiore G et al (2002) Cortical processing of noxious somatosensory stimuli in the persistent vegetative state. Neuroimage 17(2):732–41

Laureys S (ed) (2005a) The boundaries of consciousness: neurobiology and neuropathology, vol 150. Elsevier, Amsterdam

Laureys S (2005b) The neural correlate of (un)awareness: lessons from the vegetative state. Trends Cogn Sci 9(12):556–9

LeDoux JE (2000) Emotion circuits in the brain. Annu Rev Neurosci 23:155–84

Lin L, Faraco J, Li R, Kadotani H, Rogers W, Lin X et al (1999) The sleep disorder canine narcolepsy is caused by a mutation in the hypocretin (orexin) receptor 2 gene. Cell 98(3):365–76

Luppi PH, Clément O, Sapin E, Gervasoni D, Peyron C, Léger L et al (2011) The neuronal network responsible for paradoxical sleep and its dysfunctions causing narcolepsy and rapid eye movement (REM) behavior disorder. Sleep Med Rev 15(3):153–63. doi:10.1016/j.smrv.2010.08.002
Mack A, Rock I (1998) Inattentional blindness. MIT, Cambridge
Mahlios J, De la Herrán-Arita AK, Mignot E (2013) The autoimmune basis of narcolepsy. Curr Opin Neurobiol 23(5):767–73. doi:10.1016/j.conb.2013.04.013
Mendez MF, Shapira JS (2011) Loss of emotional insight in behavioral variant frontotemporal dementia or "frontal anosodiaphoria". Conscious Cogn 20(4):1690–6. doi:10.1016/j. concog.2011.09.005
Mograbi DC, Brown RG, Morris RG (2009) Anosognosia in Alzheimer's disease—the petrified self. Conscious Cogn 18(4):989–1003. doi:10.1016/j.concog.2009.07.005
Moruzzi G, Magoun HW (1949) Brain stem reticular formation and activation of the EEG. Electroencephalogr Clin Neurophysiol 1(4):455–73
Owen AM, Coleman MR, Boly M, Davis MH, Laureys S, Pickard JD (2006) Detecting awareness in the vegetative state. Science 313(5792):1402
Owen AM (2013) Detecting consciousness: a unique role for neuroimaging. Annu Rev Psychol 64:109–33. doi:10.1146/annurev-psych-113011-143729, Epub 2012 Oct 2
Panksepp J (2001) The neuro-evolutionary cusp between emotions and cognitions. Evol Cogn 7:141–163
Ravenholt RT, Foege WH (1982) 1918 Influenza, encephalitis lethargica, parkinsonism. Lancet 2(8303):860–4
Reinoso-Suarez F (2005) Neurobiologia del sueno. Rev Med Univ Navarra 49:1
Sacks O (2012) Hallucinations. Knopf, New York. ISBN 978-0307957245
Schiff ND (2012) Posterior medial corticothalamic connectivity and consciousness. Ann Neurol 72(3):305–6. doi:10.1002/ana.23671
Schultz W (2013) Updating dopamine reward signals. Curr Opin Neurobiol 23(2):229–38. doi:10.1016/j.conb.2012.11.012
Shany-Ur T, Rankin KP (2011) Personality and social cognition in neurodegenerative disease. Curr Opin Neurol 24(6):550–5. doi:10.1097/WCO.0b013e32834cd42a, Review
Silber MH, Rye DB (2001) Solving the mysteries of narcolepsy: the hypocretin story. Neurology 56(12):1616–8
Solms M, Turnbull O (2002) The Brain and the Inner World. Other Press, New York
Stam CJ, van Straaten EC (2012) The organization of physiological brain networks. Clin Neurophysiol 123(6):1067–87. doi:10.1016/j.clinph.2012.01.011
Starkstein SE, Sabe L, Chemerinski E, Jason L, Leiguarda R (1996) Two domains of anosognosia in Alzheimer's disease. J Neurol Neurosurg Psychiatry 61(5):485–90
Stern DN (1985) The interpersonal world of the infant: a view from psychoanalysis and developmental psychology. Karnac Books, London
Stern DN (2010) Forms of vitality: exploring dynamic experience in psychology and the arts. Oxford University Press, Oxford
Tononi G (2004) An information integration theory of consciousness. BMC Neurosci 5:42
Wijdicks EF (2001) The diagnosis of brain death. N Engl J Med 344(16):1215–21, Review
Young GB (2009) Coma. Ann N Y Acad Sci 1157:32–47. doi:10.1111/j.1749-6632.2009.04471.x, Review
Vaitl D, Birbaumer N, Gruzelier J, Jamieson GA, Kotchoubey B, Kübler A et al (2005) Psychobiology of altered states of consciousness. Psychol Bull 131(1):98–127
Vyazovskiy VV, Cirelli C, Pfister-Genskow M, Faraguna U, Tononi G (2008) Molecular and electrophysiological evidence for net synaptic potentiation in wake and depression in sleep. Nat Neurosci 11(2):200–8. doi:10.1038/nn2035
Wolf DS, Singer HS (2008) Pediatric movement disorders: an update. Curr Opin Neurol 21(4): 491–6. doi:10.1097/WCO.0b013e328307bf1c

# Part II

Part II

# Chapter 3
# Memory

## Introduction

Famous playwrights and writers have highlighted the critical role of memory in life. Tennessee Williams (1911–1983) said: "Life is all memory, except for the one present moment that goes by you so quickly you hardly catch it going" (1964). One of the most amazing properties of memory is its ability to transport us back in time. This is best exemplified by Marcel Proust's (1871–1922) great work, *Remembrance of Things Past* also known as *In Search of Lost Time* (1992). Proust masterly describes how suddenly a bit of our past, a bit of memory, can surge up in front of us when, for example, we smell a certain odor of childhood or we taste a long-unfamiliar food we once knew. These little stray moments can suddenly bring us back to a period of our lives we thought was lost forever.

In his book *How Proust Can Change Your Life,* De Botton (1997) states that one of the odd things about memory is that not all memories are distinct, just as not all moments of the present are clear. It is possible to remember with incredible clarity a moment that happened in early childhood, while the memory of last week seems lost in a kind of murkiness. This raises questions of how we form and retrieve memories and how we perceive time. We are drawn to the past but are urged to live in the moment.

Memorizing is the most fundamental capacity of our brain, allowing us to perform not only the simplest physical acts but also the most complex mental tasks. Memory involves storage and encoding of information. While we know the molecular mechanisms, for simple forms of memory, mainly from animal experimentation, we understand that there are a huge number of different and separate memory systems in the human brain. This view reflects the various types of memory described in great detail by psychologists, psychiatrists, and neurologists. This does not necessarily mean that all memory forms have different properties; they can use the same or similar basic mechanisms. Beyond the "how" and "where" memories are stored, we may also wonder whether memory storage is limited. Working memory is generally considered to have limited capacity. The memory span of young adults is limited to about seven elements, such as digits, letters, words, or other items (Miller 1956). However, some individuals have shown impressive increases in their memory span—up to 80 digits.

© Springer International Publishing Switzerland 2016
A. Steck, B. Steck, *Brain and Mind*, DOI 10.1007/978-3-319-21287-6_3

This can be achieved by training, but there are also heritable traits related to enhanced memory performance (Papassotiropoulos et al. 2006).

If we consider the sophistication of our mental abilities, we suspect that what is stored in memory is some sort of representation. We would like to believe that our memories are unlimited, a vision that Edelman and Tononi take up in the following way: "Our memory system has no fixed capacity limit, since it actually generates "information" by construction. In higher organisms every act of perception is to some degree an act of creation and every act of memory is to some degree an act of imagination. Biological memory is thus creative and not strictly replicative" (Edelman and Tononi 2000: p. 101).

As a matter of fact, the human brain's enormous memory capacity is processed by rate-limiting systems, such as working memory and selective attention. The capacity limits are shaped and defined by the same mechanisms generating consciousness, that is, temporal mapping and perceptual constructs. These essential bases of our memory system explain why biological memory cannot be equated to computer memory capacity. Human memory cannot be non-representational as in the case of computers. The inherent representational capacity of human memory allows the many symbolic activities that characterize our mental lives and our many skills, including foremost our language.

## Different Types of Memory

The functions of memory are very diverse, and many types of memory have been described. There has been a multidisciplinary approach culminating in the past 50 years, involving psychology, physiology, biology, genetics, and the study of patients with neurological or psychiatric disorders, to understand where and how "memories" are stored in the brain and eventually retrieved. The field has benefited from important discoveries that allow us to answer some basic questions. Foremost is the understanding that the dynamic process we call memory results from short-term or long-term changes in synaptic efficacy. Kandel and others investigated synaptic changes occurring in memory (Kandel 2001, for review see Sacktor 2012). We discuss the molecular biological aspects of memory below.

Of particular importance is the distinction between explicit or declarative and implicit or non-declarative memory (Fig. 3.1). Explicit or declarative memory typically refers to the conscious, intentional retrieval of past information or events. Major clinical studies of patients suffering from brain lesions demonstrate that damage to the hippocampus and the temporal lobe affects declarative or explicit memory (Scoville and Milner 1957). Explicit memory does not reflect a unitary function, but can be further divided into memory for facts, also called semantic memory, and memory for events, called episodic memory (Tulving 1983). Semantic memories are impersonal and devoid of autobiographical context, whereas episodic memories are personal. The following anecdote illustrates the important role of the spatiotemporal dimension in episodic memory encoding.

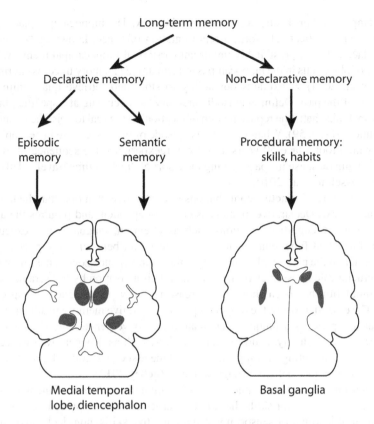

**Fig. 3.1** Memory systems. Long-term memory is divided into two broad classes: declarative or explicit memory and non-declarative or implicit memory. Declarative memory relies on hippocampal structures (medial temporal lobe) and diencephalon, while non-declarative memory depends on basal ganglia structures (Adapted from Henke 2010)

When I (Andreas) had my first course in neurophysiology in medical school, as I remember now almost 50 years later, our professor told us that the main function of the brain was learning. Learning is the acquisition of new skills, while memory is the process by which that knowledge is retained. Both are closely related, but not identical. Learning depends upon particular memory systems. In other words, learning could not exist without memory. I still vividly not only recall this particular lecture but also remember the auditorium where I was sitting as a medical student.

This recollection of past experience or events occurring at a specific time and place is called episodic memory. Recent findings, derived from both human observations and animal experiments suggest that episodic memory is a form of "detailed representation of a complex spatio-temporal trajectory on which a range of detailed items and events can be fastened" (Hasselmo 2011: p. 17). It appears that "location" is essential to episodic memory. From studies in rodents, we know that neurons are specifically activated in a particular region of space, place cells in the hippocampus, and grid cells in the entorhinal cortex. The hippocampal place cells are believed to collectively form a representation of space, known as "cognitive map." Place cells are presumably important carriers of hippocampal memory. The capacity of place cells in the hippocampus to form unique memory traces is enormous (Alme et al. 2014). It explains our ability to store and retrieve quasi-unlimited memories of the past. Defining episodic memory "as occurring at a specific place," Hasselmo thinks that: "the representation of location is essential to episodic memory" (Hasselmo 2011: p. 59). When I recall this episode of my first course in neurophysiology, which took place 50 years ago, I can reexperience the sequence of events with an exquisite sense in space, giving me a sort of "mental time travel" (Tülving, cited in Hasselmo et al. 2010).

There are other distinctive contributions to declarative memory than the temporospatial context. Declarative memory is context dependent and requires the association of many cognitive functions such as attention, language, and executive control. Important functional connectivities are found between the hippocampus, the parietal and the prefrontal cortex, a so-called convergence zone. These networks play a crucial role in associative memory, and their activation by transcranial magnetic stimulation has been shown to increase memory performance (Wang et al. 2014). The essential role of the hippocampus in declarative memory results from the fact that it represents a unique neuroanatomical convergence zone (Eichenbaum et al. 2007). Accordingly, neurological disorders, such as degenerative diseases or viral infections affecting the hippocampus and the associated cortical modules, will cause severe memory deficits (Ranganath and Ritchey 2012).

Implicit memory refers to a nonconscious, unintentional form of memory, such as the execution of motor skills that can be learned as rules or procedures. As well as procedural learning of sensorimotor and cognitive skills, non-declarative memory also includes conditioning and habituation, which are all expressed as behavioral changes and are independent of the medial temporal lobe (Henke 2010). Emotional processing of to-be-learned information enhances explicit memory, while it has little or no impact on implicit memory.

One of the major unanswered questions remains as to how and when our memories become consciously experienced. In the traditional model, the distinction between explicit and implicit memory centers on consciousness for the former and automaticity for the latter. But this dichotomy may be too simple. It is more likely that there is a continuum between these two types of memory, involving variables of cognitive processes, whether conceptually driven in the former or perceptually driven in the latter. Stimulus representation is a critical variable; when the aim is to bind together cognitive, affective, and contextual features of an event, the retrieval task involves explicit memory; on the other hand, simple information engages implicit memory. The level of intention is an important distinction between both memory types; memorizing is controlled in explicit memory, while it is more or less automatic in implicit memory (Dew and Cabeza 2011). As we discussed previously (Dehaene and Changeux 2011), consciousness is associated with activity in distributed brain areas crucially involving the prefrontal cortex. Therefore, conscious memory must involve a long-distance exchange of information across a broad cortical network, which is not the case for implicit memory.

Another important distinction of memory processes concerns the division between short- and long-term memories. Short-term memory refers to what one can hold in his mind, as stated above, about seven items, and is increasingly referred to as working memory. Working memory is involved in everyday tasks, from remembering a telephone number—while entering it in the phone—to understanding a sentence. It is also called immediate memory and represents facts or events that are currently present in one's mind. Anything lasting more than a few seconds is called long-term memory. There is a clinically important aspect to consider, a fact first reported by Théodule-Armand Ribot (1839–1916), a French psychologist who recognized that recent memories are more likely to be lost than more remote memories (Ribot 1882). This is also true in patients with brain damage due to various neurological pathologies: the more remote memories are less likely to be lost, the freshest ones being most vulnerable. The explanation of this well-established and fundamental property of memory is to be found in an essential mechanism called consolidation, a process that stabilizes a memory trace after the initial acquisition.

## The Dynamics of Memory Traces

Memory is a very dynamic phenomenon, from the moment of encoding to the time of retrieval. After encoding, labile memories undergo consolidation, that is, they are stabilized over time. This process depends on interactions between circuits located in several brain areas. It is well established that the hippocampus plays a crucial role in the initial encoding and storage of labile memories. Gradually however the neocortex becomes involved in maintenance and storage of lasting memory traces (Battaglia et al. 2011). The mechanism of consolidation is a dynamic process that can take from one to two decades to be fully formed in humans and allows memory storage for a lifetime. It is still controversial whether memories become completely independent of the hippocampus or are autonomously supported by the cortex and other structures.

Another issue is how the memory trace is transferred from the hippocampus to the neocortex. Memory is unlikely to be directly transferred from the hippocampus to the neocortex, and the current concept suggests that the hippocampus guides gradual changes in the neocortex that increase the complexity, distribution, and interconnectivity of memory storage sites[1] (Squire 2007). Memory consolidation is not necessarily a slow process. We not only learn and remember better when new material can be related to what we already know, but we can learn the new things very quickly if representations of related information have already been stored and

---

[1] A memory storage site should not be viewed as a circumscribed storage place. For example, memory encoding in the frontal cortex must involve a distributed network with a large number of connections.

stabilized in the brain. In other words, preexisting knowledge structures provide a feeling of familiarity, which will be strongly supportive of rapid consolidation of memory traces during learning.

A key feature of declarative memory is its permanence. We possess the ability to store and retrieve large amounts of information throughout our lifetime. Our inability to recall certain facts may not necessarily mean that the memory traces have been lost but rather they are inaccessible.

According to the synaptic plasticity theory described by Hebb (1949) and further developed by Kandel (2001), memory traces are stored in the form of changes in synaptic efficacy, resulting in functional modification and the formation of synapses, which get "wired together" (Bailey et al. 2000). The central dogma of the synaptic plasticity hypothesis implies that the development of a particular memory performance is the result of an activity-dependent trophic effect on the cells and synapses involved, producing an increased volume of neural tissue.

It is now well established that specific skills or performances are linked to particular brain structures. Among the many examples are longitudinal studies in children and adults, investigating specific skills such as playing an instrument or learning street maps. A study of London taxi drivers (Woollett and Maguire 2011) has been a particularly useful model to investigate memory. It illustrates the functional role of the hippocampus in specific spatial memory training, in the case of learning the complex London street lay out. These authors have convincingly shown that—with the concomitant change in memory performance—there was an associated increase in the volume of the posterior hippocampus. The fact that an environmental stimulation can promote structural changes in the brain is paramount to the notion of brain plasticity and to the realization that our brain is constantly shaped and transformed by our everyday mental activities.[2]

# The Molecular Biology of Memory

Given the evidence that all living brains store information, it is not unexpected that memory processes share common molecular mechanisms that are highly conserved in evolution. Kandel's group studies on simple learning behavior such as reflexes in a snail dissected the molecular mechanisms of memory (Kandel 2009). It is especially interesting that mechanisms of memory in invertebrates are very similar to those in mammals and basically the dynamic processes underlying either short-term or long-term memory formation are changes in synaptic efficacy or synaptic strength.

Short-term memory synaptic changes involve modifications of synaptic proteins or receptors by phosphorylation, leading to modification of synaptic connections.

---

[2] Whether the brain is only reshaped in extreme circumstances is open to discussion. Also there are compensation mechanisms: in the reported study, there was a reduced ability in non-London street-associated memory games, so there is a plasticity change in other areas, which we may not be aware of.

Long-term changes require long-lasting modifications of synapses such that complex molecular signaling cascades involving neurotransmitter receptors result in changes in synaptic strength and plasticity. This happens through the activation of transcription factors that affect the regulation of many genes. The best studied transcription factor is CREB (cAMP response element-binding protein). CREB modulates the transcription of genes coding for c-fos, BDNF (brain-derived neurotrophic factor), and several neuropeptides (Kandel 2012).

The ability of synapses to change strength, resulting in a long-lasting enhancement in signal transmission, is called long-term potentiation (LTP). As memories are encoded by modification of synaptic strengths, LTP is widely considered as one of the major cellular mechanisms underlying learning and memory processes (Lisman et al. 2012). Memory storage and consolidation involve alterations in protein synthesis, gene expression, and structural properties of neurons and synapses. The long-term synaptic changes involve activation of gene expression with the establishment of a dialog between genes and synapses (Kandel 2001). In addition epigenetic changes in gene expression can also leave unique memory traces at the molecular level.

The nature of the enduring molecular changes underlying long-term memory storage is still the subject of considerable debate. There must be some type of permanent alteration at the synaptic level to confer stability to memory storage. Any molecular basis for long-term memory formation must explain its permanence (for many years) despite the continuous turnover (every few hours) of the proteins. Other molecular switches for long-term memory include several protein kinases, so-called memory kinases (Giese and Mizuno 2013), which play an important role in memory consolidation by anchoring synaptic proteins or receptors. While we know a lot about the molecular pathways involved, an exact understanding of how the stability of the stored information is ensured is missing. Eventually memory storage involves changes in gene expression, protein synthesis, and synaptic structure and number. These different mechanisms are not mutually exclusive.

The process of memorization involves not only synaptic changes but also gene effects. Our genetic makeup determines who we are and our environment alters the way in which our DNA is expressed through epigenetic changes. There is now good evidence that epigenetic changes in gene expression can alter memory traces. Studies have shown that epigenetics influence memory and cognition in both normal and diseased brain (Saab and Mansuy 2014). Epigenetic changes consist of DNA methylation and histone modifications, but include also modification of transcription processes by microRNAs.

It is now recognized that environmental factors encountered by parents affect memory and cognition in offspring (Bohacek et al. 2014). This demonstrates the necessity to understand pathological memory processes at both genetic and environmental levels. It is still a long way off to translate basic neuroscience memory research to the clinic. However, a better understanding of these mechanisms will have implications for treatment of memory disorders caused by normal aging or diseases.

## Neurogenesis: Links to Memory and Behavior

In humans adult neurogenesis is restricted to the hippocampus, a phenomenon that takes place throughout life but diminishes with increasing age. The continuous production of new neurons is a subject of considerable interest. Bergmann and Frisen (2013) and Freund et al. (2013) propose that cognitive and behavioral development as well as formation of individuality is somehow linked to brain neurogenesis. It is well established, as we have seen above, that physical and mental activity can increase the brain's capacity for plasticity and self-repair, partly through the action of neurotrophic factors regulating neurogenesis. Neuronal activity—occurring, for example, during a mental task—is a sequential process including regulation of synaptic strength and growth. The molecular mechanism behind excitatory synapses is the NMDA (*N*-methyl-D-aspartate)-type glutamate receptor. Adult hippocampal neurogenesis allows lifelong plastic adaptation and is thought to promote successful aging (Kempermann 2008). Hippocampal networks will be shaped during lifetime by external sensory input or internal cortical computations, resulting in selective temporal and spatial activation. Psychologists have singled out two important cognitive functions, which play an important role in the storage of distinct memory and memory retrieval called "pattern completion" and "pattern separation" (Yassa and Stark 2011).

By pattern completion, we mean the ability to retrieve complete memory content when incomplete cues are given, a process that requires the rapid formation of auto-associative cellular populations. The hippocampus plays a seminal role in recruiting such large neuronal circuits.

Pattern separation on the other hand is the capacity to remember an event within a specific context. It is a critical mechanism for reducing interference among similar memory representations and not only enhances memory accuracy but is an essential element for working in a complex environment. The ability to precisely distinguish similar bits of different memory items is thought to depend to a great extent on the young neurons in the hippocampus. New neuron formation is required. These young neurons can help in the task of pattern separation because they have different electrophysiological properties from the older ones, especially as they are more sensitive to excitatory input than mature cells.

Impairment of pattern separation, resulting from diminished hippocampal neurogenesis, may underlie psychiatric disorders such as anxiety and depression (Kheirbek et al. 2012). It is speculated that patients with posttraumatic stress disorders (PTSD) may, as a consequence of decreased neurogenesis, have difficulties in distinguishing threats from similar but nonthreatening situations, a phenomenon that augments their anxiety. In this respect, it is important to understand that the behavioral effect of antidepressants may be mediated by the stimulation of neurogenesis in the hippocampus (Santarelli et al. 2003). This supports the idea that the hippocampus, through its role in contextual memory processing, is also involved in mood regulation. It appears that the hippocampus is setting up a kind of "contextual gate" to other brain regions, such as those involved in the regulation of emotional behavior. The treatment of depression and anxiety disorders may work in part by having an upregulatory effect on neurogenesis in the hippocampus and—through this mechanism—helping to restore the contextual control function of the hippocampus (Becker and Wojtowicz 2007).

As stated above, newly formed hippocampal neurons participate in encoding new memories. However, adding new neurons may affect memories already stored as the new neurons compete with the existing cells to make synapses. Thus, a high rate of hippocampal neurogenesis can induce forgetfulness (Akers et al. 2014). During infancy the markedly elevated neurogenesis that takes place around 2–3 years of age potentially renders hippocampal-dependent memories inaccessible at later time points. This may explain infantile amnesia at the neurobiological level as a type of retrograde amnesia, resulting from disrupted hippocampal-dependent memories.

# References

Akers KG, Martinez-Canabal A, Restivo L, Yiu AP, De Cristofaro A, Hsiang HL, et al. Hippocampal neurogenesis regulates forgetting during adulthood and infancy. Science. 2014;344(6184): 598–602. doi:10.1126/science.1248903.

Alme CB, Miao C, Jezek K, Treves A, Moser EI, Moser MB. Place cells in the hippocampus: eleven maps for eleven rooms. Proc Natl Acad Sci U S A. 2014. pii: 201421056.

Bailey CH, Giustetto M, Huang YY, Hawkins RD, Kandel ER. Is heterosynaptic modulation essential for stabilizing Hebbian plasticity and memory? Nat Rev Neurosci. 2000;1(1):11–20. Review.

Battaglia FP, Benchenane K, Sirota A, Pennartz CM, Wiener SI. The hippocampus: hub of brain network communication for memory. Trends Cogn Sci. 2011;15(7):310–8. doi:10.1016/j.tics.2011.05.008. Review.

Becker S, Wojtowicz JM. A model of hippocampal neurogenesis in memory and mood disorders. Trends Cogn Sci. 2007;11(2):70–6.

Bergmann O, Frisén J. Neuroscience. Why adults need new brain cells. Science. 2013; 340(6133):695–6. doi:10.1126/science.1237976.

Bohacek J, Farinelli M, Mirante O, Steiner G, Gapp K, Coiret G, et al. Pathological brain plasticity and cognition in the offspring of males subjected to postnatal traumatic stress. Mol Psychiatry. 2014. doi:10.1038/mp.2014.80.

De Botton A. How proust can change your life. London: Picador; 1997.

Dehaene S, Changeux JP. Experimental and theoretical approaches to conscious processing. Neuron. 2011;70(2):200–27. doi:10.1016/j.neuron.2011.03.018.

Dew IT, Cabeza R. The porous boundaries between explicit and implicit memory: behavioral and neural evidence. Ann N Y Acad Sci. 2011;1224:174–90. doi:10.1111/j.1749-6632.2010.05946.x. Review.

Edelman GM, Tononi G. A Universe of Consciousness. Basic Books. 2000 New York. ISBN 978-0-465-01377-7.

Eichenbaum H, Yonelinas AP, Ranganath C. The medial temporal lobe and recognition memory. Annu Rev Neurosci. 2007;30:123–52. Review.

Freund J, Brandmaier AM, Lewejohann L, Kirste I, Kritzler M, Krüger A, et al. Emergence of individuality in genetically identical mice. Science. 2013;340(6133):756–9. doi:10.1126/science.1235294.

Giese KP, Mizuno K. The roles of protein kinases in learning and memory. Learn Mem. 2013;20(10):540–52. doi:10.1101/lm.028449.112.

Hasselmo ME. How we remember: brain mechanisms of episodic memory. Cambridge: MIT Press; 2011.

Hasselmo ME, Giocomo LM, Brandon MP, Yoshida M. Cellular dynamical mechanisms for encoding the time and place of events along spatiotemporal trajectories in episodic memory. Behav Brain Res. 2010;215(2):261–74. doi:10.1016/j.bbr.2009.12.010.

Hebb DO. The organization of behavior. New York: Wiley; 1949.

Henke K. A model for memory systems based on processing modes rather than consciousness. Nat Rev Neurosci. 2010;11(7):523–32. doi:10.1038/nrn2850.

Kandel ER. The molecular biology of memory storage: a dialogue between genes and synapses. Science. 2001;294(5544):1030–8. Review.

Kandel ER. The biology of memory: a forty-year perspective. J Neurosci. 2009;29(41):12748–56. doi:10.1523/JNEUROSCI.3958-09.2009.

Kandel ER. The molecular biology of memory: cAMP, PKA, CRE, CREB-1, CREB-2, and CPEB. Mol Brain. 2012;5:14. doi:10.1186/1756-6606-5-14. Review.

Kempermann G. The neurogenic reserve hypothesis: what is adult hippocampal neurogenesis good for? Trends Neurosci. 2008;31(4):163–9. doi:10.1016/j.tins.2008.01.002.

Kheirbek MA, Klemenhagen KC, Sahay A, Hen R. Neurogenesis and generalization: a new approach to stratify and treat anxiety disorders. Nat Neurosci. 2012;15(12):1613–20. doi:10.1038/nn.3262.

Lisman J, Yasuda R, Raghavachari S. Mechanisms of CaMKII action in long-term potentiation. Nat Rev Neurosci. 2012;13(3):169–82. doi:10.1038/nrn3192. Review.

Miller GA. The magical number seven plus or minus two: some limits on our capacity for processing information. Psychol Rev. 1956;63(2):81–97.

Papassotiropoulos A, Stephan DA, Huentelman MJ, Hoerndli FJ, Craig DW, Pearson JV, et al. Common Kibra alleles are associated with human memory performance. Science. 2006; 314(5798):475–8.

Proust M. In Search of Lost Time, translated by C. K. Scott-Moncrieff, Terence Kilmartin and Andreas Mayor (Vol. 7). Revised by D.J. Enright. London: Chatto and Windus, New York: The Modern Library, 1992. Based on the French "La Pléiade" edition (1987–1989). ISBN 0-8129-6964-2

Ranganath C, Ritchey M. Two cortical systems for memory-guided behaviour. Nat Rev Neurosci. 2012;13(10):713–26. doi:10.1038/nrn3338.

Ribot T. Diseases of the memory: an essay in the positive psychology. New York: D. Appleton; 1882.

Saab BJ, Mansuy IM. Neuroepigenetics of memory formation and impairment: The role of microRNAs. Neuropharmacology. 2014;80:61–9. doi:10.1016/j.neuropharm.2014.01.026.

Sacktor TC. Memory maintenance by PKMζ--an evolutionary perspective. Mol Brain. 2012;5:31. doi:10.1186/1756-6606-5-31. Review.

Santarelli L, Saxe M, Gross C, Surget A, Battaglia F, Dulawa S, et al. Requirement of hippocampal neurogenesis for the behavioral effects of antidepressants. Science. 2003;301(5634):805–9.

Scoville WB, Milner B. Loss of recent memory after bilateral hippocampal lesions. J Neurol Neurosurg Psychiatry. 1957;20(1):11–21.

Squire LR. Neuroscience. Rapid consolidation. Science. 2007;316(5821):57–8.

Tennessee W. The milk train doesn't stop here anymore. New York: Dramatist's Play Service; 1964. ISBN 13: 978-0822207580.

Tulving E. Elements of episodic memory. New York: Oxford University Press; 1983.

Wang JX, Rogers LM, Gross EZ, Ryals AJ, Dokucu ME, Brandstatt KL, et al. Targeted enhancement of cortical-hippocampal brain networks and associative memory. Science. 2014; 345(6200):1054–7. doi:10.1126/science.1252900.

Woollett K, Maguire EA. Acquiring "the Knowledge" of London's layout drives structural brain changes. Curr Biol. 2011;21(24):2109–14. doi:10.1016/j.cub.2011.11.018.

Yassa MA, Stark CE. Pattern separation in the hippocampus. Trends Neurosci. 2011;34(10):515–25. doi:10.1016/j.tins.2011.06.006.

# Chapter 4
# Clinical View of Memory

*Our memories are the fragile but powerful products of what we recall from the past, believe about the present and imagine about the future.*

(Schacter 1996: p. 308)

## The Memory Machinery

We described in the previous chapter how synaptic changes are fundamental and essential mechanisms for inscription of memory traces in the brain. What exactly is stored remains debated. It could be that memory is laid down in a coded fashion as in a computer. This would require a static system, meaning that—when remembering—we are retrieving data from a storage bank. Memory is then equated to specific brain circuit properties. Edelman (1998) has argued for a more complex model that does not exclude these basic premises but uses the same dynamic structures underlying his theory of consciousness. He proposes that memory is a system property resulting from the "matching" at a given moment of various signals coming from the outside world, the body, and of course the brain itself. In his view, there are many more separate memory systems than the currently described clinical memory forms. What is attractive in his theory is that memory has no fixed capacity limit since it generates "information" by construction.

A scientific study of memory has to take in account the incredible richness of human recollective experience, especially if one wants to study memory disorders in neurological or psychiatric diseases. Memory is very robust, usually reliable, but can also be deceiving and fragile. These different aspects and qualities of memory can be experienced in everyday life and explain the amazingly different kinds of memory disorders that psychiatrists and neurologists have described. In real life, memories are never neutral, and this has led to the concept of "emotional memory," a topic of increasing relevance in the study of diseases like post-traumatic stress disorder or dissociative states. The fragile aspect of memory is well known. Memories of dreams often disappear after waking up. As we get older, when the aging brain begins to lose memory, if only in bits and pieces, we realize that memory

© Springer International Publishing Switzerland 2016
A. Steck, B. Steck, *Brain and Mind*, DOI 10.1007/978-3-319-21287-6_4

is what makes our lives. "Life without memory is no life at all," wrote the filmmaker Luis Bunuel (cited in Swinton 2012).

## Infantile Amnesia

Infantile or childhood amnesia was described by Freud (1901–1905, 1916–1917) as a form of amnesia, which—in the case of most people—hides the earliest life events of their childhood. Memories that exist before age 3 are at best incomplete and sketchy. He theorized that early childhood memories are actively repressed from consciousness because of their unacceptable sexual and aggressive content; in other words, early memories are held back because they could—by association—reactivate unwanted feelings, fantasies, or images.

Events occurring before the age of 3 are rarely consciously remembered. Memory traces or connections may either be lost or remain if constantly reactivated. The "use it or lose it" principle is essential in early brain development but is, according to Solms and Turnbull (2002), a lifelong process which takes place without conscious awareness. There is no need for a repression hypothesis in infantile amnesia as Freud (1915) postulated. Reactivated early childhood memories can be very strong—as, e.g., memories of traumatic events—but still consciously not retrievable as they are stored as implicit memories.

Preverbal affective and emotional experiences in the child's primary relations are stored in implicit unconscious memory (explicit memory is conscious remembering) in the amygdala (LeDoux 2000). Emotions that are expressed exclusively by the body in the form of pain, for example, often correspond to somatosensory sensations of early childhood. Traces of these experiences can be constantly reactivated and therefore influence a person's affective, emotional, sexual, and cognitive life. The frontal cortex is poorly developed in the first 2 years of life; there are two growth spurts around 2 and 5 years. Yet the frontal cortex is crucial for the retrieval of memory in a realistic, rational, and orderly way.

As the hippocampus is not fully functional in the first 2 years, memories will be implicit and procedural (bodily memory). The function of the hippocampus consists of transferring unconscious preverbal affective memories, which are above all mediated through the amygdala system, into conscious verbal memories (van der Kolk 1996; LeDoux 1996). At the time of memorization, the various aspects of memory have to be integrated according to time, location, and context (Bremner and Narayan 1998).

Current neurobiological theories suggest that there is a lower level of neurocognitive processing of memory traces in early childhood, compared to a higher level in later childhood. This transformation reflects a maturation process in memory circuits in the hippocampus and cortex. According to Pillemer (1998), the very rapid increase in narratives occurring after 3 years of age is linked to the formation of new cognitive patterns and developmental achievements such as language and the establishment of an autobiographical self.

A durable long-term autobiographical memory is dependent on social interaction. This necessitates the construction of a narrative through parent–child conversation and formation of a significant parent–child attachment. Memory development is therefore as much an external as an internal process. Memories of events experienced in infancy are expressed emotionally or behaviorally. Narrative memory appears about age 2–3, when children begin to talk about the past. Memories of early infancy may be recovered if they are "translated" from immature, mostly emotionally tainted images, to adult-like narratives. This physiological developmental perspective does not rule out the possibility of "unconscious forgetting" in the case of intense emotional trauma in early life (Pillemer 1998). The parent–child interaction plays an important role in the way painful experiences in early childhood are "remembered." Children of parents who deny these events may later manifest the traumatic experience with emotional or behavioral expressions, whereas this is not the case for children whose parents are available to engage in a supportive dialogue about the negative incident.

## Mind, Time, and Memory[1]

"The past is never dead. It's not even past" William Faulkner (1897–1962).

(Faulkner 1950)

Memories and fantasies influence our sense of time. Time is created out of our subjective experiences. Our sense of the duration of time changes; according to our feelings of joy, pain, gratification, and frustration, time passes slowly or quickly. The ancient Greeks distinguished between kairos,[2] a cyclic or mythic time, and chronos, a linear or sequential notion of time. In psychotherapeutic relationship, moments of kairos shared between patient and therapist may enhance the therapeutic relatedness, mark, and greatly enrich the therapeutic process. These so-called sacred or now moments (Bruschweiler-Stern et al. 2002) represent significant insight for patients and therapists and lead to an intimately profound understanding. They are often potentially mutative experiences and points of reference in the narrative history of a patient. Smaller and emotionally less charged modifications occur in chronos, that is, in linear time of the longitudinal treatment sequences.

---

[1] In ancient Greek, Μνημοσύνη = Mnemosyne was the goddess and personification of memory and the mother of the nine Muses.

[2] Kairos (ancient Greek: καιρός) signifies a moment of indeterminate time, a window of opportunity for change, whereas Chronos (ancient Greek: Χρόνος) "time" refers to chronological or sequential time.

## Mind and Time in Childhood and Adolescence

Child development is marked socially, in the form of birthdays, anniversaries, pre- and school entries, religious events, and other transitions. Young children try with magical effort to stop or advance time in order to prove that they are not subjected to it. One of the main tasks during adolescence is the integration of finitude—which is associated with giving up infantile omnipotent entitlement, immortality fantasies, and perfection ideals—as well as the recognition of gender and generational differences and the ubiquity and irreversibility of death. Accepting temporality as a human condition is a psychic process where the self on the one hand denies temporality and on the other accepts the reality of unilinear time (Ladame 2007). A part of the self recognizes unilinear time, another denies it.

## Retranscription of Memory

Childhood memories of the first years of life are modified or constructed at later developmental periods by the process of Nachträglichkeit,[3] that is, by means of "retrospective attribution" (Modell 2006: p. 36). Events and intrapsychic experiences of the past, which the small child was not able to accommodate, find only later meaning and interpretation. Eickhoff (2006) describes the phenomenon of "Nachträglichkeit" as a constant recontextualization of events from earlier developmental phases into later stages. The processing of events afterward introduces a special dimension to temporality: it does not influence the sequence of time but the significance of the event.

What Freud (1896,1985) called re-transcription of memory has been taken up by Edelman. For him memory is essentially a dynamic transformative process: "A memory is the enhanced ability to categorize associatively, not the storage of features or attributes as lists" (Edelman 1987: p. 241). Experiences from the time of early childhood may only later—as memories—have a traumatic impact (Freud 1893–1895). At a very young age, a child cannot react adequately to an event that will only later be understandable (Freud 1917–1919). A "repressed" memory can thus subsequently lead to traumatization. Likewise, threats endured in childhood can have pathogenic effects afterward (Freud 1909).

Earliest experiences are not stored in the form of retrievable memories. The missing engrams are often only reconstructed, sometimes starting from recurrent "acting." Unassimilated past affective experiences are brought into the present, and the compulsion to repeat represents the urge to seek re-transcription of a memory in a new context and within a meaningful relationship. Freud (1920) considered repetition as a form of memory.

---

[3] Nachträglichkeit is a term used by Freud from 1890 on, translated in English as deferred action, and in French as après-coup.

Experiences that are not inscribed in a time sequence (past–present–future) tend to repeat themselves. They appear as an everlasting presence. "… The past is not the passive container of things bygone. The past, indeed, is our very being, and it can stay alive and evolve; the present is the passage where the re-transcription and recontextualization of our past continually occur …" (Scarfone 2006: p. 814). "… for any significant mental event, there is an après-coup effect (Nachträglichkeit), a re-organizing of the mind that lets new forms show up or, conversely, that may bury ideas and affects that had emerged" (Scarfone 2011: p. 759).

## Clinical Vignette Cathleen

This vignette demonstrates how an early traumatic event is "remembered" by a child through nonverbal (emotional and behavioral) manifestations. Her symptoms disappear after she has been able to consciously memorize the event by telling her story in a psychotherapeutic relationship.

Cathleen, a 6-year-old girl, lost, at age 3 years 9 months, her then 4-month-old brother, Vincent, affected by Down syndrome, to sudden infant death (he was found dead in his crib). Since the birth of a second child—1 year ago—Cathleen sleeps only under the crib of her new brother. In kindergarten she is described as a scapegoat, letting herself be beaten by others. At home the parents experience a child who goes through cyclical periods of aggression or depression: in the depressive period, Cathleen withdraws, closes herself up entirely, and is no longer approachable. During the aggressive periods, she complains constantly, whines, cries for no reason, and commands other children.

In her second interview with the child psychiatrist, Cathleen says she wants to write a book; she draws and dictates the text: "The history of an angel. A little angel walks in heaven and meets the sun who says 'good morning' to him. Then he encounters a house." When asked who the angel is, Cathleen answers "This is my little brother, Vincent, I do not like talking about my little brother, it makes me sad, but if I had wings, I would go and get him. He must be content as there are other babies and grown-ups in heaven, in God's house. The house of God is the Church."

Cathleen has until now not been able to grieve over the loss of her brother. Feelings of anger, sadness, and pain are manifested in the behaviors described by the parents. Out of fear of repetition, Cathleen takes over a parentified role, keeping guard as close as possible over the newborn brother. The parents, burdened by severe guilt feelings, were not able to mourn their loss that is to express pain, anger, and sadness and therefore could not assist their daughter to grieve. Cathleen was able to tell her affective experience of the past and attribute meaning to her own life history. In her narration that contains not only affective memories but also imagination and fantasies, she reconfigures time, her experience of kairos (a cyclic or mythic time), and her "historical truth."

The concept of "historical truth" is highly complex, as it is the result of biological, cultural, and individual (preverbal and verbal) influences. The historical truth does not correspond to the truth of the (re)constructed story, but includes the currently valid, often rapidly-again-modified "truth," which has been elaborated by the patient and therapist. Enclosed are the reflections of the intrapsychic dialogue of the patient with himself and—in the interpersonal dialogue—the emerging and shared "certainty about the current truth," which is constantly modified by conscious and unconscious contributions of both participants leading to new insights. During the course of a psychoanalytical therapeutic process, the history of a patient is constantly created anew. The patient attempts to establish self-continuity so that in his feelings his past is connected without ruptures to the experience of his self in the present.

## Emotions and Memory

Emotional memories are the core of our personal history and life. Emotions can both enhance or disrupt memories. This duality has been referred by Schacter (1996) as memory's "fragile power." The power of emotions on memory is evident when one contemplates the many moments in our everyday life when memories suddenly overwhelm us as flashes or when past events are forgotten, repressed, or blocked, being associated with strong negative affects.

Although intrusive recollections of traumatic events can be disabling, it is also important that emotionally arousing experiences, which occur in response to dangers that can be life-threatening, persist over time and provide a basis for long-lasting memories (LeDoux 1996; McGaugh 2000). The mechanisms leading to a persistent memory have been extensively researched. Animal studies have shown that persisting emotional memories (especially fear) depend to a large extent on a specific structure in the limbic system, the amygdala, which in turn engages the frontotemporal region. The amygdala turns on the release of stress hormones such as adrenergic hormones and cortisol by way of the hypothalamic–pituitary–adrenal axis (LeDoux 1996). The humoral neuromodulation therefore involves interaction between adrenergic and glucocorticoid systems. These hormones have important positive and negative modulatory effects on memory. Adrenergic stimuli consolidate memory, in association with a hypervigilant state (Liang et al. 1986; Henckens et al. 2009). In contrast, chronic elevation of basal cortisol levels which occurs in psychiatric disorders such as depression and post-traumatic stress disorder (PTSD) results in reduced hippocampal volume and associated deficits in memory (Bremner 2006) (see Chap. 3).

## Amnesias and Memory Disorders

The distinction between explicit or declarative memory and implicit or non-declarative memory is well established on both neuropsychological and neuroscientific grounds as described before. The Swiss neurologist Edouard Claparède (1873–1940) is credited for introducing the terms "implicit" and "explicit" to the study of memory (Kihlstrom 1995). As a clinician, he believed that the study of patients provided the best way to gain insights into mental functioning. He reported a case of an amnesic patient suffering from alcoholic Korsakoff syndrome showing selective memory impairment. Claparède performed the following test with this female patient. He greeted her every day with a handshake, but each time she did not recognize him. One day he put a hidden pin in his finger that pricked her when they shook hands so that she withdrew her hand very quickly. When he wanted to shake hands with her the next day, she hesitated to give her hand while still not recognizing him. The clinical experiment demonstrated that the patient, although amnesic for the encounter with her doctor, retained a clear memory of the painful event, displaying functioning implicit or unconscious memory. While she retains a feeling of something painful, she cannot really connect this past event to herself. As we now know, an intact autobiographical self depends on a functioning explicit memory.

The implication of this observation goes beyond the study of amnesic patients. In more general terms, the distinction between implicit and explicit memory poses the problem of conscious recollection, a theme that is central to the development of modern psychology and psychoanalysis. Explicit memory—as we have seen—refers to episodes in our past life and is dependent on the integrity of the hippocampus and the medial temporal lobe. It concerns conscious experiences. Implicit memory is nonconscious and thus non-retrievable and non-verbalizable. There is evidence suggesting that perceptual (visual) implicit memory is dependent on the posterior aspects of the associative cortex of both hemispheres, in particular the right hemisphere (Gabrieli et al. 1995). As we have described, implicit memory is a term that covers diverse phenomena. It has been used in very different contexts so that wide views have emerged. Nonetheless, the concept of implicit memory follows in these different situations similar paths (Schacter 1987).

Ribot (1882)[4] wrote that the study of memory disorders will eventually complete and confirm what we know from neurophysiology and neurobiology. In his book *Diseases of Memory,* he investigates the phenomena of memory from a pathological viewpoint. He distinguishes two broad types of memory disorders: temporary or periodic amnesia (such as epileptic, transient global amnesia, and psychogenic amnesia) and progressive amnesia, where the dissolution of memory is slow and continuous resulting from a progressive brain disorder. It implies that memory depends on permanent modifications and organization of neurons and that their disorganization leads to amnesia. Indeed, amnesias arise after damage to crucial structures, such as the hippocampus, through which information has to pass before it is stored long term, but focal or widespread cortical damage also gives rise to amnestic syndromes. Ribot described an important clinical aspect in progressive diseases of memory, namely, a temporal gradient from the most recent to the oldest memories. First to be affected are recent memories. Second, personal memories disappear, "going downward to the past." Third, things acquired intellectually are lost bit by bit; last to disappear are habits and emotional memories.

---

[4] Théodule Ribot (1839–1916) is a French neuropsychologist, known for his work on retrograde amnesia.

## *Transient Global Amnesia*

Transient global amnesia (TGA) syndrome was initially described more than a century ago by Ribot (1882). The denomination "global" is not quite correct since it implies total memory loss, which is not the case as implicit memory is preserved. The key features involve an abrupt onset of anterograde amnesia that usually lasts less than 24 h, and the patient maintains personal knowledge and remote memory, but new memories cannot form. The patient typically asks repetitive questions as he always forgets the answers. After recovery, a permanent gap in memory remains, that is, the amnesia period is never recovered (Kirshner 2011). This condition has recently been the subject of interesting experimental work. Magnetic resonance imaging (MRI) data suggest that a transient perturbation in hippocampal activity is the functional correlate of TGA because high-resolution MRI shows small edema-like lesions in the CA1 sector of the hippocampus in patients during the amnestic episode (Bartsch et al. 2010) (Fig. 4.1).

The time course of these changes mimic the memory disorder and the lesions disappear as the patient recovers. It appears that hippocampal CA1 neurons are selectively vulnerable to metabolic or hypoxic stress; several studies have shown that emotional, behavioral, or physical stress plays a pivotal part in pathophysiological cascades, leading to impairment of hippocampal function during TGA. The particular susceptibility of the hippocampus with regard to stressful events might also have a role in memory deficits in other conditions such as post-traumatic stress disorders.

While MRI studies emphasize the role of dysfunctional hippocampal CA1 neurons as the neuroimaging correlate of TGA, newer studies with resting state functional MRI show in addition a bilateral reduction in functional connectivity (Peer et al. 2014). The connectivity changes were found in parts of the episodic memory network

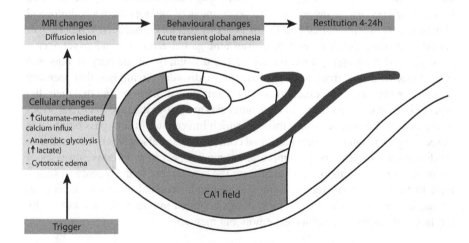

**Fig. 4.1** Model illustrating the pathophysiological changes in the CA1 (cornus ammonis) field of the hippocampus during a transient global amnestic episode (Adapted from Bartsch and Deuschl 2010)

and included mostly temporo-limbic but also frontal regions. These new data suggest that the functional changes underlying TGA are more widespread than originally believed and emphasize the necessity of bilateral dysfunction to produce amnesia.

The exact nature of the pathophysiological cascade and the cellular mechanisms that affect CA1 neurons remains unclear at present; however, an important aspect on how episodic memory works has been revealed: it can be erased transiently by a "dysmetabolic" process. When a permanent lesion occurs in pathophysiology, the resulting impairment is very different as we will see below.

## Chronic or Progressive Amnestic Disorders

The medial temporal lobe system, especially the hippocampal formation, is essential for conscious memory of facts and events. The role of the hippocampus, as it is now understood, is to consolidate the distributed elements of memory into a coherent and stable ensemble. This can be achieved because the hippocampus is reciprocally connected to all neocortical areas and has an ideal position to rapidly encode association aspects of experienced events. One can easily understand why damage to the hippocampus will have severe effects on memory.

The starting point for clinical studies of declarative memory in the 1950s was the observation of a patient known as H.M. who had undergone bilateral medial temporal lobe resection, including the hippocampus, to relieve epilepsy. After surgery he developed a profound memory defect (cited in Squire and Wixted 2011). The patient could no longer form new memories for facts and events and was unable to learn or remember new information (anterograde amnesia). Sadly he had to stay in a nursing home for the rest of his life.

Subsequent studies involving other patients have shown that damage to the medial temporal lobe impairs declarative memory, while the elements of long-term memory stored in the neocortex are not affected. Procedural learning (implicit memory) or the learning of motor functions such as bicycle riding is not disturbed.

When we remember events from our past or memorize new information, the storage takes place in a spatial and temporal context. This link or association with the target information is called contextual processing. Contextual processing is important in memory tasks, particularly in episodic learning (Kessels and Kopelman 2012), and serves also as a retrieval cue. The role of the diencephalic–hippocampal memory system in episodic forms of memory disorders has been particularly well examined in a neurological condition called Korsakoff syndrome. It was originally known as alcoholic Korsakoff syndrome because it was described in alcoholic patients (Victor et al. 1989) but has also been reported in traumatic brain injury and encephalitis.[5] The lesions in Korsakoff syndrome extend beyond the hippocampus and include the diencephalic region, a region now called the extended hippocampal circuitry.

---

[5] Korsakoff syndrome can also occur as part of Wernicke's encephalopathy, a manifestation of acute vitamin B1 deficiency in the context of alcoholism or malnutrition.

These patients have marked anterograde amnesia; they cannot create new memories. They suffer a form of contextual memory deficit with loss of temporal dating. One of the key features of Korsakoff syndrome is that these patients do not so much forget as remember inappropriately or out of context. This out of temporal sequence retrieval leads to errors and distortion of memories, a memory disturbance that is called confabulation. In Korsakoff patients, the memory deficit reflects a difficulty in dating events so that fragments of real souvenirs are mixed inappropriately. Interestingly implicit unconscious learning is little impaired in Korsakoff patients because it is presumably largely context free. In general terms, the dissociation between explicit and implicit learning is explained by the fact that these two memory systems rely on separate neural circuits. The diencephalic-hippocampal circuits are relevant for the explicit learning, while implicit learning relies on other structures such as the basal ganglia. Implicit learning depends more on perceptual processing and is data driven. Explicit memory tasks are conceptually driven as they entail analysis of meaning (Brunfaut and d'Ydewalle 1996).

Confabulation is caused by lesions in the posterior medial orbitofrontal cortex (an area damaged in patients with Korsakoff syndrome), while hippocampal lesion is responsible for the amnesia (Schnider 2013). The posterior medial orbitofrontal cortex is a structure that plays an important role in relating past events and memories to the actual context, leading to reality confusion when this filter does not function properly (Schnider 2013). It is hypothesized that the orbitofrontal cortex acts as a reality filter, checking if an incoming memory is pertaining to an ongoing reality or not. Thus, patients with a Korsakoff syndrome have difficulties to place themselves correctly in time and space.

Many other circumstances, such as viral infections, hypoxia, or carbon monoxide poisoning, lead to amnestic syndromes, though brain damage may not be restricted to the hippocampus (Markowitsch and Staniloiu 2012). In addition to organic amnesia with structural damage to the hippocampal memory system, functional deficits are thought to occur in patients with schizophrenia. Studies show that these patients present difficulties with explicit remembering, but have normal implicit memory function (Danion et al. 2001).

Memory impairment, a key feature of Alzheimer's disease (AD), shows a complex profile. The well-known retrograde memory temporal gradient impairment, with better memory for remote compared to recent events, is due to the pattern of neurodegeneration. The memory loss of recent events results from the hippocampal damage that occurs early in the disease, while remote event memory loss is related to the gradual damage of cortical areas. Memory loss in Alzheimer's disease has a striking aspect, namely, that patients lack awareness of their illness, for which Babinski coined the term anosognosia.[6] Patients with advanced Alzheimer's disease are not conscious of their deficits. Mograbi et al. (2009) propose that anosognosia

---

[6] Anosognosia is not restricted to Alzheimer's disease. Denial of other kinds of deficits such as sensorimotor functions also occurs in other neurological disorders, such as stroke and brain tumors. This is seen in lesions of the right parietal lobe, in which there is unawareness of deficits on the left side of the body.

results from missing blocks in the construction of self-representation. The self can be viewed as a constantly updated construction resulting from the integration of different functions such as autobiographical memory, somatosensory perceptions, and language. As all these processes are impaired in AD, the self is progressively "petrified" and eventually vanishes. The failure to update self representations results in a mismatch of personal evaluation capacities giving rise to an awareness deficit showing us to what extent the contents and preservation of the self is dependent on intact memory systems and other cognitive and emotional abilities. The role of memory in the development of the self has been highlighted by several authors who emphasized its importance in giving the subject a sense of a past and present and the ability to project into the future (Mograbi et al. 2009). As the self disappears in AD, the patient's personality slowly disintegrates, narrowing the scope of consciousness and barely allowing, toward the end, a glimpse of a reaction, or even a smile.

# References

Bartsch T, Deuschl G. Transient global amnesia: functional anatomy and clinical implications. Lancet Neurol. 2010;9(2):205–14. doi:10.1016/S1474-4422(09)70344-8. Review.

Bartsch T, Schönfeld R, Müller FJ, Alfke K, Leplow B, Aldenhoff J, et al. Focal lesions of human hippocampal CA1 neurons in transient global amnesia impair place memory. Science. 2010;328(5984):1412–5. doi:10.1126/science.1188160.

Bremner JD. Traumatic stress: effects on the brain. Dialogues Clin Neurosci. 2006;8(4):445–61. Review.

Bremner J, Narayan M. The effects of stress on memory and the hippocampus throughout the life cycle: Implications for childhood development and aging. Dev Psychopathol. 1998; 10:871–85.

Brunfaut E, d'Ydewalle G. A comparison of implicit memory tasks in Korsakoff and alcoholic patients. Neuropsychologia. 1996;34(12):1143–50.

Bruschweiler-Stern N, Harrison AM, Lyons-Ruth K, Morgan AC, Nahum JP, Sander LW, et al. Explicating the implicit: the local level and the microprocess of change in the analytic situation. Int J Psychoanal. 2002;83(Pt 5):1051–62.

Danion JM, Meulemans T, Kauffmann-Muller F, Vermaat H. Intact implicit learning in schizophrenia. Am J Psychiatry. 2001;158(6):944–8.

Edelman GM. Neural Darwinism. New York: Basic Books; 1987.

Edelman GM. Building a picture of the brain. Daedalus. 1998;127(2):37–70.

Eickhoff FW. On Nachträglichkeit: the modernity of an old concept. Int J Psychoanal. 2006;87(Pt 6):1453–69.

Faulkner W. Requiem for a nun. New York: Random House; 1950.

Freud S. Studies on hysteria, vol. II. SE Hogarth Press. London; 1893–1895

Freud S. A case of hysteria. Three essays on sexuality and other works, vol. VII. SE Hogarth Press; 1901–1905

Freud S. Two case histories, vol. X. London: SE Hogarth Press; 1909.

Freud S. Repression, vol. XIV. London: SE Hogarth Press; 1915. p. 146–58.

Freud S. Introductory lectures on psychoanalysis, vol. XVI. London: SE Hogarth Press; 1916–1917.

Freud S. An infantile neurosis and other works, vol. XVII. London: SE Hogarth Press; 1917–1919.

Freud S. Beyond the pleasure principle, vol. XVIII. London: SE Hogarth Press; 1920. p. 7–64.

Freud S. In: Masson JM (ed.) The complete letters of Sigmund Freud to Wilhelm Fliess,1896. Cambridge: Harvard University Press; 1985.

Gabrieli J, Fleischman D, Keane M, Reminger S, Morrell F. Double dissociation between memory systems underlying explicit and implicit memory in the human brain. Psychol Sci. 1995;6(2):76–82.

Henckens MJ, Hermans EJ, Pu Z, Joëls M, Fernández G. Stressed memories: how acute stress affects memory formation in humans. J Neurosci. 2009;29(32):10111–9. doi:10.1523/JNEUROSCI.1184-09.2009.

Kessels RP, Kopelman MD. Context memory in Korsakoff's syndrome. Neuropsychol Rev. 2012;22(2):117–31. doi:10.1007/s11065-012-9202-5.

Kihlstrom JF. Memory and consciousness: an appreciation of Claparède and recognition et moïtè. Conscious Cogn. 1995;4(4):379–86.

Kirshner HS. Transient global amnesia: a brief review and update. Curr Neurol Neurosci Rep. 2011;11(6):578–82. doi:10.1007/s11910-011-0224-9. Review.

Ladame F. Subscribing to temporality: a major issue in adolescence. EPF Bull. 2007;61:97–102.

LeDoux J. The emotional brain. New York: Simon & Schuster; 1996.

LeDoux J. Emotion circuits in the brain. Annu Rev Neurosci. 2000;23:155–84.

Liang KC, Juler RG, McGaugh JL. Modulating effects of posttraining epinephrine on memory: involvement of the amygdala noradrenergic system. Brain Res. 1986;368(1):125–33.

Markowitsch HJ, Staniloiu A. Amnesic disorders. Lancet. 2012;380(9851):1429–40. doi:10.1016/S0140-6736(11)61304-4.

McGaugh JL. Memory—a century of consolidation. Science. 2000;287(5451):248–51. Review.

Modell AH. Imagination and the meaningful brain. Cambridge: MIT Press; 2006.

Mograbi DC, Brown RG, Morris RG. Anosognosia in Alzheimer's disease—the petrified self. Conscious Cogn. 2009;18(4):989–1003. doi:10.1016/j.concog.2009.07.005.

Peer M, Nitzan M, Goldberg I, Katz J, Gomori JM, Ben-Hur T, et al. Reversible functional connectivity disturbances during transient global amnesia. Ann Neurol. 2014;75(5):634–43. doi:10.1002/ana.24137.

Pillemer DB. What is remembered about early childhood events? Clin Psychol Rev. 1998;18(8):895–913.

Ribot T. Diseases of the memory: an essay in the positive psychology. New York: D. Appleton; 1882.

Scarfone D. A matter of time: actual time and the production of the past. Psychoanal Q. 2006;75:807–34.

Scarfone D. The analyst at work. Live wires: when is the analyst at work? Int J Psychoanal. 2011;92:755–9.

Schacter DL. Implicit memory: history and current status. J Exp Psychol Learn Mem Cogn. 1987;13(3):501–18.

Schacter DL. Searching for memory: the brain, the mind, and the past. New York: Basic Books; 1996.

Schnider A. Orbitofrontal reality filtering. Front Behav Neurosci. 2013;7:67. doi:10.3389/fnbeh.2013.00067.

Solms M, Turnbull O. The brain and the inner world. New York: Other Press; 2002.

Squire LR, Wixted JT. The cognitive neuroscience of human memory since H.M. Annu Rev Neurosci. 2011;34:259–88. doi:10.1146/annurev-neuro-061010-113720.

Swinton J. Dementia, living in the memories of God. Grand Rapids: William B Eerdmans; 2012.

van der Kolk BA. Traumatic stress. London: Guilford Press; 1996.

Victor M, Adams RD, Collins GH. The Wernicke–Korsakoff syndrome. 2nd ed. Philadelphia: F.A. Davis; 1989.

# Part III

# Chapter 5
# Emotions

## Evolving Concept of the Limbic System

The brain does not function independently in the body and this is especially true for emotions, since most involve bodily responses such as rapid heart rate, sweating, and muscle tension. But emotions are more than just visceral and body changes: emotions are also positive and negative states of mind, with diverse features such as anger, anxiety, fear, panic, embarrassment, excitement, joy, and pleasure to name a few of the distinctive qualities associated with emotions.

As emotions reflect such a wide spectrum of states of mind, it is not surprising that research on the biological basis of emotions has produced a variety of different models. Over the last 50 years, anatomists, physiologists, psychologists, neurologists, and psychiatrists have tried to define and order the anatomical systems involved in processing emotions.

In 1937, an American neuroanatomist, Papez (1937), described an anatomic network that is now referred to as the Papez circuit. His basic idea was that emotions are not "a magic product but are physiologic processes dependent on anatomic mechanisms" and "emotion is such an important function that its mechanisms should be placed on a structural basis." (p. 111).

According to Papez, emotional experiences occur when the low-level subcortical areas such as the hypothalamus, the medial part of the thalamus, or the hippocampus activate the cortex, namely, the cingulate gyrus. Conversely an emotional experience also occurs when a stream of thoughts in the cortical area activates the cingulate cortex and subsequently the subcortical areas such as the hippocampus and the hypothalamus. Papez (1937) gives interesting clinical examples of patients with lesions in these anatomical regions that display a variety of disturbances in their affective and emotional behavior. In cases of viral infection affecting the hippocampus and the cerebellum, he describes how these patients are tormented by episodes of anxiety and rage. But he also identified prominent changes in memory. We now know that the Papez circuit plays an important role in memory and consciousness, and damage to parts of this circuit, for example, to the hippocampus or the mammillary bodies, produces prominent dissociation of consciousness and

© Springer International Publishing Switzerland 2016
A. Steck, B. Steck, *Brain and Mind*, DOI 10.1007/978-3-319-21287-6_5

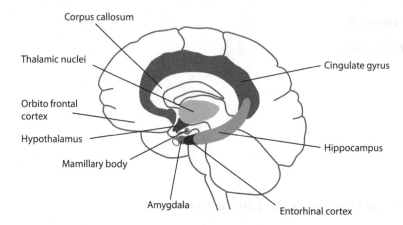

**Fig. 5.1** The limbic system includes the hypothalamus, the thalamus, the hippocampus, the amygdala, and several nearby areas. It is intimately connected to the cingulate gyrus and the orbitofrontal cortex

memory. Clinical observations reveal a fundamental role for these brain structures in organizing memory.[1]

MacLean, an American neurologist and psychiatrist, expanded Papez's original description by adding additional structures including the prefrontal cortex (PFC) and the amygdala (MacLean 1949). He named the brain circuit that channels emotions by integrating information from the body and external world the "visceral brain," later using the term limbic system (Fig. 5.1). MacLean stated: "Though our intellectual functions are carried on in the newest and most highly developed part of the brain, our affective behavior continues to be dominated by a relatively crude and primitive system. This situation provides a clue to understanding the difference between what we 'feel' and what we 'know'" (MacLean 1949: p 351).

McLean's original view has been considerably updated by studies showing widespread connection of the amygdala with the medial and PFC. Overlapping neurocircuitry was characterized in which bidirectional loops connect multiple cortical and subcortical structures, and evidence is emerging that this complex system is involved not only in emotions but also regulates mood and behavior (for review see Price and Drevets 2010). For example, a system connecting the limbic system and the medial forebrain was identified and named the mesolimbic system or medial forebrain bundle (MFB) (Fig. 5.2). This circuit is part of a reward and seeking system or motivational system that includes a key dopaminergic center, the nucleus accumbens. Another pathway, running close to the MFB, is the anterior thalamic radiation (ATR) system (Fig. 5.2). In contrast to the MFB, the ATR pathway mediates separa-

---

[1] We now know the hippocampus is primarily involved in memory processing and the amygdala more with emotions.

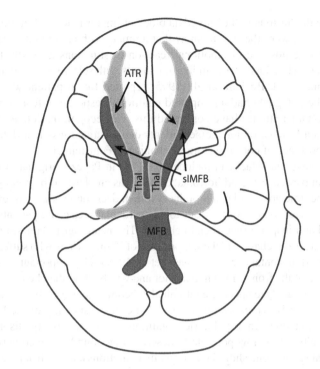

**Fig. 5.2** The medial forebrain bundle (MFB) and its superolateral branch (slMFB) run laterally to the thalamus (Thal). The anterior thalamic radiation (ATR) system runs medially and connects the thalamus to the prefrontal cortex (Adapted from Coenen et al. 2012)

tion distress and sadness (Coenen et al. 2012). The anterior cingulate cortex (ACC), to which the ATR projects, is thought to be involved in pain and sadness regulation, e.g., it plays a role in the vocalizations that infant animals make when separated from their mothers (Panksepp 2004). There is now good evidence from functional neuroimaging studies that a network involving both the cortical (PFC, ACC) and subcortical regions (amygdala, thalamus) is involved in processing emotional states (Davidson and Irwin 1999). The experience of negative emotions, such as sadness, is accompanied by marked changes in the activity of the anterior cingulate gyrus (Zubieta et al. 2003). The addition of all these networks to those originally described by Papez (1937) and MacLean (1949) enlarges the scope of emotional research. Combining different experimental approaches, including neuroimaging, demonstrates that specific types of emotions correspond indeed to a specific brain region or pathway.

The role of the amygdala in emotion and fear regulation, for example, is supported by both animal experiments and human psychopathological studies (Davis and Whalen 2001; LeDoux 1996, 2007). Researchers used a classical experimental paradigm of behavioral psychology called fear conditioning. In this experimental setting, a subject learns to associate an aversive stimulus with a neutral stimulus, so that eventually the neutral stimulus alone can trigger a fear response. Experiments clearly show that lesions in the amygdala block or impair fear conditioning. Klüver and Bucy (1939) were the first to show that animals with an amygdala lesion displayed a striking absence of emotional reaction to situations normally triggering fear or danger. In humans, a few studies of patients with selective amygdala damage have been published. Bechara et al. (1995) reported that a patient with bilateral damage to the amygdala had an impaired emotional response in fear conditioning experiments. Other studies have confirmed this fear recognition deficit in patients with amygdala lesions, though some patients demonstrated less fear deficits, suggesting the presence of compensating mechanisms (Feinstein 2013).

We saw above that MacLean included the PFC in Papez's original circuit. This region, and in particular the orbitofrontal cortex, was emphasized by neuropsychologists for some time now to play a prominent role in decision making. For example, it is known from case studies that lesions to this particular area cause patients to suffer from altered and inappropriate social behavior. The neurologist Damasio illustrated dramatic changes of behavior in the famous case of Phineas Gage who suffered severe injury to the orbitofrontal cortex (Damasio et al. 1994). This important case demonstrates the role of the frontal lobe in behavior and will be described below.

The ability to analyze specific anatomical subcomponents involved in emotional processing currently serves as a way into a better understanding of the biology of affective dysfunctions in psychiatric conditions such as anxiety disorders and depression. While it is now possible to describe functionally defined networks for emotional categories, one should not forget that emotions emerge from the interplay of a large variety of internal and external neural influences to produce the quasi-unlimited number of different brain states characterizing the human mind.

Emotions, as discussed in the chapter clinical view of consciousness, emerged early in evolution. The amygdala, a center of emotion, plays a role in fear conditioning which is a very important survival trait. It is interesting to note that—at the beginning of an emotion like fear—the amygdala is activated, but by the time feelings arise, the amygdala is suppressed. Feelings—in the context of an emotional upheaval—depend on interactions between somatosensory, attentional, and executive processes, requiring engagement of the PFC. In this context, we should note that the capacity of the PFC to suppress the amygdala will also potentially alleviate emotional distress and thus play an important role in suppressing unwanted memories (Anderson et al. 2004).[2]

What started almost 80 years ago with Papez's and MacLean's descriptions of the visceral brain is now an interdisciplinary field combining basic neuroscience with clinical disciplines such as psychiatry and psychology and is referred to as affective neuroscience. The field of affective neuroscience is relevant not only for understanding how affects play a role in learning but also how emotions influence our decision-making abilities. Similarly, exploration and knowledge of basic emotional processing mechanisms have led to better comprehension of affective dysfunctions in psychiatric disorders, for example, pathological anxiety. It also pro-

---

[2] This mechanism of active forgetting can be viewed as a biological model for Freud's theory of repression.

vides a framework for understanding the neural control of interpersonal and social behavior (Harrison and Critchley 2007).

# Emotion and Behavior

Emotion and behavior are essential parts of our mental life and as such have been intensively studied. For many years, a dichotomy prevailed with, on the one side, proponents of an objective scientific approach championed by cognitive psychology and, on the other, proponents of a more subjective view, in line with psychodynamic and psychoanalytical concepts. It is now obvious that one cannot study the mind without analyzing not only its processes but also its contents by way of an introspective approach.

To put it simply, emotions arise from the integration of sensations from the external world with information from the body. In this way, emotions can be considered as a "translation" of somatic processes. However, to be fully perceived and appreciated, an emotional experience combines high-level cortical representations with perception of bodily changes. Emotions directly shape our affective states and by nature are extremely subjective. They express a state of mind and therefore make up an important part of our conscious experience; as such we must consider emotions as important ingredients of what we call consciousness or conscious experience. In this respect, it is not surprising that the same brain structures involved in consciousness are also the structures of the emotional system. In other words, affective states are major building blocks of consciousness. The self, a basic concept of modern psychology, is an extension of self-consciousness. Emotions, reflecting the perception we have of our body, are an important ingredient in the formation of our self and our sense of being.

## *Emotional Systems*

The neuroscientist Panksepp (2011) considers emotions as basic affects present in all mammals. He emphasizes that emotions are primary processes involving subcortical brain regions. Accordingly there is an evolutionary layering of functions in the brain. Affects, at least the primary ones, are more ancient in brain/mind evolution and could thus function independently of the cognitive knowledge we consciously experience in many life situations. For Panksepp (2011) these primary emotional systems evolved to serve key adaptive purposes. In other words, emotions are specific processes that are part of an inherited neuro-mental armamentarium. These basic emotional systems include categories such as "seeking," "lust," "rage," "fear and panic," and "separation distress." This list is by no means exhaustive and these categories are derived from studies of animal behavior. They can therefore not be directly translated to human psychology. In humans there is a larger and almost infinite catalogue of emotional states and responses. They are by no means rigid, and they are open to modifications and influenced by education, learning, and life experiences.

Freud (1895) said that a real understanding of the mind and emotions should wait until neuroscience provides answers. As described above, we now assume that the neural dynamics of mental processes reflects an evolutionary layering. Primary process emotions are embedded in the lower subcortical layers, while secondary emotional processes, which arise from emotional learning like fear conditioning, engage midbrain components such as the basal ganglia. Finally tertiary affects will recruit neocortical functions, when long-range functions like planning are involved.[3] In reality however affective states are often a mixture of unconscious and conscious representations. To reflect both—unconscious and conscious representations—Panksepp proposed that emotional processes could be considered a part of "nested brain-mind hierarchies" (Panksepp 2011; Northoff et al. 2006). This can be viewed as an operational system in which higher brain/mind functions in order to properly mature have to integrate lower brain/mind processes. This system operates in two ways, bottom up and top down.

The primary emotional processes represent instinctual emotional systems. There is some evidence that the neocortex is not essential for generation of primary emotional processes such as "seeking," "lust," "rage," "fear and panic," and "separation distress." While these primary emotion responses can be triggered experimentally in animals by electric or chemical stimulation of specific subcortical structures and induce various stereotyped behaviors, the experimental paradigms utilized do not tell us what the animals are feeling. Furthermore, much of what we have learned by testing the emotional circuits in animals was undertaken in the narrow context of reward and punishment functions. It would be a mistake to hold that primary emotional feelings or behaviors are solely the construct of subcortical brain regions. Rather, emotional experiences always reflect some kind of higher-level brain sensory and associative functions. In humans, these representations are known to span large cortical areas such as the frontal, insular, and parietal cortex. These brain regions are all activated during emotional tasks.

What we need to understand is how lower-level brain circuits and higher-level cortical regions interact with each other to achieve a full working integration of the different layers. This will require a massive database that can mimic complex functional information. It is obvious that the most complex affects, the so-called third-level processes, such as hope or grief, are produced and elaborated by the engagement of large neocortical areas. Furthermore, regulation of emotions and cognitive executive activities, guided by affects, are all higher brain functions that ultimately depend on personal biographical experiences. If we consider empathy or fairness, for example, we need to take into account the existence of a personal subjective experience, which holds both cognitive and affective contents.

---

[3] Primary or core emotions are instinctual emotional processes, while secondary or tertiary emotions, or extended emotions are associated with cognitive processes depending on neocortical systems.

## The Role of the Frontal Lobe

Damasio (1996) underlines the fact that there is a strong interconnection between cognition and emotions emphasizing that emotions play a major part in decision-making abilities and behavior and points out—in accordance with MacLean's model—the tight connections between the limbic system and the prefrontal cortex (PFC). The role of emotion-related feedback in behavior and decision making is introduced.

It is well known by neurologists and neuropsychologists that patients with damage to the PFC display marked changes in personality with striking emotional and decision-making deficits. Damasio retrospectively studied the case of Phineas Gage in great detail, using modern neuronatomical reconstruction methods (Damasio et al. 1994). He showed how damage to a small region of the PFC, the ventromedial prefrontal cortex (VMPFC), had profound effects on social behavior and social functioning without inducing obvious impairments in cognitive performances. Phineas Gage was a railroad foreman who lived in the nineteenth century and suffered an accident at work, causing a relatively small unilateral damage to the VMPFC. Apparently he did not lose consciousness and made a rapid physical recovery. However, while he showed no apparent intellectual impairment, he displayed odd behavior and very poor decision-making capacity; he then lost his job and his family relations broke down. He showed features that patients with frontal lobe lesions typically display, such as difficulties in planning and decision making.

In the "somatic marker" hypothesis, Damasio (1996) postulates that decision making and behavior are influenced by signals coming from the emotional brain, the limbic system. In decision making, a signal from the limbic system generates a somatic marker.[4] This signal, which includes all kinds of sensations from our body, can be conscious or unconscious. Decision making is a two-way process combining a reasoning aspect, carrying a logical or cognitive analysis of a given action, with somatic marker signals, carrying bodily sensations. This peculiar combination helps us assess how rewarding or punishing a given action may be. The somatic marker hypothesis builds on the earlier theories of Papez and MacLean, which suggested that emotion experience is based on the perception of ever changing activities in the body. The frontal lobe has a central role in integrating this bodily information. The correct framework for body representations is dependent on critical developmental periods. This topic is reviewed in Chap. 6.

## Social Emotion and Social Norm

The way in which we connect and how we interact with other people is a subject of considerable interest for neuroscientists. Darwin formulated that a very distinctive human characteristic is the so-called "all important emotion of sympathy" (Black

---

[4] According to Damasio (1996), the marker is called somatic because it relates to body-state structure and function.

2004). Sympathy is not only a feeling or emotion ultimately aimed at helping some-body else but also represents the capacity to comprehend the feelings of others. Another word used to describe the perceptual capacity to feel or to relate to anoth-er's mental state is empathy. Both sympathy and empathy can be understood as a warm feeling for others, and this ability to feel another person's state of mind is made possible by the representations of our own body and self in our brains, images that we apply to the external world.

From a neurobiological perspective, new insights into the mechanisms of how we understand other people's feelings have come from the discovery of mirror neurons. Originally found in monkeys, these "mirror neurons" are activated when an animal acts as well when the animal observes another performing a similar action (Rizzolatti and Fabbri-Destro 2010). Since this discovery, it was speculated that the mirror neu-ron system plays an important role in our capacity to imitate or understand the inten-tion of others.[5] In other words, when we interact socially, our capacity to understand the action of others depends on the use of a "shared" neuronal network. There is still a lot of debate about a possible function of mirror neurons in humans. They can be considered as a simulating or "as if system," which helps us understand not only the actions of others but also other's emotions through the activation of a similar neuro-nal network. While the original description of mirror neurons in monkeys focused on observing an action, such as grasping for food, there is now good evidence that an emotional state observed in another person can activate the same neuronal network in the observer; the existence of such "shared" networks has been demonstrated in multiple studies of emotions in which the mere observation or imagination of some-one else's emotions triggered the same neuronal activation in the observer. For exam-ple, observing someone in pain triggers the neuronal representation subserving pain. These "shared" activation patterns were used to propose a core network for pain empathy (Singer et al. 2004) where the activated brain region contains the anterior cingulate cortex (ACC). This region is not only activated in situations of pain and empathy but also in many other emotional responses; both positive, such as happi-ness, and negative, such as fear, suggesting that the ACC is not specifically related to nociceptive mechanisms but reflects a much more general viscero-sensitive response.

We strive as individuals to achieve friendships based on mutual sympathy. Sympathy, in the philosophical sense, describes the feelings of moral sentiments. These moral sentiments are key elements that regulate social norms. How the brain generates moral sentiments is a problem that neuroscience is just beginning to address. We saw the important role of the PFC in decision making and social behav-ior. Current research is extensively investigating how fairness or selfishness guides our behavior. It is, for example, well known that we experience negative emotions, if resources such as food are unfairly distributed, while a fair distribution of goods produces positive emotions and will favor a collaborative behavior. Recent studies

---

[5] While at the beginning the role of mirror neurons was limited to the execution and control of movements, it is now well established that this system plays an important role in functions such as imitation and learning and more broadly in social interactions and communications (Rizzolatti and Fogassi 2014).

using economic exchange games involving fairness have provided interesting insights into some of the underlying neural mechanisms. For example, the lateral prefrontal cortex (LPFC) has emerged as a key area involved in fairness judgment and manipulating the LPFC with magnetic stimulation interfered with decision-making abilities of subjects involved in a decisional process in an economic game context (Ruff et al. 2013).

While these results suggest that stimulation of the LPFC, especially the right side, enhances social norm compliance in a specific game situation, generalization of these results to decision making in real life would be premature. As the authors note, increasing one type of norm compliance with brain stimulation may come at the cost of decreasing another type. Another limitation of this method of study is the fact that the experimental persons are taken as "objects," defined and limited by an experimental paradigm. The context is very much constrained, so that full development of a reflective consciousness is not possible. Decision making, at its highest level, takes place in a specific state of consciousness. It involves the whole issue of intentionality and causality, which is a fundamental aspect of our thinking mind.[6]

Behavioral economic laboratory studies have also been used to investigate how value-based or moral judgments are made (Haidt 2007). While these studies often apply hypothetical dilemmas in an artificial environment, attempts are now being made to look at moral behavior in every day's life: for example, important issues such as how morality affects people's happiness and sense of purpose are addressed in order to reveal the underlying mechanisms helping to distinguish what is "right" or "wrong" in decision making (Hofmann et al. 2014).

What is really coded or processed in areas such as the ACC or LPFC remains unresolved. It would be a gross oversimplification to call the ACC an empathy area or the LPFC a fairness center. These data confront us with the following dilemma: is it acceptable to have a modular or localizing view of brain function or is it necessary, even in a rather simple experimental paradigm, to always consider the whole brain in terms of connectivity and temporal dynamics, when interpreting mental processes such as decision making? This is especially relevant, if we want to understand not only the mechanism of social behavioral phenomena but more importantly the causal roots and the reflective states associated with decision making. We are thus still far away from having an all-encompassing brain theory for social emotions and social norms.

---

[6] It is assumed that any mental representation bears an "intentionality." Intentionality characterizes the directedness of our mind toward people, objects, and events.

# References

Anderson MC, Ochsner KN, Kuhl B, Cooper J, Robertson E, Gabrieli SW, Glover GH, Gabrieli JD. Neural systems underlying the suppression of unwanted memories. Science. 2004; 303(5655):232–5.

Bechara A, Tranel D, Damasio H, Adolphs R, Rockland C, Damasio AR. Double dissociation of conditioning and declarative knowledge relative to the amygdala and hippocampus in humans. Science. 1995;269(5227):1115–8.

Black DM. Sympathy reconfigured: some reflections on sympathy, empathy and the discovery of values. Int J Psychoanal. 2004;85(Pt 3):579–95.

Coenen VA, Panksepp J, Hurwitz TA, Urbach H, Mädler B. Human medial forebrain bundle (MFB) and anterior thalamic radiation (ATR): imaging of two major subcortical pathways and the dynamic balance of opposite affects in understanding depression. J Neuropsychiatry Clin Neurosci. 2012 Spring;24(2):223–36. doi:10.1176/appi.neuropsych.11080180

Damasio AR. The somatic marker hypothesis and the possible functions of the prefrontal cortex. Philos Trans R Soc Lond B Biol Sci. 1996;351(1346):1413–20.

Damasio H, Grabowski T, Frank R, Galaburda AM, Damasio AR. The return of Phineas Gage: clues about the brain from the skull of a famous patient. Science. 1994;264(5162):1102–5.

Davidson RJ, Irwin W. The functional neuroanatomy of emotion and affective style. Trends Cogn Sci. 1999;3(1):11–21.

Davis M, Whalen PJ. The amygdala: vigilance and emotion. Mol Psychiatry. 2001;6(1):13–34.

Feinstein JS. Lesion studies of human emotion and feeling. Curr Opin Neurobiol. 2013;23(3):304–9. doi:10.1016/j.conb.2012.12.007.

Freud S. Project for a scientific psychology, vol. I. London: Hogarth Press SE; 1895. p. 295–391.

Haidt J. The new synthesis in moral psychology. Science. 2007;316(5827):998–1002.

Harrison NA, Critchley HD. Affective neuroscience and psychiatry. Br J Psychiatry. 2007; 191:192–4.

Hofmann W, Wisneski DC, Brandt MJ, Skitka LJ. Morality in everyday life. Science. 2014;345(6202):1340–3. doi:10.1126/science.1251560.

Klüver H, Bucy PC. Preliminary analysis of functions of the temporal lobe in monkeys. Arch Neurol Psychiatry. 1939;42:979–1000.

LeDoux J. Emotional networks and motor control: a fearful view. Prog Brain Res. 1996;107:437–46. Review.

LeDoux J. The amygdala. Curr Biol. 2007;17(20):R868–74.

MacLean PD. Psychosomatic disease and the visceral brain; recent developments bearing on the Papez theory of emotion. Psychosom Med. 1949;11(6):338–53.

Northoff G, Heinzel A, de Greck M, Bermpohl F, Dobrowolny H, Panksepp J. Self-referential processing in our brain--a meta-analysis of imaging studies on the self. Neuroimage. 2006;31(1):440–57.

Panksepp J. Affective neuroscience. The foundations of human and animal emotions: Oxford University Press; 2004.

Panksepp J. Cross-species affective neuroscience decoding of the primal affective experiences of humans and related animals. PLoS One. 2011;6(9), e21236. doi:10.1371/journal.pone.0021236. Review.

Papez JW. A proposed mechanism of emotion. Arch Neurol Psychiatry. 1937;38(4):725–43.

Price JL, Drevets WC. Neurocircuitry of mood disorders. Neuropsychopharmacology. 2010;35(1):192–216. doi:10.1038/npp.2009.104. Review.

Rizzolatti G, Fabbri-Destro M. Mirror neurons: from discovery to autism. Exp Brain Res. 2010;200(3-4):223–37. doi:10.1007/s00221-009-2002-3. Review.

Rizzolatti G, Fogassi L. The mirror mechanism: recent findings and perspectives. Philos Trans R Soc Lond B Biol Sci. 2014;369(1644):20130420. doi:10.1098/rstb.2013.0420.

Ruff CC, Ugazio G, Fehr E. Changing social norm compliance with noninvasive brain stimulation. Science. 2013;342(6157):482–4. doi:10.1126/science.1241399.

Singer T, Seymour B, O'Doherty J, Kaube H, Dolan RJ, Frith CD. Empathy for pain involves the affective but not sensory components of pain. Science. 2004;303(5661):1157–62.

Zubieta JK, Ketter TA, Bueller JA, Xu Y, Kilbourn MR, Young EA, et al. Regulation of human affective responses by anterior cingulate and limbic mu-opioid neurotransmission. Arch Gen Psychiatry. 2003;60(11):1145–53.

# Chapter 6
# The Development of Self

## Brain Development and the Self

Whereas the basic wiring diagram of the brain is genetically preprogrammed, its fine-tuning throughout the different phases of infancy, childhood, adolescence, and adulthood is highly experience dependent. Early life experiences shape the specific patterns of neuronal branching and synapse formation. Neuronal connections are reorganized according to the frequency of their utilization. The sensory signals are transformed into neurochemical and cellular processes, directly impacting on the structure and function of the brain. Neuronal connections and functions are of an extraordinary plasticity at every level of the brain organization. Anatomical, physiological, and chemical changes take place throughout life in a complex interplay with the surrounding forces and continuously shape behavior, knowledge base, and skills of an individual.

Brain and environment communicate interactively and have a mutual influence on each other. Environmental factors can influence gene expression by epigenetic mechanisms directly modifying the genetic carrier substance, DNA. All mental processes correspond to biological events. Changes in states of mind are always reflected in brain modifications and vice versa (Price et al. 2000). Brain plasticity allows for great adaptability on the one hand, and on the other it can be detrimental for infants and young children who are highly vulnerable to the long-ranging impacts of adversities and traumatic events (van der Kolk et al. 1996).

For example, learning triggers neuronal changes such as synapse formation. Acquiring skills increases myelination (McKenzie et al. 2014), while social isolation or severe stress result in impaired myelination (Liu et al. 2012; Sexton et al. 2009). Currently, efforts are made to understand the molecular mechanisms of synapse stabilization or elimination, and genetic studies are linking single nucleotide polymorphisms in different genes to alterations in neuronal synapse formation.[1]

---

[1] A genetic mutation in a single nucleotide is called a single nucleotide polymorphism (SNP). While many SNPs are not associated with disorders, some are linked to diseases. Current studies looking at SNPs in bipolar disorders or schizophrenia have discovered SNPs in genes coding for synapse plasticity and regulation (Heck et al. 2014).

© Springer International Publishing Switzerland 2016
A. Steck, B. Steck, *Brain and Mind*, DOI 10.1007/978-3-319-21287-6_6

A disturbance in plasticity at critical periods of development in infancy or adolescence can lead to long-lasting behavioral changes. In adolescence the plasticity of the brain is highest. This is also the peak time for clinical onset of mental diseases, such as mood disorders or schizophrenia (Fig. 6.1, Paus et al. 2008; Lee et al. 2014).

There are important differences in age of onset, prevalence, and symptomatology in neuropsychiatric diseases. The effect of hormones on neural systems is complex and need to be better understood. During development, steroid hormones influence neuronal morphology and activity. The activation of adrenal and gonadal hormone receptors alters neurotransmitter function. Membrane-bound receptors induce short-term effects, while intraneuronal receptors can modify gene expression. "… the dramatic hormonal changes of puberty are triggered by alterations in excitatory and inhibitory inputs to gonadotropin-releasing hormone neurons in the pituitary. Behaviorally, hormonal effects drive aggression and sexual interest but their impact on impulse control, logical problem solving and other cognitive tasks has not been well established" (Giedd et al. 2008: p. 10). Sex differences emerge from different genes on the X or Y chromosomes or are the result of different hormone levels. Familial, social, and cultural variances play an important role in psychopathological manifestations. Neuroimaging allows visualizing the complex neural circuitry involved in psychopathological disorders. The typical dysphoric mood state in adolescence, for example, may involve different neural circuits than the one in anxiety disorders or depression.

As we have seen previously, advances in affective neuroscience have helped to define the key brain regions, concentrated in subcortical areas, involved in emotion processing. One has however to take into account psychosocial developmental aspects if we want to understand how affective states and emotions arise. We have to consider not only the primary affective processes going on in the brain but also the higher social–cognitive interactions already beginning in the infant at birth, where critical developmental changes occur and take place lifelong.

Perception and awareness of bodily sensations and emotions are fundamental components in the development of self-experience and self-image as well as of cognitive processes and creativity. These fundamental experience-models and -patterns are built up in the earliest relations with primary caregivers. Some areas of the nervous systems

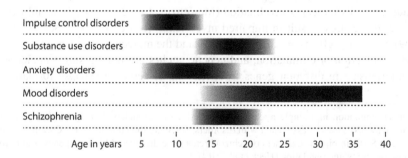

**Fig. 6.1** Ranges of onset for psychiatric disorders (Adapted from Paus et al. 2008)

need to be adequately stimulated in critical developmental phases through the interaction of a subject with his surroundings, in order to function optimally.

The discovery of critical periods in brain development or windows of opportunity goes back to the seminal experiments of Hubel and Wiesel (1970). These studies showed that if newborn kittens were prevented from using one eye for 2 weeks, this eye would remain blind. We know that the opening and closing of these windows of opportunity are regulated by genes and these regulatory genes must be turned on at a critical period of development through the activation by neurotransmitters. The regulatory genes are active in specific brain areas involved in diverse functions such as language, music, and social interactions. The proper activation of these genes during periods of susceptibility is essential for correct brain development.

From a neurobiological or psychodynamic perspective, self and personality are very complex constructs, involving many different brain systems including emotion, cognition, and motivation. These systems must be highly integrated and in constant interaction with the social context in order to generate a coherent sense of self. The development of the self in infancy is an essential process, which is subject to intensive research.

## Psychological and Self-Development

A subject is not able to construct his personal history alone; he is always anchored in a family history containing significant events prior to the life of the individual. As part of a mental transmission process, a person receives elements of cultural heritage from preceding generations. A baby inscribes himself in the longitudinal history of his mother and father. Infants need for the construction of their mental life not only a biological or genetic makeup but also a relationship history. A baby's lived experience consists of his desire for interpersonal emotional exchanges, which he can only express through nonverbal communication. The satisfaction of his vital needs is almost always linked to communicative exchange activities. Positive and negative interaction experiences are stored as corresponding relationship representations and are further elaborated by fantasy activities of the infant. The representations contain the desire and longing to continue the relationship with the caring person that is the lustful and pleasurable emotional exchange. With the help of these intrapsychic representations[2] and fantasy activities, the baby tries to bridge the separation with his mother.

The development of self and the formation of self-representations take place in a continuous process between the infant and his primary caregivers. These processes are based on interpersonal communications with all their asymmetrical needs, desires, and satisfactions. The fundamental building blocks in the development of the self and self-representation in infancy and early childhood include, "affect attunement" (Stern 1984) and "social referencing" (Klinnert et al. 1983).

---

[2] For a review of intrapsychic representations, see Bürgin (2011).

"Affect attunement" is based on the wish to build and continue a shared emotional experience in the relationship interaction between mother and infant. Both protagonists then feel perceived by the other. The term "affect attunement" has its origins in infant research and describes the phenomenon that primary caregivers assimilate—mainly by imitation—the infant's signals (the shape, the intensities, and sometimes in other sensory modalities), record them, and behave nearly identically. While the received "information" is then slightly but clearly modulated in frequency, amplitude, or even in the sensory disposition, it is still recognizable to the infant and awakes his interest. This kind of playful interactions activates a progressive discovery by the infant of his own capacities. In a social context where the infant is not able to decide on his own behavior, he—by means of "social referencing"— explores the facial expression of his mother and according to her emotional information (e.g., encouraging or warning) regulates his own behavior. Fear and uncertainty are reduced by "social referencing," thereby creating room for curiosity and exploration.

The infant "finds himself" in the facial expression of his mother, mirroring her emotional engagement, as if saying: "I am how I am perceived by you" (Winnicott 1960a). The infant's emotional self-regulation is therefore dependent on the affect-regulatory interactions with the primary caregiver, which are on the one hand influenced by the quality of the caregiver's affective states and communication behavior and on the other by the emotional feedback the infant receives through social referencing. Even in good relationships, only one third of the encounters come to a pleasurable contact; however, this is sufficient for normal development (Tronick 2007).

The infant's externalized emotions are recorded, retained, and transformed by a "good enough mother" (Winnicott 1953, 1955–1996)[3] and retransmitted to the infant. Bion[4] (1962) called this ongoing dynamic emotional interaction process containment. The internalization of holding and containing experiences constructs a system of internal relational representations. When primary caregivers lack these holding/containing functions, the infant and young child may present multiple fears and narcissistic rage,[5] which can affect the development of impulse-regulation-functions.

The cognitive integration of emotional experiences of inner and outer reality is an ongoing task from the first day of life and enables early continuity of self-experience. The more intense, differentiated, and structured the world of internal representations and skills acquired by the infant and the young child is, the greater is his autonomy from the caregivers, on both psychological and bodily levels.

---

[3] A good enough mother provides a holding environment (Winnicott 1953, 1955–1956).

[4] Winnicott's concept of holding means safeguarding and maintaining the continuity of the infant's or child's experience of being and being alive over time. Bion's term of container–contained is an emotional interaction between "dream-thoughts" (the contained) and the capacity for "dreaming" (the container). Containment is concerned with the processing of thoughts derived from lived emotional experience (Ogden 2004).

[5] Narcissistic rage (Kohut 1972) is the reactive anger following a narcissistic injury (Freud 1920), a threat to a person's self-esteem.

The capacity to differentiate but also to link internal and external reality calls for increasing regulation of impulses and emotions. In the dyadic play with a significant person, the child learns—with interpersonal communication—alternative solutions and ideas and broadens his subjective experience. Disturbances of "affect attunement" and "social referencing" can result in severe disappointment and withdrawal behavior in the infant as well as in feelings of self-depreciation, shame, and guilt. "…it is the overall quality of the emotional relationship between infant and caregiver, and its internalization as part of the representational world, which is of crucial importance for growth and development" (Bürgin 2011: p. 105).

## True and False Self

The term self is a description of subjectivity; it is the sense of feeling real, feeling in touch with others and with one's own body. Only the true self can be creative and only the true self can feel real (Winnicott 1960b).

The true self is a kind of a hereditary potential or constitutive core and permits—under suitable environmental conditions—the experience of a continuity of being. An average primary caregiver helps the infant—through proper care in the first months of his life—to experience an illusory omnipotence. This allows the true self to become alive. Disorders of mother's adaptation to a child's early needs may lead to the establishment of a "false" existence. Gradually the infant is able to acknowledge that he is not omnipotent; he is then ready for disillusionment. Disturbances in the subsequent necessary gentle disillusionment-process that leads to the recognition of the reality principle can also give rise to the formation of a false self. This is characterized by a system of "false relations." A false self means excessive docility toward latent or manifest demands of the outside world. The false self is something like a protective shell around the true self in order to hide it. Any threat to the true self is felt like an assault and causes an all-encompassing vital anxiety in early developmental stages of an infant. The formation of a false self may thus be the best possible defense against such violations of the true self, however, at an extremely high price, namely, the loss of authenticity.

There exist in the field of clinical manifestations many variations and severity-degrees of a false self. If an unsympathetic primary caregiver impacts his own intentions and desires on the infant instead of supporting the formation of the spontaneous gestures of the baby, then the ability for symbol formation is impaired and the implementation of illusion and omnipotence in play and imagination does not get started. If a child is forced into a false self or seduced into this form, he reacts with symptoms such as irritability and nutritional and functional disorders.

In developing a false self, the infant gives up his own creative gestures, imitates his caring environment, and identifies with caregivers who neither understand nor are capable of representing the infant's feelings and intentions, but replace the emotional expressions with their own mostly nonverbal communications. If the infant internalizes the defense mechanisms of his caregiver, he will not be able to adequately represent and express his own emotional experiences. An infant or young child, who internalizes emotionally non-resolved representations of the mother into his own self-image on mental and bodily levels, will develop inadequate representations of his intentional self, resulting in distorted body- and self-images. The infant or small child's experience of self and self-awareness—markedly influenced by early perceptions of thoughts and feelings of the mother—then has no connection to his present or actual emotions, feelings, and experiences. The false self is an early form of defense against impingements of the environment or against a lack of protection by the primary caregivers from outside attacks. According to Winnicott (1960b), a false self brings the child's own self-development and self-fulfillment to a standstill:

> "I always have to make a constant effort to maintain the image other person's see of me, an image—I think—they like. I am afraid they will discover that it is only an image and then—at the moment I drop my mask—they will no more love me".

This youngster's statement corresponds to his perception of a lack of personal authenticity. The formation of a false self is built up to protect the vulnerable core self. The function of a false self prevents the development of individuation and autonomy processes but allows to submit unconditionally to the real or fantasied demands of the environment and to eliminate the threat of a potential disaster of the external reality. At the time of adolescence, maintaining a false self is often no longer possible, and the collapse of the false self reveals the fact that the true self does hardly exist (Winnicott 1965).

*FANNY*, 18 years old, attempted suicide with drugs after a sentimental disappointment. She repeatedly broke off and reestablished the relationship with her lover who had for her a "protective role like a father." Subsequently she succeeded an intermediate exam at the art school, but decided to abandon her training and to suspend everything she had ever undertaken at the request of others. "I felt a trigger in myself, a trigger meaning: I Fanny." She leaves her apartment and breaks off the relationship with her adoptive mother, telling her: "I was never really your daughter and will never be." She felt "like a larva, needing affection, food, and maturation." Fanny confides to her psychotherapist her feelings of her self subsisting in a larval stage. Her suicide attempt can be understood as the destruction of her false self and her wish to preserve her true self.

Normal intrapsychic development in adolescence involves a grieving process over the loss of childhood and the transformation of mental representations; these are the primary significant relationship representations with the internalized parental figures. An adolescent has—according to his development—to renounce his internalized primary love relationships and give up the familiar experiences and functioning of his childhood. This process is associated with increased investment of the self, manifesting itself with a narcissistic retreat, and often accompanied by a depressive mood and insecurity in self-perception and feelings.

If an adolescent is not capable of containing his emotional distress resulting from personal intrapsychic conflicts, he depends even more on the attention and care of his environment. Yet adolescents—in accord with their developmental transition process—fear the dependence of adults, often lived as a submission to or an imposition of others.

Puberty is closely associated with amplification of intensive drive impulses, needs, and feelings, as well as with the reactivation of infantile conflicts. This process may lead to confrontation with narcissistic, libidinal, and aggressive impulses. Adolescents may be overwhelmed by strong emotions of anger, sadness, and pain experienced in critical life events in their early childhood. These past experiences cannot be remembered by conscious awareness and therefore cannot be expressed by words. The genital sexual maturation at the beginning of adolescence changes the relationship of the young person with his own body. This process may be associated with numerous conflicts, sometimes leading to irresponsible behavior of adolescents with respect to their own body. It includes autoaggressive behavior manifested by repetitive accidents, by substance abuse (alcohol, nicotine, drugs), by neglecting bodily care, or by promiscuity.

## Early Parent–Child Relationship

The family is the place where a child's genealogy and filiation are inscribed. This integration is required for the formation of his identity; but the family is also a place of confrontation with differences between self and others, gender, and generations. Infant research demonstrates a major influence of family relationships on child development processes. The observation of parent–child interactions in their behavioral, emotional, and phantasmatic aspects marked an important step in understanding the infant and child's self-formation and-maturation and associated disorders (Fivaz-Depeursinge and Corboz-Warnery 1999; Manzano 1996; Solis-Ponton 2002; Stern 1985, 1958).

The parents' biographical history cannot be dissociated from the child's personal history. Under certain conditions, the impact of critical events or psychic trauma can be transmitted from one generation to another. What happened in the parents' past is transmitted to the child and becomes his present reality. Transgenerational and unconscious conflictual patterns of the child's primary caregivers are—through identification with the emotional experiences of family members—internalized by the child.

In migration situations, for example, parenting can be seriously impoverished, because migration introduces manifest discontinuity in the exercise of parenthood. Migration questions the affiliation process, in other words belonging, as it is organized through identificatory movements. In migrant families parenting can lead to a crisis: the social gain is not felt as balanced with regard to the losses involved, such as separation from the families of origin and loss of generational transmission and identity.

## *Parenthood*

Parenthood represents a heritage that transcends genes. In this sense, the particularly long period of gestation will shape the offspring. In utero the fetus perceives mother's heartbeat, her voice, and the tactile contact of his constantly changing body surface with the uterine wall. As early as 16 weeks, the fetus reacts to what is around him. Prenatal exposures to voices or gustatory or olfactory experiences have long-lasting effects. At birth the baby's prenatal experience to flavors in the amniotic fluid will influence his taste for food. For a long time gustatory or olfactory senses were considered of secondary importance; flavor perception is often associated with emotionally charged memories (Beauchamp and Mennella 2011). The newborn baby is able to recognize the voice of his mother and the smell of mother's breast milk and shows it by turning his head toward her.

Parenthood according to Lebovici (Solis-Ponton 2002) is the fruit of an encounter between the biography of both parents and their baby. Parenthood is made up of parents' mental representations, affects, desires, and behaviors in the relationships with their child. The future child may only be a project of his future parents, is expected during pregnancy, or may be already born. Parenthood is based on the notion of kinship in its dual biological and social dimensions. What constitutes the parents' intrapsychic reality will unfold in fantasied and emotional interactions with the baby, then with the child, by intersubjective exchanges and interpersonal relationships and thus contribute to the attachment-modalities of the young child to his parents and family. According to Manzano et al. (1999), it is mandatory that identificatory changes take place in parents during the pregnancy period.

Psychic elaboration of each future parent's past includes a mourning process of their own internalized parental images. This process represents a period of psychic growth; if mourning does not take place, parents will not be apt to recognize and accept their child's "otherness." The child will then be the receiver of parental projective identifications.[6]

Transgenerational inheritance consists of psychic experiences—emotions, fantasies, images, and identifications—and is organized into a mythical narrative from which each individual takes up essential elements for the formation of his personal family history. The child inscribes himself in his dual maternal and paternal filiations, thus joining and belonging to his family. At the same time, he will be part of the unfolding history of his family.

Transmission of parents' unconscious desires and fantasies to their children takes place through nonverbal communication, the variants being of sensorimotor nature, tactile, visual, and auditory modalities. During breast- or bottle-feeding, for example, multiple modes of communication are used: the gaze; the respective postures of the mother and her baby and their mutual adjustment; the prosody and

---

[6] Projective identification is a process, in which—in a close relationship, such as between mother and child—an unconscious fantasy of aspects of the self or of an internal relation representation is attributed to an external person.

tonality of the dialogue; the holding, the contact, and the touch; the speech and the vocalizations; as well as gustatory and olfactory experiences[7] of the baby. The child will react to the fantasies expressed by the communicative behavior of his parents according to his own motivations, in particular his desire for communication and his need for relationship and holding, deriving from his own impulses and defenses. The newborn disposes of an important number of skills he brings into play for the "parentalization" of his parents. A baby already has the ability to establish triadic exchanges (Fivaz-Depeursinge and Corboz-Warnery 1999).

## Early Relationship Disorders

The parent's intrapsychic representations of their child will contribute to the child's self-development. Transgenerational adverse inheritance consists of raw elements that are not elaborated by previous generations, marked by traumatic experiences, bereavement, and left unspoken. The burden of the parental personal history permeates the mental development and psychic maturation of the baby. The infant builds up his inner world out of his desire for his mother or primary caregiver and out of motivation to attribute and understand meaning in the feelings and behaviors of others. The child identifies himself totally or partially with the parental representations projected onto him, which may considerably reduce his degree of freedom and sometimes alienate him (Knauer and Palacio-Espasa 2002). His mental development may be affected, leading to symptoms. These manifestations often reflect strong invested narcissistic[8] parent–child or family ties and can be considered as an indicator of transgenerational transmission of something unnamed, not-thought, revealing an unconscious alliance.

Multiple parental representations of their baby blend and alternate with the "real" baby, creating an imaginary and phantasmatic dimension of early interactions between the baby and his parents. This parent–child interaction is a complex sequence of bidirectional processes which do not develop in a closed circle, but rather in a spiral. It includes the expression of unconscious conflicts of the parents and is sometimes the source of disharmony in their relationship with the baby, who then becomes the container for projections of these conflicts.

A young couple asked for psychotherapeutic help, confronted with the sleep problems of their first born son, *JONATHAN*, now 3 years old. Since birth the boy presents a sleep disorder; he never slept through the night. Both mother and father had experienced multiple losses in their personal biographical histories. As soon as they began to share the painful emotions of their lived traumata with the help of the psychotherapist, her son slept through the night.

---

[7] The olfactory system appears to outperform other senses such as vision or audition, since it can discriminate more than one trillion different odors (Bushdid et al. 2014). By comparison, the discriminating power for color is in the order of 2–7 million, for tones about 350,000.

[8] The child serves as an essential source of the parental self-esteem.

Parenting—created by the arrival of a child—leads mother and father to identify with their own parents' parenting functions. This reidentification reactivates experiences and conflicts with internalized parental figures and may then be projected onto the child. Aspects of unresolved parental conflicts may be expressed by the child through symptomatic manifestations such as sleep-, respiratory-, or eating disorders. Communication of "unconscious to unconscious" occurs by nonverbal interactions in the mother–child relationship, as if the mother unconsciously attempts—through her child—to mourn certain losses or some critical events she experienced in her own childhood. The child—with his extreme sensitivity and responsiveness—reacts to the expressed emotions and the signs of his mother's anxiety. For parents with severe emotional disturbances, parenthood can be seriously compromised.

When there is a combination of several destabilizing factors (social precarity, unemployment, transculturation, break-up with the extended family, bereavement, illness, breakdown of the family environment), it is clear that the time, space, safety, availability, and necessary motivation fail to promote and support a child's development. Parents can be so overwhelmed by their problems that they hardly perceive the child's signals or ignore them, neglect his needs, and avoid playful contacts. They may react unpredictably or overstimulate their child until the latter rejects them. A fundamental rejection of the child may also occur in the case of a mother who is unable to identify with her maternal role. Two extreme forms of parental insensitivity are intrusion and deprivation. In the case of intrusion, for example, an infant or small child is compelled to fulfill his mother's narcissistic needs. In physical or affective deprivation, the development process and the personal life experience of an infant or small child are interrupted.

A mother may have given her baby an exceptionally good start, but cannot handle the next developmental phase, the first separation–individuation process, which she very often experiences as being rejected by her child. She is no longer able to fulfill the baby's needs. Later in his development, the child may live these extremely chaotic and unpredictable circumstances as sensations of falling, as experiences of a catastrophic breakdown. Thanks to the initial overinvestment at the baby stage—which represents a "primary maternal preoccupation" (Winnicott 1956, 1960a)—the child is sometimes able to draw enough strength to organize and defend himself with respect to his mother.

The desire of the mother to protect her child usually reflects her own traumatic separation experiences or her non-elaborated or reactivated mourning. A revival of the mother's past traumatic events during pregnancy and birth can lead to a serious failure in her primary maternal capacities. Respiratory difficulties or allergic skin manifestations, for example, may represent maternal anxieties, overprotection, and/or excessive arousal of the child. In a child with sleep disorders, one often finds an anxious mother waking her child in an attempt to reassure herself. Other disorders such as anorexia and vomiting may result from the child's opposition to the mother's intrusive behavior. The symptoms that the baby or child may present are multiple, variable, and change during development.

Mothers may select and reinforce certain of the child's expressions, which then become part of a specific mother–child communication system. For example, when a baby is expected to replace a deceased person, a brother, sister, or grandparent who's mourning has not been elaborated, he runs the risk of being a substitute. The mother's need to cling to her child, not only as a child but also as a sign of her lost love associated with the deceased person, is expressed especially through her gaze, voice, attitude, and gestures and less by what she says.

Among the rights of all children is the right to live their childhood (with protection, care, and provision of basic necessities). Parental psychopathology may deprive a child of his childhood, and we observe how children - "therapists" of their parents present often a pathological hyper-maturity, which is psychologically extremely costly and significantly reduces the degree of their developmental freedom. These signs of hyper-maturation, which consists mainly of an over-adaptation, lead to the formation of a false self and reveal extreme identification mechanisms, indicative of the child's suffering.

The too mature and precocious child manifests a serious and grave adult-like behavior and presents himself as an autonomous and hyper-controlled personality. These so-called model-children, concerned with the care and surveillance of their sick mother, show high vigilance toward a mother who is physically present, but emotionally absent, as it is the case in depressed or alcoholic mothers.

Studies of interactions between psychotic mothers and their babies have shown—at the visual level—the mother's scarcity or avoidance of eye contact. In such a situation, the child directs his gaze to a stranger. At the corporal level, one may observe scenes of rapprochement and distancing, in which holding and maintaining the baby are chaotic and followed by hyper- or hypotonic reactions. At a vocal level, interactions are poor and the mother rarely evokes and answers the baby's vocalizations. The playfulness in interactions is almost absent. The baby then lives to the rhythm of the mother's intensely unpredictable and unconscious emotional fluctuations.

The aim of preventive and therapeutic interventions is to allow parents to discover their parental role, while at the same time expressing their conflictual burdens. They need to realize their implications and meaning in the histories of their own parents and to understand the story of their own inner child. It is essential to consider the inner child in the adult person and generational dynamics, as well as the creative anticipation of the parents for their own children (Lamour and Maury 2000).

# References

Beauchamp GK, Mennella JA. Flavor perception in human infants: development and functional significance. Digestion. 2011;83 Suppl 1:1–6. doi:10.1159/000323397.

Bion WR. Learning from experience. London: Heinemann; 1962.

Bürgin D. From outside to inside to outside: comments on intrapsychic representations and interpersonal interactions. Infant Ment Health J. 2011;32(1):95–114. doi:10.1002/imhj.20285.

Bushdid C, Magnasco MO, Vosshall LB, Keller A. Humans can discriminate more than 1 trillion olfactory stimuli. Science. 2014;343(6177):1370–2. doi:10.1126/science.1249168.

Fivaz-Depeursinge E, Corboz-Warnery A. The primary triangle. New York: Basic Behavioral Science; 1999.

Freud S. Beyond the pleasure principle. In: Complete psychological works, standard ed, vol. 18. London: Hogarth Press; 1920, p. 7–64. Reprinted in 1955.

Giedd JN, Keshavan M, Paus T. Why do many psychiatric disorders emerge during adolescence? Nat Rev Neurosci. 2008;9(12):947–57. doi:10.1038/nrn2513.

Heck A, Fastenrath M, Ackermann S, Auschra B, Bickel H, Coynel D, et al. Converging genetic and functional brain imaging evidence links neuronal excitability to working memory, psychiatric disease, and brain activity. Neuron. 2014;81(5):1203–13. doi:10.1016/j.neuron.2014.01.010.

Hubel DH, Wiesel TN. The period of susceptibility to the physiological effects of unilateral eye closure in kittens. J Physiol. 1970;206(2):419–36.

Klinnert MD, Campos JJ, Sorce JF, Emde RN, Svejda M. Emotions as behavior regulations: Social referencing in infancy. In: Plutchhick R, Kellermann H, editors. Emotion: theory, research, and experience. New York: Academic; 1983.

Knauer D, Palacio-Espasa F. Interventions précoces parents-enfants: Avantages et limites. Psychiatrie de l'enfant. 2002;XLV:103–32.

Kohut H. Thoughts on narcissism and narcissistic rage. Psychoanal Study Child. 1972;27:360–400.

Lamour M, Maury M. Alliance autour du bébé. PUF, Paris: Monographie de la psychiatrie enfant; 2000.

Lee H, Brott BK, Kirkby LA, Adelson JD, Cheng S, Feller MB, et al. Synapse elimination and learning rules co-regulated by MHC class I H2-Db. Nature. 2014;509(7499):195–200. doi:10.1038/nature13154.

Liu J, Dietz K, DeLoyht JM, Pedre X, Kelkar D, Kaur J, et al. Impaired adult myelination in the prefrontal cortex of socially isolated mice. Nat Neurosci. 2012;15(12):1621–3. doi:10.1038/nn.3263.

Manzano J. Les relations précoces parents-enfants et leurs troubles. Suisse: Médecine et Hygiène. Chêne-Bourg; 1996.

Manzano J, Palacio Espasa F, Zilkha N. Les scenarios narcissiques de la parentalite, clinique de la consultation therapeutique. Paris: PUF. Le Fil Rouge; 1999.

McKenzie IA, Ohayon D, Li H, de Faria JP, Emery B, Tohyama K, et al. Motor skill learning requires active central myelination. Science. 2014;346(6207):318–22. doi:10.1126/science.1254960.

Ogden TH. On holding and containing, being and dreaming. Int J Psychoanal. 2004;85(Pt 6):1349–64.

Paus T, Keshavan M, Giedd JN. Why do many psychiatric disorders emerge during adolescence? Nat Rev Neurosci. 2008;9(12):947–57. doi:10.1038/nrn2513. Epub 2008 Nov 12. Review.

Price BH, Adams RD, Coyle JT. Neurology and psychiatry, closing the great divide. Neurology. 2000;54:8–14.

Sexton CE, Mackay CE, Ebmeier KP. A systematic review of diffusion tensor imaging studies in affective disorders. Biol Psychiatry. 2009;66(9):814–23. doi:10.1016/j.biopsych.2009.05.024.

Solis-Ponton L. La parentalité. Paris: Un hommage international à Serge Lebovici. Le fil rouge. PUF; 2002.

Stern DN. Affect attunement. In: Call JD, Galenson E, Tyson RL, editors. Frontiers of infant psychiatry, vol. 2. New York: Basic Books; 1984. p. 3–14.

Stern D. The interpersonal world of the infant. New York: Basic Books; 1985. ISBN 978-0-465-09589-6.

Tronick EZ. The neurobehavioral and social-emotional development of infants and children. New York: Norton; 2007.

Van der Kolk BA, McFarlane AC, Weisaeth L. Traumatic stress. New York: Guilford Press; 1996.

Winnicott DW. Transitional objects and transitional phenomena. Int J Psychoanal. 1953;34:89–97.

Winnicott DW. Collected papers: through pediatrics to psychoanalysis. 1st ed. London: Tavistock; 1958.

Winnicott DW. The maturational process and the facilitating environment: studies in the theory of emotional development. New York: International UP; 1965. p. 140–52.

Winnicott DW. Clinical varieties of transference. 1955–1966. In: Collected papers. Through pediatrics to psychoanalysis. London: Tavistock; 1958.

Winnicott DW. Ego distortion in terms of true and false self. In: The maturational process and the facilitating environment: studies in the theory of emotional development. New York: International UP; 1960b, p. 140–52. Reprinted in 1965.

Winnicott DW. The theory of the parent-infant relationship. Int J Psychoanal. 1960a; 41:585-595

Winnicott DW. Primary maternal preoccupation. 1956. In: Winnicott DW. Through pediatrics to psychoanalysis. London: Tavistock; 1958, p. 300–5.

# Part IV

# Chapter 7
# Language

## The Evolutionary Origin of Language

Before human language development arose about 100,000 years ago, a number of important morphological changes took place in early hominids, such as bipedalism, prehensile grasp, and a reshaped neurocranium (Miyagawa et al. 2013). Notably, the surface area of the cortex and in particular the frontal lobe expanded many folds in early hominids giving them new potentialities that eventually gave rise to language acquisition. Our ancestors must have initially used gestures for social interaction, gaining a selective advantage in their daily activities such as hunting, looking for food, and defending themselves against predators. Humans have a strong motivation to communicate, a quasi-instinctive drive.

Because of the many parallels of how children learn to speak and young birds learn to sing, the investigation of the origin of language has centered on neurodevelopmental, behavioral, and genetic aspects. In his book *Descent of Man*, Darwin (1871, 1809–1882) already proposed that human language derives from songs. Darwin's theory has gained support from neurolinguistic studies on the emergence of human language syntax. Recent studies suggest that the full semantic and syntaxic capabilities of humans result from the integration of two older communication systems, used by birds or monkeys (Miyagawa et al. 2013). Songbirds seem to communicate using an expressive structure: songs and prosody. In humans prosody processing is localized in the right hemisphere. On the other hand, the naming of lexical abilities that can be found in monkey's alarm calls is typical left-brain activity. A dominant view among linguists today considers that human language evolved from the combination of two preexisting systems, a lexical layer, meaning the words we use, and an expression structure (prosody) involved in organizing these words.

Language relies not only on cortical sensory and motor areas but also on the function of subcortical structures such as the basal ganglia, to regulate motor and sequencing functions. The basal ganglia allow automatization of many processes, including walking or talking, so that these motor activities take place without conscious thought (Lieberman 2013). It is therefore not surprising, given the shared

© Springer International Publishing Switzerland 2016
A. Steck, B. Steck, *Brain and Mind*, DOI 10.1007/978-3-319-21287-6_7

regulation of locomotion and speech, that language capacities and bipedalism appeared concurrently in evolution (Lieberman 2002).

Obviously language has been shaped by natural selection and genetic mutations. Contrary to the idea that children learn language by simple imitation and trial and error, Chomsky (2005) proposed that language abilities are universal and preprogrammed in the brain. Thus, any child has the biological capacity to learn any language. In the same line, Lieberman (2013) argues that language is a learned skill, based on a functional language system distributed across numerous cortical and subcortical structures. These circuits constitute a genetically predetermined set that defines the characteristics of language.

The development of cortical brain regions such as Broca's area, one of the major language centers, is under genetic control. Studies demonstrate that the capacity for speech acquisition and language derives from the activation of specific genes (Bae et al. 2014). One gene, called FOXP2, is of particular interest (Marcus and Fisher 2003). A mutation in this gene was described in a family who displayed severe articulation difficulty that affected many aspects of grammar and language abilities over several generations (Vargha-Khadem et al. 1995). FOXP2 is one of many genes involved in human communication and is thought to regulate circuits tied to coordinating vocal sequences allowing fluent speech. This is achieved by regulating synaptogenesis in language-related neural circuits (Sia et al. 2013). Neuroimaging studies demonstrate that individuals with FOXP2 mutations show significant underactivation of Broca's area, accounting for their difficulties in speech production. Higher expression of FOXP2 was shown in girls compared to boys, which could explain the general observation that girls learn language faster and earlier than boys (Bowers et al. 2013).

"Humanization" of FOXP2 is thought to have played a key role in the development of spoken language, marking the emergence of modern humans. This development may have arisen as part of a selection advantage. Alternatively, as cultural exchange provides a large selective advantage, culturally derived evolution could occur via epigenetic mechanisms, i.e., genetic change is in this case stimulated by cultural innovation. This idea is in keeping with the concept that human evolution is culturally driven, resulting in an accelerating process of behaviorally acquired characteristics (Fisher and Ridley 2013). The theory is arguable but in line with a role of epigenetic mechanisms in the transmission of behavioral traits (Heard and Martienssen 2014). This is particularly true for the last ten millennia. Social gains are not necessarily recorded in the genome but are added epigenetically, kept as cultural heritage, and transmitted from generation to generation by tradition, arts, speech, writing, and symbolic representations and today by modern electronic means of dissemination.

## The Classical Language Regions

The historical identification of brain areas involved in language and speech processing goes back to the seminal observation by the French neurologist Paul Broca (1861, 1824–1880). He used the clinical–anatomical method to demonstrate that loss of speech was related to a lesion in the posterior part of the left frontal area,

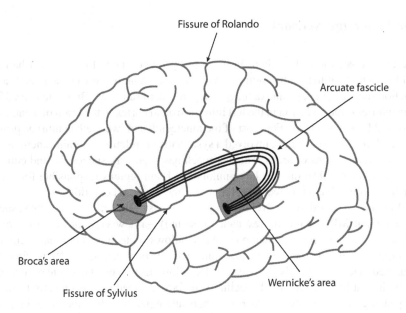

**Fig. 7.1** The classical language loop: at the caudal end lies in the temporal lobe Wernicke's area associated with the understanding of spoken words and at the other end in the frontal lobe, Broca's area associated with the production of language. The arcuate fascicle connects Wernicke's area with Broca's area

later called Broca's region (Fig. 7.1). Broca's observation was truly revolutionary because he showed that loss of articulated speech, which he called aphemia, did not affect other mental capacities. He thus provided the first strong evidence for the localization of language and also demonstrated a hemispheric localization because in most people language is localized in the left hemisphere. Broca's contribution was the starting point of neuroscientific research in language.

The other historical reference is Karl Wernicke (1848–1905), a German psychiatrist, who described that damage to the superior posterior part of the left temporal lobe, later known as Wernicke's area (Fig. 7.1), resulted in a deficit in speech comprehension (Geschwind 1967). These two discoveries laid the groundwork for modern conceptualization of brain–language relations. While this classical model relied entirely on clinical–anatomical methods, modern research is now dominated by noninvasive functional brain imaging. This technique has markedly improved the resolution with which we can investigate the neuronal foundation of language processing (Poeppel et al. 2012). Other areas of research including genetic, psychophysical,[1] linguistic, and computational models also contribute to a better understanding of the neural basis of language.

---

[1] Psychophysics is the science that analyzes in a quantitative manner the relationship between a physical stimulus and its subjective perception.

## The Language Network

The clinical–anatomical method, introduced by French neurologists like Charcot and Broca in the nineteenth century, is based on a correlation between a given brain function such as language and damage to a particular brain area. Broca described in a postmortem study a lesion in the left inferior frontal cortex in the brain of a patient, who could no more speak. For most of the nineteenth and twentieth centuries, progress in clinical neurosciences involved a systematic correlation of brain functions to specific brain regions or areas. This approach has been very successful and culminated in the identification of a large number of brain regions responsible for such functions as movement, perception, language, memory, and emotion.

With the introduction of novel imaging techniques of the brain in the 1990s, such as functional MRI (magnetic resonance imaging)—a new view of how the brain functions has emerged. Functional MRI allows detecting neuronal activity noninvasively throughout the brain. Brain activity in functional MRI is directly measured in terms of pixels or voxels.[2] fMRI allows us to look at discrete regions of the brain that have a functional specificity and are engaged in a given activity such as speaking or playing music. As researchers attempted to define the mental representations of language, it became clear that—when speaking—we engage not only the brain areas described by nineteenth-century neurologists as the specific language areas but also a much larger "nonlinguistic network." It is now obvious that specialized regions do not work in isolation, and therefore it is increasingly important to understand how regions work together. The emerging picture from newer studies points to the fact that neuronal representations are not only widely distributed across brain regions but depend on a dynamic interactions between regions (Zatorre 2013; Turk-Browne 2013). For adequate language comprehension and production, a wide network including the left inferior frontal gyrus, a large part of the superior middle temporal cortex, the inferior parietal cortex, the basal ganglia, and the cerebellum is involved. In addition to the left hemisphere, homotopic regions in the right hemisphere are also involved.

Classical models of language impairment, based primarily on the study of patients with cerebrovascular lesions, showed that aphasias differ in their manifestations depending on lesion location. The language network is much more extended than the classical language regions of Broca and Wernicke. While the early neurological concept of language made the distinction mainly between comprehension impairment (Wernicke's aphasia) and production impairment (Broca's aphasia), advances in linguistics lead to the concept that the language network is organized into a multistage operating system, constituted by a dual stream (Fig. 7.2, Saur et al. 2008). One stream, the dorsal stream (Hickok and Poeppel 2004), deals with the conversion of sensory information such as speech sound into a format suitable for linguistic computation. This is the most basic system of the language network and is also referred to as an acoustic–phonetic processing system. How this system is

---

[2] A pixel is the smallest element in a digital picture. Voxels are images that correspond to a neuronal activation in a given volume of the brain.

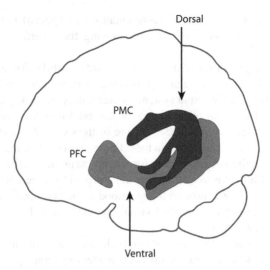

**Fig. 7.2** Ventral and dorsal pathways for language. The dorsal pathway (*black*) corresponds to the classical arcuate fascicle and is concerned with the mapping of the phonemic representation on the articulatory maps in Broca's region in the premotor cortex. The ventral stream (*gray*) connects the temporal Wernicke's area and the prefrontal cortex and deals with the semantic representation of speech. *PFC* prefrontal cortex, *PMC* premotor cortex. These pathways are visualized by combining fMRI with tractography (Adapted from Saur et al. 2008)

organized, that is, how sound is transformed into a phonetic representation is not yet known in detail. A second stream, the ventral stream, deals with the transformation of the phonetic representation into a conceptual semantic representation. This system can be viewed as a sound–meaning interface and is embedded in Wernicke's area, where classically speech comprehension is localized. The precise nature of speech sound representation is still a matter of debate, and we lack a clear understanding of the cellular mechanisms pertaining to a neural code for mental storing and processing of speech.

Language processing can be viewed as a set of transformations between an acoustic signal and a conceptual representation leading to a motor output that is speech production. This sensorimotor integration is at the root of language production. In order to function properly, there must be very tight integration between the sensory aspects of language and the motor aspects of speech production. This can be best appreciated with the example of how a child learns to speak. In order for the child to articulate correctly, a sensory representation of speech must exist, allowing him to retain what he has heard. These stored sensory speech representations will help the child shape his future articulation attempts, and experiences show that children display a certain degree of mismatch in their speech output, for example, when a toddler says "pastic" instead of "plastic," until—with rehearsal—the articulation will be perfected. According to Baddeley (1992), the tight auditory–motor integration is part of a phonological loop, a verbal working memory. This system supports a storage component (sound-based representations of speech) together with the articulatory output component of speech, allowing for a perfect auditory–motor adjustment.

The functional organization of the language system is still work in progress compared to the visual system where comprehension of visual perception is at a much more advanced stage. In the visual system the machinery extending from the retinal receptors through the visual pathways to the occipital cortex is well known. The optical elements of the eye produce an image of the external world on the retina. The patterned excitation of receptors in the retina is processed and transmitted to the neuronal network in the visual cortex to form a representation of the external world. Our knowledge of how this visual input is transformed to represent shape, orientation, movements, or color is now well understood at the organizational and cellular levels so that it is possible to implant visual prosthesis to help patients with profound vision loss (da Cruz et al. 2013).

The perceptual system required for comprehension in sign language is vision, not audition. Though sign language differs considerably from spoken language, it has been shown that visual–manual modalities activate the same iconic-phonological structures in the left frontotemporal region as spoken language (Poeppel et al. 2012). The fact, that spoken and signed language share neuronal structures, points to a modality independence of neurocognitive processing of human language.

## The Neural Basis of Speech Perception and Language

Many areas of the cortex and subcortical structures, not only Broca's and Wernicke's areas, confer speech perception and language ability, including phonetic processing, syntax, vocabulary, and speech production. Using high-resolution, fast computational methods and neural recording devices, it is now possible to investigate the microcircuitry of language areas with respect to phonological and grammatical aspects of linguistic processing (Sahin et al. 2009; Mesgarani et al. 2014). The linguistic machinery is organized around distinct neuronal sets for lexical, grammatical, and phonological processing.

While it was previously assumed that neurons in the high-order speech perception area of the superior temporal gyrus or Wernicke's region responded to phonemes,[3] it is now thought that more elemental acoustic properties are recognized in these neurons. These basic elements of speech recognition include articulatory and acoustic features, reflecting where the sound is generated, for example, in the oral cavity or the vocal cords. The feature-based algorithm used by our brain to identify speech sounds is not yet completely understood, but there is an analogy to

---

[3] A phoneme is a perceptually distinct phonological unit that distinguishes one word from another, for example, bad and bat.

the visual system: In the visual system, images are not directly recognized but are reconstructed with an algorithm based on shape and edge recognition.

Language processing in Broca's area is embedded in distinct circuits giving rise to a finely distributed spatiotemporal network. Thus, the ability to make words, combine them grammatically, and articulate the corresponding sounds involves a specific, finely tuned neurocircuitry. However, it should not be seen as a rigid connectionist model. Modern representation of brain circuits considers these networks as having a high degree of plasticity; they should not be viewed as an innate fixed system but as preformed molds, which can be altered by training. This explains that children have the biological capacity to learn any language. On the other hand when specific components of the language network are damaged such as Broca's region, following a brain injury, alternate brain regions can only partially compensate the language disability.

It is clear that the role of Broca's region is not limited to language processing, but is a component involved in other cognitive networks. For example, Broca's area is activated in fine motor actions from movement preparation to production of action, as well as in visual and auditory functions. Broca's area serves as a convergence zone for many tasks. It is, for example, bilaterally activated as part of the mirror neuron system (Iacoboni and Dapretto 2006), a very important system in learning by watching and imitating others. While Broca's role in supporting grammatical and articulatory processing of language is clearly established, studies have shown that Broca's area has also an important functional role in regulating perceptive and attentional functions. In other words Broca's region should be considered as part of the larger executive control network, a network that regulates and guides cognitive processes in sensory and motor systems. According to the prevalent neurobehavioral view, language and executive functions should not be separated but considered as part of a larger cognitive network (Ye and Zhou 2009). For example, when we speak, we have to constantly select the right word over competing synonyms. As listeners, we are also confronted with selecting different interpretations as we decipher a sentence. Thus executive control, which is necessary to manage our thoughts and actions, is deeply involved in language processing.

When we speak or listen, large-scale networks are activated such as frontal and posterior regions of the cortex. Broca's area is not the only syntaxic organ: when we process words, it activates our memory system, especially the verbal working memory (Baddeley 1992). This system is highly dynamic and—depending on the difficulty of the linguistic task—recruits additional resources in the frontoparietal cortex and anterior cingulate gyrus. Full human speech capability relies on an extensive large-scale neurocognitive network. Language—one of the most complex mental activities—is dependent on conceptual knowledge stored in vast regions of the brain, associated with sensory and motor control.

## Language Learning Disorders

Communication disorders such as language impairment or reading disability are complex and have multiple causes. They are among the most common developmental disorders. As their behavioral and genetic backgrounds are better understood, identification of children at risk will help implement program for early intervention (Smith et al. 2010).

Developmental stuttering (DS) is a speech fluency disorder that begins during the childhood years of rapid speech development. It manifests itself as intermittent interruptions of words, taking the form of repetition or prolongation of sounds and syllables (Viswanath et al. 2003). The majority of children with DS recover spontaneously; those who continue to stutter into adulthood make up about 1 % of the general population. The etiology of DS is still unclear, and besides environmental factors, there is evidence for a strong genetic component (Rautakoski et al. 2012).

Genetic studies show mutations in genes with high expression in the hippocampus and cerebellum (Kang and Drayna 2011), structures associated with memory, emotions, and motor functions. While the discovered susceptibility genes for stuttering explain only a small percentage of subjects affected by stuttering, they should help us better understand the functioning of the neural structures generating speech.

Brain imaging studies found that multiple neural systems involved in speech production are affected in DS; it is often difficult to differentiate between changes that are responsible for stuttering from those that are the result of compensation mechanisms. One of the current models suggests that DS is related to a dysfunction of sensory motor integration with impaired ability of the basal ganglia to give the appropriate motor timing cues (Alm 2004). In support of this idea are reports that damage to the basal ganglia can cause stuttering (Tani and Sakai 2011). However, we know that fluency can be improved in stutterers therapeutically by choral reading techniques. In this technique others speak the same discourse as the stutterer, which helps to reestablish his fluency. This experience suggests that there is a sensorimotor mismatch in stuttering, and when the sensory system is flooded with external acoustic input, the motor error can be corrected (Hickok et al. 2011). In other words DS may result from a failure of sensorimotor integration, either from a mismatch on the sensory side or alternatively on the motor side of the control loop.

Reading difficulties in children not suffering from vision-, hearing-, or intelligence deficiencies are called dyslexia (Vellutino et al. 2004). Dyslexia is common among the specific learning disabilities, affecting 5–10 % of the general population (Butterworth and Kovas 2013). Reading is primarily a linguistic skill, including phonological and syntactic competence. It has been assumed for a long time that most dyslexic children suffer from a phonological deficit in coding that is a difficulty in the processing or representation of speech sounds or phonemes. The core deficit seems to be difficulties in mapping letters and sounds resulting in impaired speech processing. Brain imaging studies show reduced activity in the area linking letters to speech sounds, in particular in the left middle temporal gyrus, though the changes may be more functional than structural (Paulesu et al. 2001). Additional evidence shows that subjects with dyslexia have impaired brain connections in the regions processing phonemes, including Broca's area, rendering them slower in accessing phonetic representations (Boets 2013). Like most neurocognitive developmental disorders, reading difficulties present as a continuum. The cause of dyslexia is likely multifactorial, involving mutations in different genes affecting neural migration and axonal guidance as well as environmental factors (Peterson and Pennington 2012).

# References

Alm PA. Stuttering and the basal ganglia circuits: a critical review of possible relations. J Commun Disord. 2004;37(4):325–69. Review.

Baddeley A. Working memory. Science. 1992;255(5044):556–9.

Bae BI, Tietjen I, Atabay KD, Evrony GD, Johnson MB, Asare E, et al. Evolutionarily dynamic alternative splicing of GPR56 regulates regional cerebral cortical patterning. Science. 2014;343(6172):764–8. doi:10.1126/science.1244392.

Boets B, Op de Beeck HP, Vandermosten M, Scott SK, Gillebert CR, Mantini D, et al. Intact but less accessible phonetic representations in adults with dyslexia. Science. 2013;;342(6163):1251–4. doi:10.1126/science.1244333.

Bowers JM, Perez-Pouchoulen M, Edwards NS, McCarthy MM. Foxp2 mediates sex differences in ultrasonic vocalization by rat pups and directs order of maternal retrieval. J Neurosci. 2013;33(8):3276–83. doi:10.1523/JNEUROSCI.0425-12.2013.

Broca P. Perte de la parole, ramollissement chronique et destruction partielle du lobe antérieur gauche. Bull de la Société d'Anthropol. 1861;2:235–8.

Butterworth B, Kovas Y. Understanding neurocognitive developmental disorders can improve education for all. Science. 2013;340(6130):300–5. doi:10.1126/science.1231022.

Chomsky N. Universals of human nature. Psychother Psychosom. 2005;74(5):263–8.

da Cruz L, Coley BF, Dorn J, Merlini F, Filley E, Christopher P, et al. Argus II Study Group. The Argus II epiretinal prosthesis system allows letter and word reading and long-term function in patients with profound vision loss. Br J Ophthalmol. 2013;97(5):632–6. doi:10.1136/bjophthalmol-2012-301525.

Darwin C. The descent of man and selection in relation to sex. London John Murray. 1871.

Fisher SE, Ridley M. Evolution. Culture, genes, and the human revolution. Science. 2013;340(6135):929–30. doi:10.1126/science.1236171.

Geschwind N. Wernicke's contribution to the study of aphasia. Cortex. 1967;3(4):449–63.

Heard E, Martienssen RA. Transgenerational epigenetic inheritance: myths and mechanisms. Cell. 2014;157(1):95–109. doi:10.1016/j.cell.2014.02.045.

Hickok G, Poeppel D. Dorsal and ventral streams: a framework for understanding aspects of the functional anatomy of language. Cognition. 2004;92(1-2):67–99.

Hickok G, Houde J, Rong F. Sensorimotor integration in speech processing: computational basis and neural organization. Neuron. 2011;69(3):407–22. doi:10.1016/j.neuron.2011.

Iacoboni M, Dapretto M. The mirror neuron system and the consequences of its dysfunction. Nat Rev Neurosci. 2006;7(12):942–51. Review.

Kang C, Drayna D. Genetics of speech and language disorders. Annu Rev Genomics Hum Genet. 2011;12:145–64. doi:10.1146/annurev-genom-090810-183119. Review.

Lieberman P. On the nature and evolution of the neural bases of human language. Yearb Phys Anthropol. 2002;45:36–62.

Lieberman P. Synapses, language, and being. Hum Sci. 2013;342:944. doi:10.1126/science.1247515.

Marcus GF, Fisher SE. FOXP2 in focus: what can genes tell us about speech and language? Trends Cogn Sci. 2003;7(6):257–62.

Mesgarani N, Cheung C, Johnson K, Chang EF. Phonetic feature encoding in human superior temporal gyrus. Science. 2014;343(6174):1006–10. doi:10.1126/science.1245994.

Miyagawa S, Berwick RC, Okanoya K. The emergence of hierarchical structure in human language. Front Psychol. 2013;4:71. doi:10.3389/fpsyg.2013.

Paulesu E, Démonet JF, Fazio F, McCrory E, Chanoine V, Brunswick N, et al. Dyslexia: cultural diversity and biological unity. Science. 2001;291(5511):2165–7.

Peterson RL, Pennington BF. Developmental dyslexia. Lancet. 2012;379(9830):1997-2007. doi: 10.1016/S0140-6736(12)60198-6. Review.

Poeppel D, Emmorey K, Hickok G, Pylkkänen L. Towards a new neurobiology of language. J Neurosci. 2012;32(41):14125–31. doi:10.1523/JNEUROSCI.3244-12.2012. Review.

Rautakoski P, Hannus T, Simberg S, Sandnabba NK, Santtila P. Genetic and environmental effects on stuttering: a twin study from Finland. J Fluency Disord. 2012;37(3):202–10. doi:10.1016/j.jfludis.2011.12.003.

Sahin NT, Pinker S, Cash SS, Schomer D, Halgren E. Sequential processing of lexical, grammatical, and phonological information within Broca's area. Science. 2009;326(5951):445–9. doi:10.1126/science.1174481.

Saur D, Kreher BW, Schnell S, Kümmerer D, Kellmeyer P, Vry MS, et al. Ventral and dorsal pathways for language. Proc Natl Acad Sci U S A. 2008;105(46):18035–40.

Sia GM, Clem RL, Huganir RL. The human language-associated gene SRPX2 regulates synapse formation and vocalization in mice. Science. 2013;342(6161):987–91. doi:10.1126/science.1245079.

Smith SD, Grigorenko E, Willcutt E, Pennington BF, Olson RK, DeFries JC. Etiologies and molecular mechanisms of communication disorders. J Dev Behav Pediatr. 2010;31(7):555–63. doi:10.1097/DBP.0b013e3181ee3d9e.

Tani T, Sakai Y. Analysis of five cases with neurogenic stuttering following brain injury in the basal ganglia. J Fluency Disord. 2011;36(1):1–16. doi:10.1016/j.jfludis.2010.12.002.

Turk-Browne NB. Functional interactions as big data in the human brain. Science. 2013;342(6158):580–4. doi:10.1126/science.1238409. Review.

Vargha-Khadem F, Watkins K, Alcock K, Fletcher P, Passingham R. Praxic and nonverbal cognitive deficits in a large family with a genetically transmitted speech and language disorder. Proc Natl Acad Sci U S A. 1995;92(3):930–3.

Vellutino FR, Fletcher JM, Snowling MJ, Scanlon DM. Specific reading disability (dyslexia): what have we learned in the past four decades? J Child Psychol Psychiatry. 2004;45(1):2–40.

Viswanath NS, Karmonik C, King D, Rosenfield DB, Mawad M. Functional magnetic resonance imaging (fMRI) of a stutterer's brain during overt speech. J Neuroimaging. 2003;13(3):280–1.

Ye Z, Zhou X. Executive control in language processing. Neurosci Biobehav Rev. 2009;33(8):1168–77. doi:10.1016/j.neubiorev.2009.03.003. Review.

Zatorre RJ. Predispositions and plasticity in music and speech learning: neural correlates and implications. Science. 2013;342(6158):585–9. doi:10.1126/science.1238414. Review.

# Chapter 8
# Communication

## Introduction

Why do babies communicate at all? They signal intentions and wishes to care persons hoping that they will satisfy their drives, desires, and physical needs. A common cultural background facilitates this process of exchange. Communication between humans is based on cooperative structures and shared intentionality (Tomasello 1999, 2005). The ability to collaborate with others on commonly shared goals is a typical human way of cooperation. The players of the social activities and intentions are a plural subject, a "we." The interaction is part of a joint intention and attention, and includes the social motivation to help each other and to share with others.

Declarative communication directs the attention, demanding something in an imperative manner. Altruistic communication serves the other person, helps her to achieve a goal. When a mother arouses the attention of her baby in an imperative manner, the baby probably perceives her message quite differently than if she invites her baby in an altruistic manner to mutual pleasure and play (Tomasello et al. 2005).

The person who wishes to receive the communication usually signals his communication intention. Both sender and receiver work together to ensure the success of their communication act. Conventions of communication can only be built on commonly shared conceptual and mostly cultural backgrounds. Often there are besides communication expectations also more or less explicit social norms such as courtesy and respect. For the building of communication conventions, shared learning by imitation and by role exchanges is necessary. Mutual imitation is a way to get to "know" each other and represents at the same time the basis for reciprocal social exchanges.

## Gestural Communication

Both gestures and language are learned within a shared intentionality. Only if we understand what and why a person does something can we develop common goals on the basis of shared attention, such as a common visual focus on potential

© Springer International Publishing Switzerland 2016
A. Steck, B. Steck, *Brain and Mind*, DOI 10.1007/978-3-319-21287-6_8

reference objects. Already at 1 year, a child can—in simple common activities—switch roles and at 14 months is able to build common goals with others.

When adults suddenly stop communication, toddlers react strongly as the "still face experiment" shows (Tomasello et al. 2007, 2008). The still face experiment refers to a phenomenon in which, after 3 minutes of interaction with a nonresponsive expressionless mother, an infant sobers and looks wary. He attempts repeatedly by smiling briefly at his mother to get the interaction back to its shared reciprocal pattern. When these attempts fail, "the infant withdraws, orients his face and body away from his mother with hopeless facial expression and stays turned away from her" (Tronick et al. 1978: p.8).

Gestures, which are used for full communication acts, occurred in evolution before language. Pointing gestures and play gestures as "natural" communications are easily understood. Human gestures intend to direct the attention of the receiver to something in the immediate vicinity or guide the imagination of the receiver to something by simulating an action, relationship, or object through a particular behavior. Each gesture can represent a referential or social intention. The wider the common social background, the easier the understanding of the social intention.

Within the first few months of life, infants are able to obtain what they wish from their primary care persons, e.g., by crying, a kind of vocal intentional movement. Months later they begin with communicative pointing gestures, which can already be seen in 3-month-old infants. Pointing is established around the first year: children's pointing may be imperative to request an object or declarative to draw attention. Pointing occurs with fingers or with the chin. Pointing gestures of infants occur within the same social norms or out of the same motives as those of adults, namely, sharing, informing, and requesting.

Nine-month-old infants are able to see the other person as an intentional player and begin to understand that others have their own goals. At about 12 months, there is a real understanding of the goals of others. Between 12 and 14 months, toddlers begin to develop own intentions and common goals. They represent absent objects and actions symbolically for playful purposes and share these with adults in a pretend play. Infants understand the most important aspects of the functioning of human cooperative communication, that is, to help others and to inform about relevant things. They consider the intentional states of others clearly and relate to a common conceptual background.

## Social Interactions or Proto-Conversations

From the moment of birth, infants are social beings. They immediately participate in social interaction, in which caregiver and infant focus their attention on each other; infants often vocalize to express their basic moods, begin to share behavioral interactions, and are able to change roles (so-called proto-conversations according to Tomasello et al. 2005). They mimic body movements of adults such as face expression, mouth opening, and head movement and begin to identify themselves with their care persons. They begin to learn about themselves through interaction with the physical and social environment.

Infants' self-awareness proceeds from birth on, particularly through their own actions. Young children's understanding of others probably increases in analogy to their own self, that is, from their experiences of self-induced actions. They learn that external things give in or resist to their goal-directed actions and that inanimate objects do not react with emotion and are therefore not like them.

Trevarthen (1979, 1993) assumes that children—in the sense of a primary inter-subjectivity—are born with a model of dialogue, with an inborn sense of the "virtual" other; they only need to acquire the motor skills to express this "knowing" in behavior.[1] As a result of his active exploration of his environment, an infant constructs "reality" with sensory and motor information. Already at age 3–4 months, an infant has an understanding of objects as independent entities: an object cannot be found in two different places. Human cognitive and emotional skills are based on the disposition and capacity of the individual to identify with others. Infants identify themselves early with their parents or caregivers. This ability seems to be very limited in autistic children.

## Speech and Language

Hearing ability evolves from the fifth fetal month onward. Among all sounds, human speech is particularly attractive for the infant. Neural memory traces are formed by auditory learning before birth. The infant is notably receptive to mother's "language" (Partanen et al. 2013). In response to being addressed, infants smile earlier to the specific language of the primary caregiver than to his facial stimulus. Infants' affective perceptions are stimulated by the primary caregiver's sounds and the awareness of his face. They will soon be merged through the transmodal sensory properties of the infant. Not later than 4 months, the activation of motor functions follows the linguistic rhythm and intonation of adults. Primary caregivers regulate the wake and attention of the infant through their language (tone, intensity, melody).

The ability to learn to speak is innate and the initiation is dependent on the language provision of the environment. The right hemisphere seems to be mostly involved in prosody, the emotional melody of speech. Language facilitates the building of time-structures, for example, "turn taking", and carries—in parallel to the cognitive information—emotions, and affect-regulation. There are key factors and functions to be considered at every speech event: words and speech are directed to another person; establish and maintain a contact; are related to conscious or unconscious content of the past, the present, or the future; and contain a variety of emotional messages (Jakobson 1990).

Language acquisition (Bruner 1983) begins with the first interactions, immediately after birth. The infant is able to recognize and imitate the facial expressions of

---

[1] For a review on infant's intersubjectivity, see Trevarthen and Aitken (2001).

another person and to save and recall this form of exchange over a period of 1 week (Meltzoff and Moore 1994). An infant is genetically equipped with the ability to record interpersonal relationships; from birth on he tries to order his experiences, dividing them—according to pleasure and unpleasure—into those whose repetition he aspires and those he seeks to avoid.

According to Chomsky (2000), a genetic disposition for language learning ability exists, which he called the "language acquisition device" (LAD). Infants and toddlers are able to bring this language learning system into action, if an interaction framework by relevant persons in their environment is provided. The core of this system consists of the innate understanding of a universal grammar or a "linguistic deep structure." The LAD allows the child to recognize words and sentences of each of the over 6000 spoken languages, in whatever language the child is born. Chomsky thus postulated a relationship between a human's innate universal grammar and the grammar of any natural language. The child is capable to produce properly formed expressions of the local language and avoid improperly shaped expressions. The innate mental structure contains the universal grammatical categories. The significant care persons offer an additional support system for the acquisition of language. According to Bruner (1983), this is the language acquisition support system (LASS).

The development of language acquisition depends on the appropriation of functions, which exist not only in genes but are also rooted in the local culture. Children gain a working knowledge of their world before they acquire language. Such knowledge provides them with semantic goals and distinctions, which can be further differentiated by language. The LASS is not only linguistic in nature but also represents a central part of the transmission of culture. The child learns in a communicative, prelinguistic context how to speak and simultaneously learns what is customary and reasonable in the particular social setting and what is valued by his adult interaction partners. Parents play a far more active role than just being a language model in their child's language acquisition. They are speaking partners who basically agree to negotiate with the child, to make their intentions clear, and to adapt their linguistic expressions to the historical, social, and cultural conditions.

Children have a special talent to combine activities, to "make more out of less." They and their caregivers constantly combine elements in many ways to create new meanings, assign fresh interpretations, and open up unusual intentions of the other person. Children initially learn to use language (or its preverbal precursor) to achieve their goals, to play with adults, and to stay connected with the persons they depend on. They meet the standards set by cultural conditions and are confronted by their parents' rules and restrictions. Language is a systematic procedure to communicate with others, to influence foreign and own behavior, to draw attention, and to create shared "realities" with other persons.

For example, a child may cry when it refuses food. Later the conventional "no" replaces early negative sounds. The context stays about the same, but has been refined through the use of gestures and language. Natural contexts are transferred to conventional forms. Formats are routinely repeated interactions of adults and children performing certain activities together. Formats fulfill important functions in language acquisition as they enclose the communicative intentions of a child in a cultural matrix; they thus serve both the transmission of culture and language. Since formats have a sequential structure and a history, they enable the child to form elementary temporal concepts. They also provide a context for the interpretation of the communication in the here and now.

Perhaps the most important reason for developing children's oral language is that all learning depends on the ability to question, reason, formulate ideas, pose hypotheses, and exchange ideas with others. These are not just oral language skills; they are thinking skills (Browne 2009).

# References

Browne A. Developing language and literacy 3-8. London: Sage; 2009.

Bruner J. Child's talk: learning to use language. New York: Norton; 1983.

Chomsky N. New horizon in the study of language and mind. New York: Cambridge University Press; 2000.

Jakobson R. The speech event and the function of language. In: Waugh LR, Monville-Burston M, editors. On language. Cambridge: Harvard University Press; 1990.

Meltzoff AN, Moore MK. Imitation, memory and the representation of persons. Infant Behav Dev. 1994;17:83–99.

Partanen E, Kujala T, Näätänen R, Liitola A, Sambeth A, Huotilainen M. Learning-induced neural plasticity of speech processing before birth. Proc Natl Acad Sci U S A. 2013;110(37):15145–50. doi:10.1073/pnas.1302159110.

Tomasello M. The cultural origins of human cognition. London: Harvard University Press; 1999. ISBN 0-674-00582-1.

Tomasello M. Origins of human communication. Cambridge: MIT; 2008. ISBN 978-0-262-20177-3.

Tomasello M, Carpenter M, Call J, Behne T, Moll H. Understanding and sharing intentions: the origins of cultural cognition. Behav Brain Sci. 2005;28(5):675–91; discussion 691–735. Review.

Tomasello M, Carpenter M, Liszkowski U. A new look at infant pointing. Child Dev. 2007;78(3):705–22.

Trevarthen C. Instincts for human understanding and for cultural cooperation: their development in infancy. In: von Cranach M, Foppa K, Lepenies W, Ploog D, editors. Human ethology. Claims and limits of a new discipline. Cambridge: Cambridge University Press; 1979.

Trevarthen C. Predispositions to cultural learning in young infants. Behav Brain Sci. 1993;16:534–5.

Trevarthen C, Aitken JA. Infant's intersubjectivity: research, theory, and clinical application. J Child Psychol Psychiatry. 2001;42(1):3–48.

Tronick E, Als H, Adamson L, Wise S, Brazelton TB. The infant's response to entrapment between contradictory messages in face-to-face interaction. J Am Acad Child Psychiatry. 1978 Winter;17(1):1–13.

# Chapter 9
# Music

*Music expresses that which cannot be said and on which it is
impossible to be silent (Victor Hugo 1802–1885).*

## Introduction

From a neuroscientific point of view, music has strong links with speech.
Neuroimaging studies show that music and speech engage similar overlapping brain
regions such as the temporal, parietal, and inferior-frontal areas, including the
speech centers of Broca and Wernicke described above. Music and language are
communication systems that utilize similar acoustic cues such as tone, pitch, and
rhythm and are perceived as a temporal sequence. Speech and especially music cannot however be reduced to a simple sensorimotor processing system. In language
the musical contribution is important, especially in children where speech melody
and intonation play such an essential role. Music relates more strongly to emotion
than speech. According to Panksepp and Bernatzky (2002), music has particularly
strong influences on subcortical emotional systems. The effect of music on our
brain results in the interplay of many brain areas. Music has great emotional power
and evokes bodily movements. The strong link between music and movement is
thought to derive from subcortical areas such as the basal ganglia and the cerebellum. Music is much more suited to induce synchronous movements than speech and
fosters a tight coupling between sound and movement. It can act as a coordinating
force at a group level, thus promoting social bonding (Dalla Bella et al. 2013). The
origin of music is rooted in social experiences. It goes back to the early interactions
between mother and child, where musical aspects of speech such as rhythm and
melody are the first means of communication (Dalla Bella et al. 2013).

## Music and the Brain

According to Oliver Sacks (2007), music involves more areas of the human brain than
language. Current research exploring the interrelations between music and language
pinpoints both similarities and differences. When processing music and language,
separate brain mechanisms are involved; but music and language also share important
neural connections (Patel 2008). While there is a clear overlap in the brain networks

© Springer International Publishing Switzerland 2016
A. Steck, B. Steck, *Brain and Mind*, DOI 10.1007/978-3-319-21287-6_9

processing acoustic features, music puts a higher demand on the auditory system than ordinary speech. Patel (2014) stresses two aspects that are particularly important for music perception. The first is that music is much more demanding in terms of precision, timing, and temporal processing. Music, for example, requires a much higher precision in tone or pitch perception and in timing than speech. On the other hand, speech communication is not so dependent on subtle acoustic constraints, because it relies on semantic and syntactic content. The second feature of music is its very close connections to emotional systems, such as the mesolimbic circuit and in particular the nucleus accumbens (Blood and Zatorre 2001). The strong interaction between the auditory system and the dopaminergic mesolimbic circuitry is at the root of the rewarding aspect and aesthetic sensation when listening to music (Salimpoor et al. 2013).

There is evidence that musical training can affect neural plasticity in speech processing and thus could be helpful to ameliorate speech perception, for example, in cochlear implant users (Patel 2014). Given the high affective impact of music and its direct interaction with the dopaminergic reward system, it is no surprise that music—since ages—has been part of therapeutic approaches to mental disorders. The realization, that passive listening to music or music making has marked effects on neural plasticity, helps to develop better educational and rehabilitation strategies (Herholz and Zatorre 2012).

Synesthesia or fusion of senses is a field of neuroscientific investigation already explored in the nineteenth century. Synesthesia results from coactivation of two or more sensory areas (e.g., visual and auditory) of the cerebral cortex (Sacks 2007). The senses of newborns are not sufficiently differentiated; only after a few months, distinction of the senses may—with cortical maturation—take place. In persons with synesthesia, one postulates a genetic change, hindering the process of segregation, thus leaving a hyper-connectivity in place (Sacks 2007).

Synesthesia seems to be more frequent in children and disappears in adolescence. Loss of vision is a cause of acquired synesthesia, especially in childhood (Sacks 2007). Visual images may then paradoxically increase. Increasing visual impairment may lead to visual hallucinations, as increasing deafness is associated with musical hallucinations. In hearing music, visual colored hallucinations may even dominate over the perception of music. Such acquired synesthesia can be of great nuisance and leads to painful situations. It is of course different to subjects born with color–music synesthesia; in this case color–music synesthesia is considered as belonging to them like any other characteristics of their personality (Sacks 2007).

Due to plasticity of the cortex, we know now that there are possibilities of reallocations of specific brain areas: in congenitally deaf people, the auditory cortex can serve for visual processes, whereas in blind individuals, the visual cortex takes over auditory and tactile functions. Even more surprising is the discovery that the right hemisphere can be trained to perform linguistic capacities with the help of music (Sacks 2007).

Various sensations may accompany listeners of music and the individual intensity varies greatly from being indifferent or annoyed to being passionately touched by music (Sacks 2007). In most people music initiates profound resonance, often accompanied by a desire to dance and to sing. It has also a great influence on mood, for example, soothing tensions and motivating to work.

Music is the art of sounds, not ideas, and sounds affect our feelings more than our cognition and intelligence. Music is neither speech nor language. Unlike linguistic signs, music is universal, affects our body and mind, and moves us by the emotion it expresses. It lets us feel a more humane and harmonious world than the one we ordinarily inhabit.

## Music in Early Human Development

Children are sensitive to music from a very young age: they dance and sing to music and are able to distinguish happy from sad feelings in music (Peretz 2006). Musical memories are particularly long-lasting. What a child hears at an early age seems to be "engraved" for the rest of his life (Sacks 2007). Music reaches the earliest emotional experiences encoded in memories. Human fetuses can detect "pseudowords" in the third to fifth trimester of pregnancy and remember them in the days after birth, demonstrating that memory traces are already formed before birth. Prenatal experiences enable newborns to generate specific language behavior and eventually also language acquisition during infancy (Partanen et al. 2013).

The first developed sensory system is the auditory organ. Tactile and auditory perceptions are the fetus' main sensory modes in the interaction with his mother. Thanks to his motility, the fetus is able to come in contact with the uterine wall. Hearing to the contrary is passively receiving sounds. The fetus has no means to influence his mother's voice, but is probably apt to recognize or differentiate the emotional state of his mother's mind. Does her voice express joy or sorrow? The question arises how the infant perceives the voice of, for example, a depressed mother. Only at and after birth is the infant capable to cry and to create and evoke sounds (Maiello 2001).

The listening fetus is embedded in an internal sonorous continuum created by his mother's heart sounds and her voice. The steady rhythm of the heart sounds represents an existential beat, whereas mother's prosody imprints the fetal ear with her melodic dialect. At the moment of birth, the infant discovers that mother's heartbeat and familiar voice are silenced. He will miss the sounds of his first continuous intimacy and will try through music to rediscover mother's sonorous presence. According to Sloterdijk (2014), the road to music is inseparable from the retrieval of individual and intimate hearing.

> "What so attracts the infant are not the parents' words, but their musical qualities: rhythm, variations in intonation and tonal ranges at a particular pitch … across cultures parents, intuitively sensing this, automatically exaggerate the musical features of speech, speaking or sing-songing to the infant in a higher and more variable pitch than in adult conversation. Before linguistic exchanges are established, the earliest communication system is then primarily an affective one …" (Rose in Sabbadini 2002: p. 265).

Affects are the matrix of pleasurable or unpleasurable feelings. Attributing meaning to life events relies more on emotions than on words. According to Rose

(2004:p. 97). "… music is a representation of the emotional quality of subjective, lived time made audible—an auditory apparition of felt-time."

The fetus and then the infant recognize the maternal voice, its prosodic features, and the mother's response to the infant's emotional condition. This happens well before the understanding of cognitive and semantic meaning of speech. Rizutto (cited in Etchegoyen 2004:p.1479) considers that the mother's voice mirroring the infant's internal affective state is as important as the mother's mirroring of the baby's face, a well-known concept of Winnicott (1971). Anzieu (1976) described the "sound envelope of the self," a kind of sound mirror between the voices of the baby and his mother. The baby is held in the arms; tightened to the body of the mother of whom he feels her warmth, smell, and movements; carried; handled; rubbed; washed; and caressed, all usually accompanied by a bath of words and humming (Anzieu 1974). Studies demonstrate that 6-month-old infants show preference to mother's singing than to mother's speaking voice (Nakata et al. 2004).

## The Emotional Power of Music

The ancient Greek chorus accompanied and commented the drama of the hero in epic poetry. Alcibiades, in Plato's Symposium, compared Socrates great wisdom to the satyr Marsyas, whose flute song's great charm produced a state of inebriation.

"If a human being wants to say something he cannot, he takes the language of sounds" wrote Robert Schumann (1810–1856). It is as if music expresses what a subject feels: somatic, kinesthetic, or aesthetic sensations. Music is an essential mean to express never verbalized, but felt emotions in traumatic experiences. It is an attempt to overcome silence, one of the most characteristic aspects of lived traumatic events.

LAURA, a young female patient in psychotherapy (whose father died 3 years ago, when the patient, living abroad, came back for the funeral), tells sobbing:

> "Yesterday was the birthday of my father. Everything I lived on my journey back home caught up with me: I heard the same music as I was listening to then, I saw the stars, even the smell came back. Everything remembers me the death of my father. I cried for hours. It is as if I have to return to all that in order to finally find peace …"

> "Music can serve compound defensive or coping functions in transforming our perceptual and sensory experience of time to evoke temporally distant events or reminiscences, provoke a heightened or accelerated anticipation of a future moment, induce or relax states of tension, or seeming to altogether suspend time's ineluctable forward movement. Music's discursive narrativism engenders a sense of time's passage, of a beginning traveling toward an end" (Stein 2004: p. 763).

"The mediator of the inexpressible is the work of art" wrote Wolfgang Goethe (1749–1832). Creation is born out of suffering as artists testify. Any art may bear witness of unspoken traumatic experiences. When Pyotr Ilyich Tchaikovsky (1840–1893) was recovering from a depressive episode, he composed the violin concerto in D major op.35, one of the most emotionally moving concerts.

*IRENE* tells her analyst:

"When I am listening to Tchaikovsky's violin concert it feels like singing of blissful peace and mournful nostalgia, as raging tempestuously in a thunderstorm and rejoicing and exulting in jubilating triumph. Tchaikovsky knows best to give expression to melancholy, to inner struggling and finally to victory in overcoming psychic pain, despair, sadness".

Music may influence perception of time, appears in dreaming, creates meaning for emotional states, contributes to conscious awareness, and is helpful in mourning.

# References

Anzieu D. Le moi-peau. Nouvelle Revue de Psychanalyse, 9, Le dedans et le dehors. Paris: Gallimard; 1974, p.195–208.

Anzieu D. L'enveloppe sonore du Soi. Nouvelle Revue de Psychanalyse, 13, Narcisses. Paris: Gallimard; 1976, p.161–79.

Blood AJ, Zatorre RJ. Intensely pleasurable responses to music correlate with activity in brain regions implicated in reward and emotion. Proc Natl Acad Sci U S A. 2001;98(20):11818–23.

Dalla Bella S, Białuńska A, Sowiński J. Why movement is captured by music, but less by speech: role of temporal regularity. PLoS One. 2013;8(8), e71945. doi:10.1371/journal.pone.0071945. Print 2013.

Etchegoyen L. Language and affects in the analytic practice. Int J Psychoanal. 2004;85(Pt 6): 1479–83.

Herholz SC, Zatorre RJ. Musical training as a framework for brain plasticity: behavior, function, and structure. Neuron. 2012;76(3):486–502. doi:10.1016/j.neuron.2012.10.011. Review.

Maiello S. Prenatal trauma and autism. J Child Psychother. 2001;27(2):107–24. doi:10.1080/00754170110056661.

Nakata T, Sandra E, Trehubb SE. Infants' responsiveness to maternal speech and singing. Infant Behav Dev. 2004;27:455–64.

Panksepp J, Bernatzky G. Emotional sounds and the brain: the neuro-affective foundations of musical appreciation. Behav Processes. 2002;60(2):133–55.

Partanen E, Kujala T, Tervaniemi M, Huotilainen M. Prenatal music exposure induces long-term neural effects. PLoS One. 2013;8(10), e78946. doi:10.1371/journal.pone.0078946. eCollection 2013.

Patel AD. Music, language, and the brain. Oxford: Oxford University Press; 2008.

Patel AD. Can nonlinguistic musical training change the way the brain processes speech? The expanded OPERA hypothesis. Hear Res. 2014;308:98–108. doi:10.1016/j.heares.2013.08.011. Review.

Peretz I. The nature of music from a biological perspective. Cognition. 2006;100(1):1–32.

Rose GJ. Between couch and piano: Psychoanalysis, music, art, and neuroscience. Brunner-Routledge: Hove; 2004.

Sabbadini A. Colour and music: voices of the unconscious. Int J Psychoanal. 2002;83(Pt 1): 263–6.

Sacks O. Musicophilia, Picador. London 2007 xi, xii

Salimpoor VN, van den Bosch I, Kovacevic N, McIntosh AR, Dagher A, Zatorre RJ. Interactions between the nucleus accumbens and auditory cortices predict music reward value. Science. 2013;340(6129):216–9. doi:10.1126/science.1231059.

Sloterdijk P. Der ästhetische Imperativ. Suhrkamp Taschenbuch 4529. Berlin: Suhrkamp; 2014.

Stein A. Music and trauma in Polanski's The pianist (2002). Int J Psychoanal. 2004;85:755–65.

Winnicott DW. Playing and reality. London: Tavistock; 1971.

# Part V

Part V

# Chapter 10
# Stress and Trauma

## Stress and the Brain

From a biological perspective, the brain is the central organ for adaptation. At the most basic level, the brain processes our experiences involving the physical environment as part of a homeostatic regulation to maintain personal and bodily integrity. In a broader perspective, the brain not only processes events in the physical environment but also our experiences involving social interactions. As a result, the social and physical environment in which we live has a huge effect upon our mental state (McEwen 2012).

We know that life experiences change brain structure and function and these changes are called adaptive plasticity. When we encounter critical life events—the so-called stressors—we respond by a coordinated and energizing reaction to help maintain our physical integrity and mental well-being. The entire field of stress research has seen an enormous development, which we summarize here.

It is the brain that determines what is threatening and therefore potentially stressful, as well as initiating the physiological, emotional, and behavioral responses to the stressors. These responses can be either adaptive or damaging. Stress always involves a bidirectional communication between the brain and the cardiovascular, immune, and metabolic systems through the autonomic nervous system and by endocrine mechanisms. The complex effects of these different systems will eventually lead to positive or negative changes in the brain and the body (Fig. 10.1).

## Neurobiological Responses to Stress

The central components of the stress system are located in the hypothalamus and the brain stem. They are part of a major neuroendocrine control system called the hypothalamic–pituitary–adrenal (HPA) axis (Fig. 10.2). The stress system has two major operative modes. The immediate mode involving the fight-or-flight response[1] results from rapid activation of the sympathetic nervous system through release of adrenaline. In parallel, the HPA axis is stimulated: The two important hormones released from the hypothalamus and the pituitary are corticotropin-releasing hormone (CRH) and adreno-corticotropic hormone (ACTH). They help to coordinate the fast behavioral and metabolic response to stress. Glucocorticoids are released by ACTH action on the adrenal gland and are responsible for many of the behavioral and physical responses occurring during the acute stress response. The other mode consists of a more long-lasting modulation of social behavior and is thought to play a key role in our dealing with "every day" social stress. It involves a variety of circuits in the limbic system, and CRH plays an important role in modulating behaviors accompanying chronic stress (Hostetler and Ryabinin 2013).

The stress response is aimed at rapidly answering to unexpected situations, thereby maintaining adequate control over external events. If the stress reaction is excessive or prolonged as in chronic stress, it triggers an inappropriate response that may induce stress-related dysfunctions. It is well established that traumatic experiences in early life will affect the capacity of an individual to cope with stressful events (de Kloet et al. 2005). Failure to cope is accompanied by a number of changes that appear to reflect abnormal HPA axis activity and altered limbic functions. The neurobiological consequences are reflected by molecular and cellular changes not only in the limbic system, in particular in the amygdala and the hippocampus, but also in the prefrontal cortex. While the exact molecular mechanism responsible for

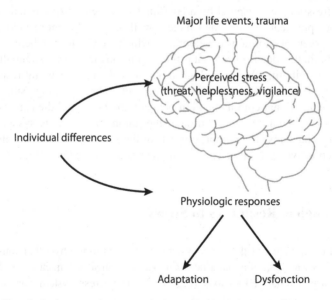

**Fig. 10.1** How the brain responds to stress is determined by individual differences. The physiological and behavioral response can be adaptive or dysfunctional (Adapted from McEwen 1998)

---

[1] The fight-or-flight response was first described by the American physiologist Walter Cannon (1871–1945) as a reaction in animals to a threatening event. The response may also lead to a freezing reaction.

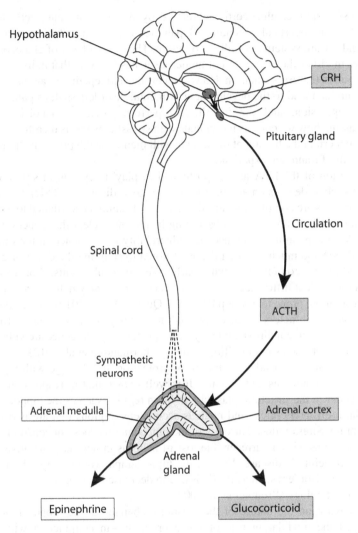

**Fig. 10.2** The activation of the sympathetic nervous system leads to epinephrine release (immediate) and the activation of the hypothalamus–pituitary–adrenal axis leads to glucocorticoids release (short term)

stress-induced cognitive impairment is not yet known, there is evidence to suggest that changes in the anchoring properties of synapses by cell adhesion molecules may be involved: It has been shown that dysregulation of synaptic adhesion molecules by stress results in spine loss at synapses and memory deficits (Wang et al. 2013). Stress events at early age such as bereavements will impair hippocampal integrity resulting in diminished cognitive performance. Several observations show that early life stress leads to an increase in amygdala function (Coplan et al. 2014). As part of a functional adaptation, an increased amygdala volume was reported in children with early life stress such as severe deprivation (Mehta et al. 2009).

In stress response, glucocorticoid release by the adrenal gland activates the mesolimbic, mesocortical ascending dopaminergic system, which controls the motor- and reward systems as well as cognition. The rapid release of glucocorticoid hormones modifies the expression of numerous genes in a way that individuals can best respond to the stress situation. However, chronic and repetitive traumatic stressful exposure can lead to the development of mental disorders such as pathological anxiety, depression, and the inability to perform socially (Sapolsky 2005). Understanding how we cope as individuals with stressful events is therefore a major clinical concern in the treatment of patients with mental health problems thought to be the result of traumatic experiences.

Dysfunction of the HPA axis is postulated to play a key role in stress-related disorders such as depression and post-traumatic stress disorder (PTSD). Of course, these conditions are complex and multifactorial and cannot be attributed to a simple dysfunction of the HPA axis. It is becoming increasingly clear that genetic factors play a role in explaining differences in vulnerability or resilience in the development of PTSD and much research is now devoted to studying the effect of genetic predisposition in combination with early life stressful events. For example, genotype-dependent differences in memory performance may help to identify subjects that are more prone to develop PTSD (de Quervain et al. 2012). Developmental and environmental factors are also involved in the programming of an appropriate response to stressful conditions. Infancy, childhood, and adolescence are vulnerable periods with increased susceptibility to stress (Charmandari et al. 2012).

It is important to consider the notion of protection and damage with regard to recent studies in animals and humans. It is well known that in response to stress changes occur in the structural plasticity in brain regions such as the hippocampus, amygdala, prefrontal cortex, and nucleus accumbens, regions that are part of our visceral brain. Stress-induced atrophy of the hippocampus does not constitute brain damage per se as with the irreversible loss of neurons in neurodegenerative disorders like Alzheimer's disease. In fact, the hippocampal volume loss observed in chronic stress disorders such as PTSD is due to decreased neurogenesis and altered dendritic morphology (Bremner et al. 2008).

Recent work on the nature of the plasticity changes in the hippocampus has emphasized the modulating role of glucocorticoids—in conjunction with other mediators such as oxytocin and brain-derived nerve growth factor (BDNF)—on the regulation of neurogenesis and remodeling of dendrites and synapses (Aimone et al. 2014). For example, hippocampal volume loss in chronic stress has been attributed to reduced BDNF, leading to the hypothesis that stress-related learning deficits result from suppressed hippocampal neurogenesis. These changes are reversible and individual differences in vulnerability to stress can be viewed on a biological level as the distinctive ability to recover from stress-induced modifications in brain circuitry and functions.

The hippocampus is exposed to stress-induced changes during activation of the HPA axis. However it is also important to appreciate the fact that elevated cortisol just prior to a stressful event may also be protective of stress-induced changes in the amygdala. The overall view is that the effects of glucocorticoids and BDNF vary

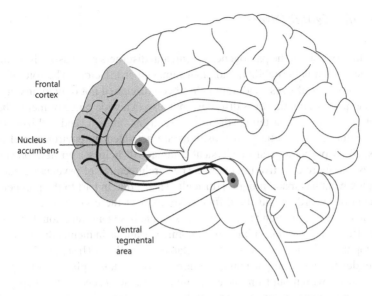

**Fig. 10.3** Glucocorticoids released in a stress response activate the ventral tegmental area and the nucleus accumbens that are parts of the ascending dopaminergic system, which controls the motor system, but also the reward system and more generally cognition and behavior (shaded area corresponds to activation of the frontal cortex). (Adapted from McEwen 2013)

greatly depending on the specific brain region, timing and duration. In other words, regulation of the HPA axis in response to stress is highly complex and involves distinct aspects, whether stress is acute or chronic. Neurotransmitters and neurotrophic factors act together with BDNF to modulate the dynamic response to stress (for review, see Gray et al. 2013).

When mobilized in reaction to an acute challenge, the brain's stress response is adaptive, organizing not only mental processes, but also bodily energy. Chronic stress eventually affects the entire body with increased risk of developing cardiovascular disorders, insulin-resistant diabetes, immune suppression, and reproductive impairments. The endogenous mechanisms of these underlying stress-related changes are becoming better understood, although the exact molecular mechanisms remain unclear. The current idea is that in a chronic stress situation following a traumatic experience, the long-lasting glucocorticoid elevation leads to an adverse epigenetic modulation of the mesocortical dopaminergic system (Fig. 10.3, McEwen 2013). These molecular changes appear to be dependent on genetic risk variants (Niwa et al. 2013). It is also known that epigenetic changes can be transmitted to the next generation, reproducing the metabolic and behavioral alterations in the offspring. Thus, exposure to stress can alter behavior across generations (Franklin et al. 2010). While much of the research involving stress-induced epigenetic control of dopaminergic neurons by glucocorticoids has been performed in animals, the biological alterations found in these experimental models may open new approaches for the understanding of chronic stress in humans.

## Stress and Mental Disorders

Modern theories about the pathogenesis of mental disorders emphasize the dual role of genetic, which is heritability, and environmental risk factors. The role of acute and chronic forms of stress and trauma has been discussed not only in anxiety disorders and post-traumatic stress disorders, but also in a wide range of mental health diseases including devastating disorders such as autism and schizophrenia. Understanding how genetic predispositions are activated by environmental influences such as psychological or physical trauma will help set up new preventive strategies and more effective treatments. The "architecture" of psychiatric genetics is complex what has made progress difficult. This is due in part to the polygenicity of psychiatric disorders and the difficulty to connect these genes (Sullivan et al. 2012). In addition, common variants, such as single base pair mutation, have only a modest effect on risk. Thus, numerous genomic variations in mental disorders, such as schizophrenia or depression, confer a relatively small risk (Insel 2012).

Brain development, in particular the human cortex, takes place mostly postnatally in concert with input from the environment. It is well accepted that epigenetic changes and rearrangements occur through a wide variety of mechanisms resulting in changes in gene expression and synaptic or neuronal development (Gabel and Greenberg 2013). Mental disorders cannot be reduced to a simple genetic or molecular level, but should be understood as a dysfunction of large-scale brain circuits, therefore adding another level of complexity to the pathogenesis of these conditions. We know that brain structures essential for the development of the self, thus shaping behavior and personality, are progressively established during childhood and adolescence. Therefore, a valid framework for approaching brain development and psychiatric disorders has to not only consider brain genetics and chemistry but should also take into account the complex environmental factors and personal life experiences that lead to acute or chronic emotional distress (Solms 2004).

## New Avenues for Treatment

Current studies dissecting the dopaminergic and serotoninergic circuits for their contribution to stress-related disorders offer new insight into how subcortical regions such as the nucleus accumbens and cortical regions such as the medial prefrontal cortex (MPFC) interact. It is particularly relevant for psychiatric disorders as we know that long-lasting stress can lead, for example, to depression. Brain-imaging studies have shown that the MPFC is underactive in depression and stimulation of the MPFC may alleviate the symptoms of severe depressive states (Mayberg et al. 2005).

A dysregulated fear response is a hallmark of traumatic experience and anxiety disorders (Parsons and Ressler 2013). The amygdala is the most critical brain site for fear learning. As mechanisms modulating fear memory acquisition are being better understood, new pharmacological treatments, often in conjunction with psychotherapeutic approaches, are being developed. Classically treatment of fear-related disorders was based on modulating monoaminergic circuits with anti-depressants or enhancing inhibitory gamma-aminobutyric acid (GABA) activity with benzodiazepines. However, these approaches are not very selective. More specific pharmacologic manipulations are now emerging from animal experiments, consisting of a direct modulation of memory circuits (Redondo et al. 2014). Admittedly, these findings are not yet applicable to a clinical setting, but they give us a better understanding of the function of defined memory circuits. We know that traumatic experiences are encoded in parallel in different memory systems, such as in declarative and implicit memory, where they are embedded in emotional and motor pathways. Ideally we should be able to selectively target and block the distressful part of the traumatic memory, leaving the declarative memory trace intact. In other words, the fearful part of the traumatic memory should be replaced by a simple "bad" memory.

As pathways determining responsiveness to stress and factors reducing the ability to cope are being identified, selective therapeutic agents may become available. Since the BDNF system is critical in the regulation of emotional learning and memory, it would be logical to use enhancers of fear extinction, that is molecules targeting BDNF signaling. The development of small molecule agonists or antagonists of the BDNF system or related pathways should provide new possibilities for the treatment of stress- and fear-related disorders (Andero and Ressler 2012). Drugs currently in trials are partial $N$-methyl-D-aspartate (NMDA) receptor agonists such as D-cyclo-serine, which are thought to increase extinction of traumatic memories. However, one has to keep in mind that extrapolating approaches used for fear extinction in animal models of PTSD to clinical pathology will remain an enormous challenge. Artificially removing painful memories without interfering with memory functions as a whole—considering that we are subjects dependent on lifelong learning—may only be feasible if we are able to specifically and momentarily limit awareness of unwanted memories occurring in the aftermath of a trauma (Benoit and Anderson 2012).

## Psychic Trauma

The significance of psychic trauma in the development of diseases has always been rooted in human consciousness, as the epic poems—Iliad and Odyssey—of Homer, the ancient Greek poet, already testified. Homer described the traumatic reactions and the ways of coping of the hero Achilles, who was subjected to the traumatization of wartime experience.

Every epoch has a need to conceptualize clinical manifestations; this is especially true for what is today called psycho-traumatology. The concept of traumatic neurosis was developed in the 19th century and extended in World War I when psychiatrists began dealing with victims of war neurosis.[2] A further important evolution took place during the Vietnam War, when a connection between wartime trauma and the inability of coping with these events was realized, leading to the concept of PTSD.

Psychic trauma (in Greek the word τραύμα means wound) results in no objectively seen lesions—in contrast to an organic lesion—but often leaves "wounds"— that is memory traces—which will not heal and may unexpectedly begin to "bleed" again.[3] These memory traces are imprinted in the personal life of an individual, even if they are no longer part of his conscious awareness.

Trauma is "an event in the subject's life defined by its intensity, the subject's incapacity to respond adequately to it, and by the upheaval and long-lasting effects that it brings about in the psychic organization" (Laplanche and Pontalis 1973: p.465). The notion of trauma represents a conceptual bridge between an event and its impacts. It tries to connect the external reality, the life events, with their consequences on the inner world of an individual, and thus establishes a relationship between external and internal reality. The interest of psychiatry in the cause of trauma was originally focused on whether it is of organic or psychological nature. Today, the major issues are how mental harm leads to physical consequences and how somatic illnesses have mental impacts. In addition, familial, social, and cultural environments play an important role.

In 1889 Janet, a contemporary of Freud and Charcot described the relationship between symptoms and unprocessed memories of traumatic events: Certain events leave indelible and frightening memories, to which the affected person continuously returns and is tormented by day and night. During his scientific work, Sigmund Freud (1895, 1932–1936, 1937, 1937–1939) dealt repetitively with the question of whether external influences or the phantasmatic configuration and the individual meaning of the lived reality were responsible for the psychic consequences. He came to the conclusion that not the trauma itself, but its subsequent processing, retranscription of memory, can result in pathogenic effects, e.g., when early childhood traumatic experiences remain non-assimilated in the present.

Winnicott (1965a) considered trauma as any event disrupting the continuous living experience of an individual. For Shengold (1989), an overwhelming psychological trauma is synonymous with soul murder, while Nathan (1986) considered that the unthinkable and unspeakable loss of one's cultural environment is in itself a psychic trauma, as each individual relies on his cultural environment to decipher reality. Khan developed the concept of cumulative trauma (1974). He considered

---

[2] Freud (1919) and psychoanalysts used the term traumatic neurosis to describe symptoms such as tremors, paralyzes, and recurrent nightmares related to war exposure. Today, we use the term "post-traumatic stress disorder."

[3] What is revealed from the hidden (ληθη, laethae in Greek), the Greeks called ἀλήθεια, a-laetheia, meaning truth. For Parmenides, the ancient Greek philosopher, truth is well rounded, ἀλήθεια ευκυκλέος, alaetheia eukukleos, a circle without beginning or end, just like the psychic trauma repeats itself; neither its origin is seen, nor its end is predictable (Kirk et al. 1994).

the lack of the motherly shield function as especially traumatic. He hypothesized a kind of short-circuiting between mind and body. What cannot be integrated mentally is imprinted in the body and manifests itself in psychosomatic symptoms, which are constantly repeated. It is as if the body "remembers" and the subject inscribes into his body, what is unbearable to feel, what is psychologically intolerable.

For Barrois (1988) psychic trauma is conceived as the result of an emotional overflow which cannot be mastered by the individual mind or a panic anxiety, generated by a given situation. A psychic trauma can establish a kind of "psychic crypt." An individual has no interest to repeat emotionally overwhelming experiences. He splits—whenever possible—such experiences from conscious awareness, "hiding" them—by means of encapsulation—in the form of crypts. According to Abraham and Torok (1994) whenever the loss of a loved person is denied, the subject—via incorporation of the lost one—turns into a crypt carrier.

Traumatic experience is defined as a vital experience of discrepancy between threatening situational factors and individual coping abilities, which is accompanied by feelings of helplessness, abandonment, and defenselessness (Fischer and Riedesser 1999). Some individuals cannot accomplish trauma-processing work: The nightmare of the past is lived in the present and is the unique perspective of the future.

## Psychic Trauma in Children

The child psychiatrists Donovan and McIntyre (1990) proposed in their publication *Healing the hurt child* a developmental–contextual approach to trauma when describing psychic injuries in children. The occurrence of post-traumatic disorders in children—as a result of serious mental distress—has been recognized only in the nineties (Udwin 1993).

There are important questions to address, which—due to the complexity of human nature itself, also considering the individual genetic makeup and the manifold connectivity to the environment in which the child grows up—may not be answered definitively: What external or internal factors are crucial for traumatization to arise? What are the short-term and long-term effects of traumatic events? What do children experience and how do they try to deal with a psychic trauma? Why is it that some children exposed to severe psychic traumatization for many years, seem psychically less affected than other children, who are seemingly traumatized by less serious experiences?

The following comments are limited to psychic traumas that occur within the family framework. These include: abuse, neglect and deprivation, loss of loved ones through separation or death, multiple placements, chronic somatic or mental illness of a parent, accidents, operations or own chronic illness, witnessing cruel acts and cultural uprooting. According to the Child Maltreatment 2012 report of the US

National Child Abuse and Neglect Data System,[4] the majority of victims (78.3 %) suffered neglect defined as "a type of maltreatment that refers to the failure by the caregiver to provide needed, age-appropriate care although financially able to do so or offered financial or other means to do so" (http://www.acf.hhs.gov/programs/cb/research-data-technology/statistics-research/child-maltreatment).

The consequences of human aggression and atrocities such as war and terrorism, disasters caused by human error in technical matters, e.g., aircraft accidents, industrial disasters, and finally also natural disasters such as earthquakes and floods belong to the traumata occurring outside the family framework, not discussed here.

## Psychobiological Aspects

Adverse experiences at critical or sensitive developmental phases during early childhood influence to a great degree brain development and may have long-lasting impacts, but brain development maintains its malleability until adulthood (Weder and Kaufman 2011; Weder et al. 2014). Traumatic events in early childhood, leading to epigenetic modifications that alter gene expression, play an important role in the development of stress-related psychiatric illnesses and other health problems in later life. These changes are often enduring, but do not have to be permanent (Nemeroff and Binder 2014; Weder et al. 2014). Some neurobiological changes can be reversed by treatment interventions, for example, in providing secure attachment relationships. Various studies demonstrate that the negative consequences of early environmental stress or traumatic exposure, such as psychopathological disorders, can be alleviated by preventive interventions offering among others, a continuous and meaningful relationship with alternative care persons, as well as addressing parent–child psychopathology and creating environmental opportunities (see resilience Chap. 13). These interventions show their efficiency up to adult life.

Early childhood traumatic experiences affect the normal development of the cerebral cortex and the limbic system and lead to long-term changes in multiple neurotransmitter systems. Certain areas of the brain must be adequately stimulated at crucial stages of development, so they can function optimally later. The specific design of the dendritic branching and neuronal synapses are shaped in accordance to the frequency in which they are used. "The thalamus, amygdala, hippocampus and prefrontal cortex are all involved in the stepwise integration and interpretation of incoming sensory information. This integration can be disrupted by high levels of arousal: moderate to high activation of the amygdala enhances the long term potentiation of declarative memory, mediated by the hippocampus, while extreme arousal

---

[4] Child Abuse and Neglect is defined as "any recent act or failure to act on the part of a parent or caretaker which results in death, serious physical or emotional harm, sexual abuse or exploitation; or an act or failure to act, which presents an imminent risk of serious harm."

disrupts hippocampal functioning, leaving the memories to be stored as affective states or in sensory-motor modalities, as somatic sensations and visual images" (van der Kolk et al. 2007: p. 294). Adequate assessment and integration of emotional experiences do not take place. Therefore, trauma-related memories remain timeless and self-alien.

Even if children have a great capacity to adapt, traumatic experiences can alter the mental and biological balance of a child, thus impeding him to accomplish his developmental steps in the present. The plasticity of the brain allows considerable adaptability, but at the same time leaves infants and young children particularly vulnerable to long-term impacts of disturbing influences. Perception and awareness of body sensations and emotions are fundamental building blocks in the development of self-experience and self-image, as well as of cognitive processes and creativity. These basic experience patterns are built up in the earliest relationships with primary caregivers. Any disturbance in the early adaptation of the primary caregivers to the infant's needs or any event that interrupts the continuity of the child's experience and development can present a risk factor for psychic traumatization.

A study of over 2000 children aged 2–9 (Turner et al. 2012) confirmed that emotional maltreatment (without physical aggression) and hostile, rejecting or inconsistent parenting are among the highest risk factors for children's physical and mental development. In addition, various negative impacts have subsequently cumulative effects. The most lasting mental consequences of traumatic events are the inability to regulate arousal states, to control and verbally express feelings of anger, fear, and sadness, to perceive stimuli appropriately and to adapt to the environment. The younger the child at the time of traumatization and the longer the trauma lasts, the greater is his relevant risk (van der Kolk 1996).

Multiple or repeated traumatization (cumulative traumata) in childhood have severe outcomes and affect multiple developmental domains such as regulation of affect and impulses, memory, attention, consciousness, self-perception, interpersonal relations, somatization, and systems of meaning. They result in complex symptoms and disorders also in adulthood (D'Andrea et al. 2012; Cloitre et al. 2009; van der Kolk et al. 2005).

Children are particularly vulnerable to compulsively reenacting traumatic experiences, as they have no conscious memory of the traumatic event(s), leading to repeated suffering either for themselves as victims or for others as perpetrators. Their behavior can be traced back to adversities encountered with primary caregivers in infancy or early childhood. If caregivers are absent or their reliance is existentially failing, children experience extremes of under-stimulation and hyperarousal, longing for and fearing the caregiver's presence and intimacy. Violence and hostility of caregivers overwhelm infants or young children's inner lives, which are then filled with chronic anxiety, wariness, rage, anger, and finally retaliation (van der Kolk 1989).

## Psychodynamic Aspects

In the traumatic situation, a child suffers a personal loss of love, affection, and protection, which represent existential and essential needs for a child in his dependency and vulnerability. The "good enough maternal or parental holding"[5] (Winnicott 1964, 1965b) creates a feeling of reliance on the human environment as a guarantee for the continuity of the child's personal experience. A child is deprived when it has not known this reliance experience, when the continuity in his life and development has been interrupted. The experience of rejection or abandonment by his parents leads to feelings of being exposed to threatening circumstances and deprived of their fundamental love. This is often described as the most important factor for childhood psychic trauma.

Subsequently—as the communication is interrupted—the child cannot share his experience of the traumatic event. The infant and the small child do not possess the necessary perception functions and perception structures to record and organize an experience associated with overwhelming feelings. But also the older child is overwhelmed by feelings of helplessness, powerlessness, and despair and plunges into an emotional state of annihilation, consternation, and confusion.

As Ferenczi already described in 1933,[6] a child expects tender play in his exchanges with the adult caregiver, yet the adult sometimes responds with sexual or aggressive impulses. Anxiety and fear compel the child to surrender to the adult, to identify with the aggressor, and to introject the guilt feelings of the adult.[7] "The most important change, produced in the mind of the child by the anxiety-fear-ridden identification with the adult partner, is the introjection of the guilt feelings of the adult..." (Ferenczi 1949).

Subsequently, the child tries to build up a fantasy world, which serves as a kind of survival strategy. The fantasies the child creates after the traumatic experience can be understood as an attempt to find meaning for what happened to him. The child searches—on a fantasy level—for an explanation in order to understand the event. These fantasy formations may lead to intrapsychic conflicts, which are often expressed through symptoms. The meaning and significance the child attributes to the traumatic challenge by his affective response form the basis of his post-traumatic adjustment.

---

[5] Winnicott's concept of holding means safeguarding and maintaining the continuity of the infant's or child's experience of being and being alive over time.

[6] The original paper was *The Passions of Adults and their Influence on the Sexual and Character Development of Children* published in Int. Z. f. Psa. (1933; 19: p. 5–15).

[7] Through an identification process called introjection, the aggressor disappears as part of the external reality and becomes intra- instead of extra-psychic.

**Clinical Vignette Aurelia**

An adoptive mother required a child psychiatric consultation for her 8-year-old girl who was taken out of her country of origin for adoption at the age of 2. Aurelia's symptoms consisted of opposition behavior, slowness and apathy, masturbation, eating- and learning disorders—she refused to learn to read. Aurelia did not speak in the first encounter with the child psychiatrist, but played, and commented her play-scene summarized as follows: This is a poor family that does not have enough money, and the children have nothing to eat. The oldest girl left with other people to get money; she will come back. Her mother (placed in the play-scene on a terrace) looks at her and knows that she will come back. To the question "when" Aurelia answers: "The girl will have the same height, when she comes back with a lot of money."

The adoptive parents were shocked when told their girl's play-scene and informed the psychiatrist that the biological mother waved from a balcony to her daughter when they took the girl with them for adoption. Aurelia lost her biological mother, her first love relationship. What happened to her in the final moments of separation from her mother, why her mother abandoned her, she was never able to ask as the communication with her mother was definitively interrupted. Her personal fantasy construction of this traumatic experience, "the girl will have the same height" was pathogenic for Aurelia, prohibiting her to grow up, which she expressed by a symptomatology of eating- and learning disorders. Simultaneously—thanks to her fantasies—Aurelia maintained her loyal attachment to the biological mother. This example shows that traumatic experiences, even if they are not consciously remembered, leave unconscious memory traces.

## *Symptoms and Phases of Psychic Trauma*

The interactions of developmental processes and traumatic stress are complex; therefore, the assessment of a child's traumatic situation is essential. His cognitive and affective development has to be evaluated as well as his interpersonal relationship, his familial- and social situation. Maturity of defense strategies and coping mechanisms, resources such as temperament, humor, and good cognitive skills, which affect the meaning—attribution of traumatic experiences, are considered as protective factors. In contrast, preexisting physical and emotional vulnerability are risk factors. Often multiple causes and circumstances are involved in a traumatic event. Various traumatic events or conditions may interact simultaneously or successively. Acute events are distinguished from prolonged life circumstances and psychosocial stress is differentiated depending on its severity.

Terr (1991) summarizes the characteristics of childhood trauma as follows: (a) recurrent, intrusive memories (most often visual, but also auditory, tactile, and olfactory); (b) repetitive behaviors: the traumatic experience is repeated in playing and some aspects of the traumatic experience are (re)enacted in behaviors; (c) trauma-specific fears, which are linked to the original traumatic situation; (d) the attitude towards others, life and the future is changed; expectations are negative and confidence is lost. The child is terrified by feelings of helplessness, horror, and despair. The younger the child or the greater his vulnerability, the more he will be overwhelmed by annihilation- and death anxieties.

Fischer and Riedesser (1999) describe four phases of traumatic reactions and the subsequent states of experience. They are not always sequential, but can exist simultaneously. Trauma processes are influenced by coping and adaptive skills, as well as by age, developmental-phase, defense mechanisms, and critical life events.

*Phase I* corresponds to the situation of the traumatic experience: emotional disorders are characterized by hyperarousal with manifestations of motor hyperactivity, explosive aggression-, or panic anxiety states. Subsequently (*phase II*), the traumatic event is denied, banned from the waking consciousness, the memory of the event displaced or repressed. The original feelings of fear, helplessness, and despair are split off. Children are emotionally upset, withdraw, and appear apathetic and joyless. At the same time, the child is often very alert in an attempt to anticipate threatening situations. Children try to keep emotional distance and avoid emotionally charged situations, which could relate to the trauma.

The transition to the intrusion phase (*phase III*) may occur with decreasing defenses; representations and thoughts associated with the traumatic experience are imposed on the child's mind. Since the memory traces are not extinguished, they appear as spontaneous images, sounds, and nightmares. *CHANTAL*, a 10-year-old girl, for example, sees—in her nightmares—her parents as monsters.

In playing and storytelling, children try to cope with and overcome the traumatic experience (*phase IV*). The child's play is characterized by repetitive scenes of the trauma. Children lack the ability—in pretend play—to try out interactive social roles and situations and to tell corresponding stories. Traumatized children's narratives are often chaotic and involve threatening topics. Working through—for instance, in a psychotherapeutic process—facilitates the integration of the traumatic experience. The cognitive integration of emotionally lived inner and outer reality is a sustained task from the first day of life, allowing already very early to live continuity in self-experience. As more and more complex integrations take place, more intensely and differentiated will the perception of one's own self-continuity be experienced.

In stressful situations at later stages, e.g., entering adolescence or the outbreak of a serious illness, children or adolescents react with the emotional intensity they felt at the time of the traumatic experience, as if the traumatic event would repeat itself. They are not able to understand what is happening to them, as the biographical reference is unconscious. Long-standing traumatic situations coupled with further injury or loss, lead to long-lasting pathological grief or chronic depression, which may be associated with feelings of emptiness, meaninglessness, and lifelessness.

**Clinical Vignette Antoine**

Eleven-year-old Antoine came to Switzerland for adoption after several institutional and foster care placements. His adoptive family was unable to deal with his enormous behavioral problems and Antoine was reintegrated into an institution. He was afraid of his recurring dream: He knocks at the house where he once lived, and no one answers him. The whole village has been abandoned by its inhabitants. In his nightmare, Antoine expresses the feelings of abandonment he experienced in his multiple ruptures with significant persons in his past. He draws an oblique detached house which—as he comments his drawing—will soon fall into the water. All attempts to save the house with a ship, aircraft, parachute, or crane will fail. "The house will fall and smash everything to pieces, because it is very menacing, what one did not notice when the house was built." Antoine feels his inner-psychic "house" as so dangerous that it can only destroy or be destroyed. He refuses psychotherapeutic help because—as he says—no one can help him. Antoine draws two trees. The trees have the same outline: the first is entirely and richly filled with branches and leaves in different colors, while the second is completely bare. The boy comments: "These are the trees of my life; the first at the beginning of my life, the second now."

## Familial Aspects

Families where maltreatment occurs have certain common features of family dynamics, relationship structures, and intergenerational transmission mechanisms (Boszormenyi-Nagy and Framo 1985; Minuchin and Fishman 2004; Stierlin et al. 1980).

In families where children are exposed to traumatic situations, the parents themselves often experienced traumatic events as children. Components of such experiences are—in the next generation—parts of the functional modalities of family life. Intergenerational triangulations are the resulting consequence. In family therapy terminology, triangulation means that the parents include the child in their conflict. If adults do not overcome their couple conflicts and tensions, these are often displaced onto a child; the classic example is the "scapegoat child." Generally, it is the child who is most closely identified with the parent; he often reminds the parent of his own, unacceptable impulses or character traits. The child, on the other hand, takes it upon himself to be blamed and thinks he deserves punishment. In situations of abuse, there is often a reversal of role functions. In the hierarchy, the child is placed at the level of the parents, and in a hidden way becomes the ally of one parent against the other. The so-called parentified child takes over parental functions, for example, for a parent who suffers from depression or drug addiction. The child can also assume substitute roles, for example, as a father or mother for siblings, or as a sexual partner in incest relationships. Children are parentified delegates[8] when they are trying—through the process of introjection[9]—to fulfill unconscious missions from their parents.

Triangulation can occur when parental functions are inadequate or when the outbreak of a hidden marital conflict has to be prevented. Parents project specific mental representations and nonintegrated, e.g., aggressive drives onto the child, who tries to suppress his own feelings in order to help the incompetent adult. If interpersonal boundaries are violated again and again, the child does not learn to set his own limits or to feel his own emotions and needs and is therefore unable to express his feelings. The development of a false self (see Chap. 6) as an adaptive structure will allow the child to behave loyally towards his parents, because the false self protects the true self like a shield, yet prevents its development (Winnicott 1958). Traumatized and traumatizing families rely heavily on defense mechanisms such as denial, trivialization, and avoidance in order to protect themselves from traumatic experiences. Family members commit themselves to remain silent and keep secrets, often under the influence of blackmail, threats of retaliation or coercion.

The dread of revelation with regard to the surroundings is apparently so enormous because of fears of a familial or individual breakdown. The apprehension of disclosure revealing humiliating secrets can already trigger an explosive crisis as shown in the following vignette.

*JEROME*, 10 years old, expressed suicidal threats. His drug- and alcohol-dependent depressed mother required her son to buy alcohol behind his father's back. In the first interview with the child psychiatrist, Jerome said that he had attempted everything to help his mother in her depression, to be vigilant and to prevent her addiction behavior.

Jerome was highly parentified. He felt responsible for saving his mother from her depression and drug and alcohol dependence. But Jerome's mother obliged him to be her alcohol supplier, thus building a secret coalition relationship, directed against the father. Jerome broke down with tremendous guilt- and loyalty feelings. He directed his anger and aggressiveness against himself.


## Trauma Related Psychopathology

Maltreatments that constitute acute physical or psychic aggression and threaten the child with feelings of abandonment and destruction have to be differentiated from chronic trauma forms such as neglect and deprivation. In the first situation, the excessive stress exceeds the coping capabilities of the subject. In the second situation, the lack of essential caring attention and emotional reliance fails to meet the basic developmental needs of a child.

Psychic trauma can impact all developmental areas leading to growth arrest, developmental delays, functional disturbances, and structural changes, involving

---

[8] Children are delegated to serve the emotional or physical needs of their parents.

[9] Unconscious internalization of aspects of another person within the self.

body, brain, and mind. Trauma-related psychopathology results from an overload on different systems including a dysregulation of the hippocampus–hypothalamus–pituitary–adrenal axis (Cirulli and Alleva 2009).

The *SEPARATION* of an infant from his mother leads to long-lasting neurobiological changes specifically of neurotransmitters, such as serotonin and catecholamines, with disturbances in heart rhythm, body temperature, and sleep, and changes in neurohormones such as oxytocin, known to increase empathy and bonding. That oxytocin plays a central role in stress regulation is underlined by the demonstration that application of oxytocin in psychosocial stress situations reduces anxiety (Heinrichs et al. 2003). Children who experienced traumatic separations remain vulnerable because disturbances in neurotransmitters and neuroendocrine systems are long-lasting and can be reactivated later in other stressful situations, such as the loss of affective relationships.

Children who have lived traumatic separations are more prone to physical disorders and especially to infectious diseases. The child's body seems to take over the function of expressing the unbearable emotions. The somatic symptoms must be taken seriously as a cry for help and often have symbolic meaning, such as the occurrence of asthma attacks or flare-ups of skin manifestations (eczema) in the context of traumatic or painful separation experiences.

*MICHEL*, 8 years old, lived separately from his mother with his remarried father. Before each meeting with his mother, his eczema flared up massively. The boy lived in anticipatory anxiety of the recurrence of the overwhelming emotions he felt at the moment of his traumatic separation from his mother as an infant.

Anzieu (1989) speaks of a "toxic function" of the skin-ego; he considers the outburst of eczema as an attempt of the subject to feel from the outside the somatic surface layer of the self, torn in a most painful, self-destructive conflict. Separation anxiety disorders in childhood are a risk factor for developing panic- or anxiety disorders in adults (Kossowsky et al. 2012).

Based on psychotherapeutic observations of abused infants and young children, Green (1983) described the occurrence of developmental disorders. He noted that these children avoided eye contact with their parents, kept a distance, and approached parents only from the side or behind. They sat around, often immobile, but highly alert. This higher state of alertness prevents normal language and motor skill learning.

Children, who are abused when they cry or even vocalize, learn to suppress their verbal expressions, what delays and inhibits language development. They speak and articulate later and commonly show expression difficulties. In a similar way, they abstain from motor activities such as crawling and climbing if this behavior disturbs their caregivers. This can lead to transitory motor and coordination disorders. These children are often very clumsy and hurt themselves easily.

Two-year-and-a-half-old *CHRISTINE* still does not vocalize any sounds. Her pediatrician—fearing she might be an autistic child—requests an evaluation. In the first encounter with the child psychotherapist and the separate living parents, Christine starts babbling, vocalizing, and crawls on all fours towards the psychotherapist to the stupefaction of her parents.

The *EMOTIONAL RESPONSE* to psychological traumas such as kidnapping, abuse, deprivation, or incest has been described as biphasic: first characterized by hyperarousal and overwhelming of emotions, then by apathetic encapsulation and emotional seclusion. Any emotional and sensory stimulus can subsequently arouse and overwhelm a child so that he responds with motor hyperactivity, explosive hetero- and/or auto-aggressiveness or a panic fright reaction, less frequently with weeping and crying crises. Deprived children are incapable of regulating their feelings of fear and aggression against others or themselves and unable to modulate their excitability and hyperarousal state. Infants and young children, who are left alone in a state of extreme anxiety and helplessness, finally cry themselves to sleep out of exhaustion, what can be regarded as a physiological protection mechanism, an avoidance of "psychic death."

A relationship between persistent intolerable affect- and arousal states and the risk of developing drug dependency in adolescence is postulated. Deprivation in childhood can lead to various addictive behaviors. Opiates have the ability to mitigate feelings of separation and alienation by decreasing feelings of pain. Children, who have experienced early childhood separation anxiety, later try to behave in a way that will stimulate their opiate system to calm their excitement and intolerable anxiety states. It is well known that stressors elevate endogenous opiates (Cohen et al. 1982). This can lead to compulsive behaviors in which children have a tendency to repeatedly expose themselves to traumatic situations, a phenomenon that clinicians have known for a long time (Green 1978, 1988).

Another inner response of the child is his state of nonparticipation and sadness: a state of anhedonia. Trauma or overwhelming stress increases endorphin secretion and triggers numbing of certain feelings (Glover 1992). This leads to emotional numbness and dissociated emotions: namely the feeling to be cut off from life and from concern for others. Children are dysphoric, isolate themselves, and withdraw affectively; they are apathetic, but simultaneously over alert—a state called frozen watchfulness—and thus remain in a "frozen state of alertness."

*THOMAS*, 8-year-old, draws himself with eyes all over his body and spare eyes: he comments his drawing: "I will always be able to see, even with my back and when asleep."

In the first encounter with the child psychiatrist, *SABINE*, 8-year-old, shows an opaque mask-like face, remains sitting, entirely stiff in her body, motionless and hardly responds, or with "I do not know." She starts with great difficulty several times to draw houses, which are "cut into two parts and burning." Sabine comments: "No one will come out alive from these houses, except a cat." She would like to be this cat. Sabine's greatest fear is to be blind, that is no longer able to foresee and control the imminent disasters she has to face, namely the return of unbearable terrifying feelings of past traumatic experiences. Sabine was 18 months old when hospitalized for the first time in a serious state of neglect; her development was delayed by 1 year.

One considers—as a significant feature of a post-traumatic condition—the behavior of a child that no longer smiles, nor responds to laughter, nor initiates a smile and is unable to engage with others in exchanges of joy, pleasure, and gratification. Behind this affective self-encapsulation one often finds a chronic depressive state and/or intense feelings of anger and hatred. Children are incapable of sustaining an affective tonality; their affective communications are unpredictable, marked by high ambivalence and ambiguity and very often superficial. The question is not always easy to answer whether neglect and abuse create disturbed affective communications, or whether this affective climate favors neglect and abuse to happen. Both parents and children are in a relation of "malignant embrace" (Stierlin et al. 1980), which they are unable to change.

The developmental delays in COGNITIVE FUNCTIONS are the result of acoustic and visual perception disorders. Traumatized children are not able to use mental images that are essential for problem solving, but have to rely on sensory-motor acting in order to manage changes. Distinctive signs are the missing flexibility of cognitive structures and functions so that dynamic changes no longer take place. Autonomic nervous system alertness and the permanent anxiety state prevent planning and playing with alternative options. Children show a lack of essential learning curiosity, which is necessary for exploratory behavior and learning opportunities. Traumatized children function by far the worst in perception and awareness of themselves and others compared to control groups. For example they have great difficulties and feel no joy in storytelling. The content of their narratives often reflects terrifying events such as murder, kidnapping, abandonment, and rejection and rarely has happy ends, as it is the case of control groups.

The longer the traumatic situation lasts, the less the child can adapt to its environment and the more energy he will spend creating an inner world with multiple omnipotent identities, a world in which the child is no longer confronted with the reality of the outside world and where he no longer receives criticism or judgment.

LUC, an 11-year-old adopted boy, speaks in an infantile language with his "clown" who dictates him with a quiet voice requests that Luc must absolutely fulfill. It's the clown, says Luc, who commits all the follies for which he is unjustly accused. The clown also communicates with the significant persons Luc knew in his country of origin. Luc has been sexually abused in childhood. What he experienced as a powerless victim, he now reenacts as an active perpetrator with his clown and is able to express his feelings of rage and retaliation, in identification with the aggressor. The dissociation allows Luc to maintain his desire to be a kind and loved child.

Chronically traumatized children give the impression of shadow figures. "The excess of the trauma is accompanied by its shadow, the silence of the unspeakable." (Barrois 1988: p. 195). These children are also described as machines or robots. Having cut off their memories of the past, they live without joy into the day, apparently in a kind of continuous present—seeking to exclude any "absence," whether separation, loss, or death—and without any kind of wishes for the future. The sooner children suffering from psychic trauma receive help, the greater their chance of not becoming "shadow children."

Seven-year-old CYNTHIA tells the following story about a caterpillar: "The caterpillar was cut by evil people, so it was blind. Birds brought the caterpillar to the village" (where the girl lives with her adoptive parents). "There the caterpillar promised never wanting to see again, but to stay blind forever, adoring the feeling of never being able to see again." The caterpillar should never again feel and perceive the horror it had experienced in its country of origin. Cynthia was able to use psychotherapeutic help to "transform herself into a seeing butterfly."

Children deal differently with their great fear to be confronted again with their lived traumatic experiences as the vignettes of Sabine, Thomas, and Cynthia demonstrate: Whereas Sabine and Thomas want to see, that is anticipate an eventual recurrence of traumatization, Cynthia wishes to remain blind, hoping that in this way she could protect herself.

The consequences of severely psychic trauma can—under certain circumstances—be transmitted from one generation to another like a cultural heritage. The history of the parents is not separable from the personal history of their child. The past of the parents becomes the present for the child. With children one has always to keep in mind that symptoms may be the expression of intergenerational transmission of unresolved and unintegrated traumatic events of the parents. The fact that certain feelings cannot be expressed by the parents may have the consequence that the emotions of the parents cannot be integrated by their child. What the parents are not able to express takes an unimaginable dimension for their children. The fears and feelings associated with the parent's traumatic experience are transferred by nonverbal communication (voice, gestures, and gaze) to the child. As a substitute, the child expresses the parent's fears with symptoms and also by symbolization in play and drawings, sometimes on the anniversary of the parental trauma (see section "Transgenerational Transmission of Traumatic Events" in Chap. 14).

### Clinical Vignette Roberto

The parents ask for a child psychiatric consultation for their 6-year-old son, who suffers from school phobia, intense anxieties, and fears and does not want to grow up. In the first individual interview with the child psychiatrist, Roberto tells of his recurrent nightmare of a white ghost. Later, his mother informs the psychotherapist that—on the anniversary of the death of her father, which occurred 4 years ago—Roberto drew a skeleton in a coffin. Her son had never known his grandfather. When the mother asked who was lying in the coffin, Roberto answered: "My grandfather" and wanted to know the cause of his grandfather's death.

The boy's symptomatology disappeared as soon as the mother was able to engage in a psychotherapeutic process, which lasted 6 years. The psychotherapy revealed that her father, who suffered from bipolar psychosis, was no longer able to keep up his farm and piled up depts. He finally committed suicide. The maternal grandmother of Roberto was affected by syphilis. It is in this particularly dramatic context that Roberto's mother—already as a child and then as teenager—endured long-lasting sexual abuse, first by her paternal grandfather then by the paternal uncle, who had taken over the farm and ensured the financial existence of her family.

Roberto's mother had never been able to talk about her cumulative traumatic childhood and adolescence experiences. She kept her overwhelming emotions of shame, guilt, fear, and despair secret; a mourning process for the loss of her father and her traumatic experiences never took place.

# Post-Traumatic Stress Disorder

PTSD—a recent name for an old condition—entered the classification of mental disorders in 1980. It has however a long medical history. Charcot, the French neurologist spoke of traumatic memories as "parasites of the mind" (van der Kolk 1996), while Freud referred to traumatic memories as "traumatic neurosis." PTSD is a disorder occurring after exposure to traumatic events associated with a significant stress response. A genetic susceptibility seems to play an important role in building particular persisting memories, and an increased risk of developing symptoms of PTSD has been linked to genetic traits predisposing the formation of a strong aversive memory (de Quervain et al. 2012).

The response to traumatic events has many individual facets. Jones et al. (2003) emphasizes the fact that response to trauma has changed over time and is clearly influenced by culture. The predominance of somatic symptoms such as tics, movement disorders, or paralysis was common in the early part of the twentieth century. These symptoms have now been replaced by neuropsychiatric symptoms where flashbacks[10] or involuntary overwhelming recollections of traumatic scenes are predominant. This changing symptomatology has led to the idea that PTSD symptoms are not invariant but should be viewed in the context of a continually evolving picture of human reaction to adversity (Young 2001). Persistence of negative or intrusive memories is a sign of anxiety disorders and depression. Individuals with dysphoric moods are often experiencing persistent negative memories or flashbacks.

We like to think that a rational mind can organize and take care of our feelings and impulses. Intense emotions, particularly triggered by traumatic exposure activate distinct brain regions such as the amygdala, hippocampus, anterior cingulate gyrus, orbitofrontal and prefrontal cortex. The amygdala is one of the structures that determine the emotional significance of an incoming stimulus. The "rational" brain before reacting to an emotional challenge will contextualize the information by comparing it to an existing internal map. In a "normal" situation, we are able to deal with our feelings and respond in an appropriate and flexible manner. In contrast, children and adults confronted with acute or chronic psychic trauma lose the capacity to handle their emotions and feelings in an appropriate way and as van der Kolk rightfully says; people who suffer from PTSD "seem to lose their way in the world" (van der Kolk 2006: p. 280).

The neurobiological disturbances of PTSD involve many of the stress-induced changes that we reviewed above such as alterations in the limbic system, especially the amygdala (Charney et al. 1993). Significant changes also arise in the locus coeruleus, which regulates the release of catecholamines and mobilizes the body for an emergency situation. If PTSD is already present, there is overreaction by parts of the limbic system with symptoms of fear, anxiety, hypervigilance, irritability, and

---

[10] Flashbacks, a form of dissociative state, are defined as involuntary, vivid images that occur in the waking state.

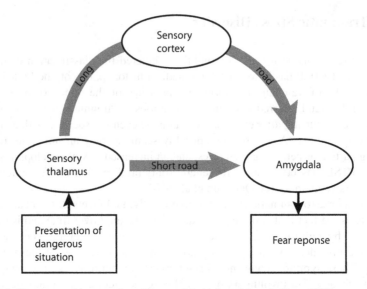

**Fig. 10.4**  The short and long roads to the amygdala (Adapted from LeDoux 1996)

readiness to fight or flee. "Victims of a devastating trauma may never be the same biologically." "It does not matter if it was the incessant terror of combat, torture, or repeated abuse in childhood, or a one-time experience, like being trapped in a hurricane or nearly dying in an auto accident. All uncontrollable stress can have the same biological impact." (Charney, cited in Goleman 1990).

The amygdala holds a privileged position as emotional guard (LeDoux 2000). It is a hub for emotions and for emotional memories. Sensory, visual, or auditory signals arrive first to the thalamus and then the cortex; the signal then passes to the amygdala and activates the emotional centers. Alternatively—in an extreme threatening situation—a portion of the original signal passes directly from the thalamus to the amygdala, bypassing the cortex. This transmission is faster allowing a quicker, although less accurate response. In this way, the amygdala can trigger a reaction even before the cortical centers have fully understood what is going on (Fig. 10.4, LeDoux 1996).

Recent findings suggest that when an old fear memory is recalled, a separate brain pathway from the one originally engaged is used (Do-Monte et al. 2015). Specifically memory retrieval then involves a different circuit—from the prefrontal cortex to the paraventricular region of the thalamus—a region known to activate fear expression in the amygdala (Courtin et al. 2014). This shift of memory recall over time may explain why in patients with PTSD fear experiences remain so vivid and unpleasant.

## *Post-Traumatic Stress Disorders in Children*

Children, unlike adults, do not have the same skills to understand and manage stress. The child's post-traumatic consequences result from complex dynamic interactions between inner and outer worlds, facts and their subjective meanings, and between the traumatic event and the post-traumatic processing capabilities. They are always in relation to the child's developmental stage and the familial and social context. Increased vulnerability, chronic persistent anxiety, and emotional numbness are all features of PTSD in children.

Research in the field of post-traumatic consequences of cumulative traumata or poly-victimization of children and youth has centered on the developmental aspects and family context in order to assess the multiple and serious mental health problems in children, youth, and adults[11] and to propose earlier preventive and therapeutic measures (Cloitre et al. 2009; van der Kolk et al. 2005; D'Andrea et al. 2012; Finkelhor et al. 2009; Turner et al. 2012).

A national survey of trauma exposure and PTSD in adolescents in Switzerland came to the conclusion that, in the general population, about half of the adolescents had experienced at least one traumatic event. Higher risk of trauma exposure was found in adolescents who did not live with both biological parents, who were not of Swiss origin or who had parents with lower education. The occurrence of PTSD was higher in females. Adolescents having witnessed domestic violence had the highest occurrence of PTSD (Landolt et al. 2013).

Boys and girls show different mental trends and behaviors. Girls tend to suffer from depression and show self-destructive behavior, identifying with the victim position. They are more vulnerable, manifest chronic feelings of helplessness, and the danger is considerable that they will be exploited and victimized again. Boys identify themselves more with the aggressor position; they behave destructively as far as committing delinquent acts. In their relationship with younger children, they are aggressive and let the weaker ones suffer what they had to endure.

If psychological traumata are not integrated into a subject's life experiences, the victim remains with fixed memories to the trauma. Splitting, a major defense mechanism, allows exteriorizing the traumatic experiences from conscious awareness, repressing the memory of the event and cleaving the initial feelings of fear, helplessness, and despair. In later stress situations, children react with the emotional intensity they felt at the time of traumatization, as if the traumatic event would be

---

[11] Adults who have experienced multiple or cumulative traumata in early childhood often present not only symptoms of PTSD, but additional symptoms, including difficulties in affective and interpersonal situations and disturbances in self-regulation skills. Psychotherapeutic interventions for adults with such complex symptomatology have therefore to take into account failures of reliance in early relationships with primary care persons and the resulting developmental, emotional, and interpersonal problems.

repeated. They are not able to understand what is happening to them because the historical, biographical references remain unconscious. Even if children try to keep an emotional distance and avoid emotional situations associated with the trauma, memory traces cannot be erased. Often split-off elements of the traumatic experience emerge again, triggered by memory traces, such as nightmares, but also by spontaneous images, sometimes by sounds or even a smell.

Transition periods such as adolescence, and life events such as a first love relationship, a loss, or other stressful situations, can reactivate traumatic infantile events; this can lead to an outburst of such overwhelming feelings that a mental breakdown may follow. The consequences are: panic anxiety, escape reactions, confusion- and depersonalization- or severe depressive states with hetero- or auto-aggressive behavior.

## Risk for Psychic Traumatization

Among the multiple risk factors for psychic traumatization of children, we discuss two situations, which may represent a psychic trauma for a child: A psychic or a somatic illness of a parent and the rupture of filiation in adoption. A parent's severe mental or somatic illness is a risk factor for psychiatric disorders in children, as Rutter, an English psychiatrist, already noticed in 1966. A significant disease in a parent has an impact on the child's development and psychosocial functioning. Adoption constitutes a potential risk situation for psychic traumatization. For the child adoption represents the rupture of his relationship with biological parents and the creation of a new relationship with adoptive parents.

### Children of Mentally Ill Parents

In his long-term study of offspring of schizophrenic patients, the Swiss psychiatrist Eugen Bleuler (1857–1939) emphasized that three quarter of them remained healthy. He underlined that there is no absolute obstacle to healthy development in the offspring, despite their genetic predisposition and family burden (1972). Bleuer's study gave a decisive impulse for modern research on resilience[12] (Rutter 2012).

Bipolar disorders and schizophrenia have shared genetic risk factors (Berrettini 2000). Large studies of heritability in twins have shown that the risk is higher for schizophrenia than bipolar disorders (Kendler et al. 2006; Giusti-Rodríguez and Sullivan 2013). Major depression, often coexisting with anxiety, represents a disease which is etiologically heterogeneous with regard to genetic and environmental

---

[12] Garmezy (1974, 1985), a pioneer of resilience research, was influenced by Bleuler's study of schizophrenic mothers offspring.

factors.[13] Offspring of mothers with major depression and antisocial life history are exposed to multiple adverse experiences and have a greater risk for early onset psychopathology compared to children of mothers with depression without antisocial history (Kim-Cohen et al. 2006; Kozhimannil and Kim 2014).

When assessing risk, one has to take into account the genotype–environment interaction. Thus, heritability estimates have not a fixed value. According to Plomin (2004), identical twins are only in 45 % concordant for schizophrenia. This means that environmental determinants, including psychosocial factors play an important role in triggering clinical manifestations. Multiple studies deal with the gene–environmental interplay in the origin of psychopathology (Rutter et al. 2006a, b). The interaction of genetic and environmental influences on psychosocial disorders of adoptees revealed that genetic predispositions are above all expressed when they are activated by environmental factors. Thus, children of biological parents with proven mental illnesses such as schizophrenia are at higher risk of developing the parental mental illness when they grow up in dysfunctional adoptive families (Rutter et al. 1999). A long-term follow-up study of Finnish adoptees (Tienari et al. 2004; Wahlberg et al. 2004) confirms that genetic factors affect susceptibility to environmentally mediated risks. In adoptees at high genetic risk of schizophrenia (having a biological mother with a diagnosis of a schizophrenia spectrum disorder), but not in those at low genetic risk (having a biological mother with a non-schizophrenia spectrum psychiatric diagnosis or no psychiatric diagnosis), dysfunctional adoptive-family rearing was a significant predictor of schizophrenia spectrum disorders in adoptees at long-term follow-up. Adoptees at high genetic risk are significantly more sensitive to adverse rearing patterns than adoptees at low genetic risk. In the higher risk group, the postulated genotype seems to be "sensitive" to family environment, both to dysfunctional as well as to protective factors.

Parental and offspring factors are decisive for how the parental illness affects the parent–child relationship. The socioeconomic situation of the parents, the quality of the parental couple relationship and the social contacts with the extended family also play important roles. Offspring's preexisting physical or emotional vulnerabilities represent risk factors. In a complex interplay, these factors ultimately determine if a child develops age appropriately and whether his coping with the stressful situation may even strengthen his social ability and responsibility; or if the long-lasting stressful situation exceeds the child's coping competence and results in mental disorders.

Children and adolescents are often severely parentified, taking over adult roles and functions for parents or siblings. The long-lasting emotional distress impairs developmental processes. Precocious behavior and—at the same time—emotional dependency and immaturity are possible consequences. Children also show great adjustment efforts putting aside their own needs, problems, and fears. A child fears nothing as much as the loss of a parent, i.e., abandonment. The parent's mental illness represents a special kind of loss for the child: even if the parent is

---

[13] For a review of *The Genetics of Major Depression*, see Flint and Kendler (2014).

physically present, the father or mother remains inaccessible. The ill and with-drawn parent is not able to devote affective attention to the child that is longing for tenderness and approval.

There is ample evidence of the association between parental mental disorders and children's adjustment (Beardslee et al. 1998; Davies and Windle 1997; Olfson et al. 2003). The quality of the healthy parent's emotional availability may how-ever compensate for the ill parent's inattentiveness. In their studies of parents with mental health problems and the psychosocial impact on children, Leinonen et al. (2003) show that effects of parental mental health on child adjustment are mostly mediated through the healthy parent's quality parenting. Children of severely men-tally ill parents can cope with the stressful situation if they have the ability to develop social ties with other family members or alternative relationships outside the family. Offspring need to accept the inadequate parental relationship as an expression of the disease and not as a personal shortcoming, or as a result of malicious feelings of their parents towards them (Rutter 1987). The emotional availability of the healthy parent or an alternative significant relationship protects against negative chain reactions.

Studies observing parental interaction patterns show that in contacts with their children depressed mothers demonstrate less interest and emotional participation and have great difficulties to empathize with their children; their communications are poor; they are less responsive and behave more passively. They appear irritable, hostile, and critical (Field 1992). As a result, children have a tendency to be self-critical and have difficulties controlling their emotions. The combination of nega-tive self-image and insufficient regulation of negative feelings leads to difficulties in coping with stressful events. The erratic behavior of parents suffering from psycho-sis or addiction may be lived by the child as unpredictable and unreliable, for exam-ple, during a psychotic-, alcohol-, or drug-intoxication episode. Children then perceive the disease as something scary, which takes possession of their parent and become frightened by feelings of anxiety and loss. The attitude of the surroundings, such as rejection and social exclusion of children with mentally ill parents, influ-ence their social behavior. Their careful and cautious interaction with peers and classmates demonstrates their anxiety to be hurt or depreciated. Hiding and conceal-ment states at home as well as shame- and guilt feelings, hinder cheerful and open contact and often lead to the isolation of children with mentally ill parents. Survival guilt refers to conflicts of loyalty and guilt feelings that arise from the wish to meet their own needs, on the one hand, and the obvious need for supporting the critically ill parent on the other (Dunn 1993).

The encounter and living with a sick parent undergoing fundamental changes is frightening, e.g., psychotic parents' hallucinations and delusions or addicted par-ents' behavioral and personality changes, as well as witnessing violence in alco-holic or psychotic parents. Children no longer recognize their father or mother and are confused and uncertain as to whether the parent still recognizes them. Reality is no longer reliable and children even doubt their perception of reality and lose trust in their parents. The parent–child relationship is dominated by mutual fears and fantasies. Due to the ill parents' lack of consistency and continuity in thinking, feeling, and acting, the child perceives the father or mother as unstable, unreliable, and doubtful in their personality and identity, complicating the child's identity-development and -formation.

Another childhood event that many children of mentally ill parents have to witness is the compulsory commitment or "protective custody" of their father or mother. The forced hospitalization, sometimes in highly dramatic circumstances, may often trigger contradictory feelings in children: shock, anger (which is also directed against the healthy parent who does not prevent the hospitalization), pity, shame, and guilt, but also relief that the chaotic, stressful life from which children cannot escape, takes a more normal path. Children observe not only their sick parent's personality loss but also their loss of autonomy and authority. This painful experience often represents a traumatic experience for the child who hardly recognizes his mother or father.

## Clinical Vignette Reto and Heidy

During a 3-year period of child psychotherapeutic intervention in a family with the mother suffering from schizophrenia, the main difficulty was the ill mother's rejection of outpatient and drug treatment, leading to repeated hospitalizations because of psychotic episodes. The father established a caring relationship with his two children of 2- and 11 years old. Day care with individual psychotherapy for both children, as well as monthly family meetings were installed, yet the mother refused to take part. The father accepted psychiatric help himself, but declined placements for his children. The high degree of stress was differently expressed by the children. Reto presented psychosomatic symptoms, concentration- and school performance difficulties with a severe self-esteem- and depressive disorder. He cared solicitously for his little sister Heidy, who manifested existential fears, regressive and depressive behavior, and a developmental arrest. Reto was asked to draw a tree: the roots of his tree grow over a large stone. Reto seems to perceive and be aware of how heavy, hard, and durable his situation is, represented in his drawing by the stone, restraining and hampering his development.

Research findings in families with mentally ill parents show that infants and young children are particularly vulnerable to traumatization caused by serious parental illness. Preventive measures are therefore of great importance including joint admissions and treatment of mother–infant or parent–child in adult psychiatric or child and adolescent psychiatric clinics, as well as mother–child care in day clinics. This will help to avoid mother–child separation and maintain the bond between mother and child to promote good early mother–child relationships (Field 2010). For child and mother intrapsychic self-regulation, it is important to ease the emotional strain on the mother–child interaction. Studies show that mother and child separation prolongs the disease process, while shared care favorably influences disease course. For mentally ill mothers, early parenting represents a special time of hope, motivation to change, insight into their illness, and accepting help because mothers want to do the best for their child. "Mothers can be helped to appreciate the importance of their own—and their infant's—stability and predictability, which can be facilitated through educational, interpretive and imaging strategies." (Beebe et al. 2012: p. 403).

## Children of Somatically Ill Parents

Somatic illness in a parent is also a risk factor for psychiatric disorders in children (Rutter 1966, 1989; Romer et al. 2002). A parent's significant physical disease has an impact on children's development and psychosocial functioning (Bogosian et al. 2010). Stressful life events require coping strategies from both parents and children. Coping and long-term adjustment to a chronic illness include the effort and time needed for each individual, and the family as a group, to integrate the physical, psychological, and social consequences of the disease into the inner-psychic and interpersonal reality (Steck 2002). The task children face is to find meaning of their experience of parental illness and to integrate the experience in an adaptive way into their ongoing development. Chronic somatic disease, as for example multiple sclerosis, confronts patients, partners and their children to a wide array of challenges. In addition to physical symptoms, cognitive dysfunction, depression, or personality changes may occur. Changes in family roles, loss of work, income and social status as well as caregiver burnout are common in these families. Thus, a severe somatic illness represents a condition that has the potential to affect the partner and children in a number of ways.

How a person copes with a disease depends on intrapsychic factors such as life history, personality, critical life events, as well as on the diagnosis, course, and severity of the disease. The subjective experience of an illness differs greatly and is characterized by the importance and meaning attributed to the disease, as well as by external factors, such as partnership, family, and social support. To actively confront the disease and its consequences and appropriately adjust to it is a long and difficult process for both patients and relatives. For sick parents and their family, the unpredictability of the disease course and the uncertain future represent a great psychological burden and a continual stress, often described as a Damocles' sword situation.

Adjustment to a chronic disease is a process of remitting loss, grief, and adaptation. Both patient and partner need to mourn the losses of health, future goals, such as pursuing a professional career or to have a family with several children, of independence and self-identity. Thus, a chronic disease represents a condition that has the potential to affect the patient's children in a number of ways.

Numerous studies of somatically ill parents and their offspring have evaluated the coping process of all family members and analyzed disease variables, parental factors, and family situations, favoring or aggravating the coping process of children, resulting in serious consequences for their psychosocial development (Steck et al. 2007b). Studies on patient and family coping show the mutual influences between the parental couple as well as between the parents and their children.

*Parental Coping*: There are significant mutual interactions between the patient and his or her partner in terms of their coping and associated depression. Studies show that high perceived illness uncertainty increases depression and negatively affects coping behavior (Kroencke et al. 2001). Chwastiak et al. (2002) studied the relationship of depressive symptoms with severity, duration, and course of multiple sclerosis in over 700 patients and concluded that the severity of illness was strongly associated with depressive symptoms. O'Neill's and Morrow's (2001) literature review of 4084 patients with chronic illnesses shows that illness severity, age, and available resources such as social support are influential in coping; positive social support has a protective effect, while interpersonal conflict and dissention have a negative effect. The quality of the couple's relationship seems to be crucial in the mutual coping process of patient and partner. Psychological distress affects not only the chronically ill patient but also the caregiver and according to Pakenham (2002), the positive interpersonal relationship between patient and spouse is associated with better coping in caregiving.

*Children's Coping*: The ability of children to cope with a parent's chronic somatic disease seems to be determined by the healthy parent's coping style. Identification with the healthy parent is essential for the child's development. The healthy parent is the most important person for imitation and role modeling. Identification with the ill parent's symptoms may lead to offspring's expression of psychosomatic symptoms and hypochondrial complaints. These manifestations are often accompanied by regressive wishes, associated with difficulties in own physical and sexual development. The child's or adolescent's identification with the injured or damaged parent's physical integrity may result in the formation of an impaired body self-image.

Multiple fears of loss, death, separation, disease-transmission as well as depression, learning problems, and relationship difficulties are other frequent symptoms of children and adolescents with a parent affected by a somatic illness. Seven-year-old *LUCILE* draws her mother in a wheelchair: her body is transparent, without consistency, her father without hands (helpless), herself without feet, but with hands and a big thumb. Her comment: I have to be self-reliant.

If multiple psychosocial distress factors come together, the impact on the child's psychological development may be traumatizing. Main factors aggravating children's burden and impeding their coping process are: parental depression, single parenthood, and social isolation of the family, parental communication incapacity, and unresolved traumatic experience in the parents' own past history. The latter may be associated with the parents' feelings of being victimized and a tendency to focus their life around the disease. Such an attitude interferes with the parent's capacity to perceive and be available to the child's developmental and affective needs, leading eventually to his emotional or in rare cases physical abuse. In this context, social isolation may operate as a more or less important factor. If parents experience the illness as a traumatic event, children are then confronted with despair, hopelessness, and helplessness and a threatening, unpredictable future. Somatization and hypochondrial fears are more frequent manifestations—evolving through identification with the ill parent—in children of somatically ill parents than in children of healthy parents.

"I want to get the disease because my mother has it." The message of 9-year-old *NICOLAS*, who suffered from multiple somatic pains, shows his extreme identification with his mother's illness. His only preoccupation was how he could best help her. He dreamed almost every night that his mother was throwing away wheelchair and crutches. When asked about his own plans, he answered astonishingly: "Until now I was only thinking of my mother."

The quality of the child's relationship with compensatory caregiver(s) may be a key variable that allows the child some respite and perhaps even some escape from risk (Drotar 1994). Children who have both the ability and opportunity to develop significant relationships with alternative persons experience their parents' illness very differently than children who have exclusive, negative, and/or conflictual relationships with overburdened parents.

Against the background of the disease course, family dynamics and life phase, the coping process of each family and its individual members varies greatly. There is clearly no right or wrong way of coping; to understand the very particular meaning, each family attributes to the disease is of fundamental importance to professional helpers. The importance of the family of the ill parent, the function and competence of the parental couple, and the welfare of the children have to be analyzed most carefully before the possibility of preventive and/or therapeutic intervention can be introduced (Steck et al. 2005). Helping families to express and share their grief seems to be a way to enhance psychological development—an essential feature of comprehensive care.

## Psychotherapeutic Interventions

Often the care of ill parents and their families is difficult because families experience offers of help as interference, additional stress, or even a threat (e.g., professionals could take away their children). Most children are able to integrate parental illness experience in their development. Yet, some children develop psychopathological symptoms and need help (Steck et al. 2007a). The aim is to enable children of ill parents to develop the necessary psychosocial skills to master the stressful situation and in doing so to mature. Therefore, it is important to integrate the family—from the beginning of the parent's illness—into the care process, so that the specific risks and needs of the family, of both sick and healthy parents and especially of the children of different ages (high risk for infants and young children) can be evaluated more effectively (Pakenham and Cox 2012; Horner 2013; Dennison et al. 2013).

Age-specific and continuous information for children and young people about the disease helps them to distinguish between fantasied causes (e.g., to be responsible for the illness of a parent), and the real causes of the disease. The objective information about illness and death—by an adequate individual approach and adapted to the understanding capacity of the child—supports conscious processing and facilitates the separation between fantasy and reality. For children, it is important that their emotional and developmental needs are met, that their own interests and activities, as well as alternative meaningful relationships are respected. An open dialogue about the disease and the recognition of the social and psychological impact of the disease on their children, as well as the knowledge that their parents are supported in a social network, are decisive in contributing to the healthy development of the child. Social or psychotherapeutic support—of the ill parent, the healthy parent, or the family—may play an important role in coping with the stress for the whole family.

Relief efforts of interinstitutional and interdisciplinary collaboration should be tailored to the situation of ill parents and their children. The cooperation of all parties and involved professionals is necessary and must be supported by factual and mutual personal respect. Often, it is best that one contact person of the family coordinates the various services.

Parents and children should be informed about the available assistance and whenever possible be able to express their wishes regarding the therapeutic interventions. Professional assistance is there to help sick parents and their families make competent decisions themselves by strengthening their skills but never patronizing or incapacitating them. In addition to the therapeutic measures for the ill parent, help for the family, children's nurseries, foster or day care should be considered on an outpatient basis. Sometimes, early intervention and special schooling is necessary. With sick parents and families, it is desirable to plan the action to be taken in acute situations or in the event of a relapse. This includes any hospitalization of the ill parent, taking care of the children, the support of healthy parents, and the necessary information.

## Adopted Children

The adopted child stands out with a dual position: to be an exposed and at the same time, chosen child. This is already a theme in ancient mythologies, as the legend of Moses shows, first exposed on the Nile and then reared by the daughter of the Pharaoh. Adoption belongs—as this is the case for existential events—to the unpredictable since it is associated with many—partly unconscious—personal and familial variables. Therefore, adoption may bear fateful outcomes. While adoption is a potential risk factor for psychic traumatization, it is also a child protection measure, a successful natural intervention for helping deprived children, enhancing their psychosocial development (Stams et al. 2002; van Ijzendoorn and Juffer 2006).

*Rupture and Creation of Filiation*: Adoption constitutes a potential risk situation for psychic traumatization. For the child, adoption represents the rupture of his relationship with biological parents and the creation of a new relationship with adoptive parents. The relationship dynamics can be considered as a lifelong process for the persons involved in this triangle of birth parents, adoptive parents, and the child. In international adoptions, the child also loses his ethnic, cultural, and linguistic ties. Children experience this relationship constellation as a psychic trauma, particularly when they are not able to cope with their feelings of having been abandoned or rejected by biological parents (Brodzinsky and Schechter 1990; Steck 2007). This psychic injury affects the child's self-worth or self-esteem. Ethnological-, cultural-, and language differences are associated with feelings of being a stranger, of having been excluded, which impairs adopted children's integration into the culture of their adoptive parents.

Both the child and the adopting parents experience—in mirror fashion—an interruption of temporal continuity, lived as a breakdown. Adoption too often takes the form of repetition of this traumatic situation, the unconscious hope being to succeed in mastering this event at last and to reestablish a continuity in the self-representation, so that the experience can be remembered and become "history" (Winnicott 1974). For the child, the breakdown is the void of origin, a non-experience of its genesis, the absence of a mirror image, which includes the self. For the adopting couple, the procreative impotence prevents them from projecting themselves into the future, from inserting themselves in the biological cycle of birth–procreation–death and from making the generational leap from the role of son–daughter to that of parents.

*Consequences of Traumatic Losses*: Children try to cope with the adoption event by building an inner world of fantasies "explaining" what has happened to them. In the inner world of an adopted child, real events such as relationship rupture, obtained information, and above all own fantasies are combined to often confusing and conflictual family–romance representations, which a child may express in a variety of (preverbal) psychic or psychosomatic symptoms. In the adoption situation, not only family romance fantasies of the parents and the child are part of the interpersonal family dynamics, but also fantasies of the adoptive parents and the adopted child concerning birth- and or foster parents. The real existence of birth or foster parents seems to play an important role in the integration of family romance fantasies for adoptive parents and adopted children. The origin problem is shared by both.

Fantasy stories, also called narratives, are revised repeatedly by the child in the course of his development. Storytelling serves to attribute meaning and significance to life events that have interrupted the continuity of the child's lived experience. Adopted children's symbolic repetitive play with birth, babies, and their mothers represent often not only their own preoccupation, but also the non-accomplished grief of the adoptive parent's failure to have a biological child. In the play-scenes of lost and found babies, the child tries—through yet nonverbal narratives—to find an explanation for his loss. If he is a lost baby, then the birth- and foster mother have no responsibility and can be idealized as innocent mother figures: the child is taking responsibility for having been lost; if he is a baby stolen by adoptive parents, then they can be incriminated and the child is entitled to be angry at them. The fantasies of being stolen reestablish a self-representation of being wanted and valued.

*NOAH* came at the age of 6 years from an Indian prison to Switzerland for adoption. He accuses his adoptive parents to have stolen him. He thinks that his mother did not care for him because he was an ugly baby. Fantasies include numerous questions about guilt and responsibility for the loss of biological parents and at the same time wishes for reunification with them and for restitution, an unconscious desire to make things right again.

Eight-year-old *SARAH*, adopted, brings a sad parrot (a stuffed animal) to the first interview with the child psychiatrist. His sadness is a secret that only Sarah knows. She reveals to the psychotherapist her "big dream": "A baby bird has flown away and is lost. The father finds the baby bird and brings it back as a surprise to his mother who waits for her baby." The dream contains the phantasm of having lost her biological parents through her own fault and the wish to be reunited with them. The wish for reunion with the biological parents is often expressed in the fantasy that the parents are searching for their child, thus confirming the child's narcissistic worth.

Somatic and behavioral expressions may also result from the child's belief of being an unwanted child. Children bear fantasies of having been bad, dirty, or monstrous. "I am not desired" appears in the self-representation as being rejected. The adopted child's unconscious hope is that, for instance, his regressive or aggressive manifestations will not be disowned, but accepted by his adoptive parents. He expects that the adoptive parents recognize his past identity and help him to preserve it. Fears of death or even suicide attempts are based on fantasied wishes to reunite with the lost parent, but can also express a need for punishment. "Abandonment is murder" said an adopted adolescent girl. In identifying with the aggressor, these fantasies are acted out against the adoptive parents or significant other persons, as they cannot be directed against absent birth- or foster parents. Adopted children have a tendency to anticipate and act out potential separation situations, e.g., by running away in order to avoid painful feelings, experienced in previous separations.

Children understand the meaning of being adopted only around 10 years (Brodzinsky et al. 1986). The revelation by adoptive parents of the child's state of adoption is a continuous process over years, being inscribed in the child's developmental history. Announcement of being adopted in the period of life when the distinction between fantasy and reality is not clearly differentiated can lead to fantasies of the actuality of abandonment. Often children get preoccupied with questions and the meaning of their adoption when another child arrives for adoption. At this moment, the child "loses" the continuous tie to his adoptive mother, experiencing the integration of a new sibling as re-traumatization.

Representations of the biological parents and particularly of giving up their child become translated into aspects of self-representation. This shadow of the past leaves the child vulnerable. Heredity says Guyotat (1980) is an absolute necessity; if transmission is not possible, the necessity of inheritance is replaced by chronology. He considers the loss of the emotional bonds between mother and child as a loss of what the mother could have transmitted to her child. The traumatic moment of this situation is then incorporated and reappears at a crucial moment, for example, as re-traumatization at the arrival of a sister or brother for adoption.

*Mourning*: At first, children may integrate the adoptive family without problems, adjusting continuously to their expectations. They are apparently able to transfer their attachment from biological or foster mother or parents, to a substitute, the adoptive mother or parents, but this transfer to another person is not mourning, only adaptation. Children tend to keep secret their imaginary parent, their fantasied tie to the lost parent. Adopted children often show great and continuing difficulty to engage in a relationship and build up meaningful relatedness, due to threatening fears of separation, meaning abandonment and loss and reexperience of painful feelings associated with the traumatic events in the past.

The grieving process for the loss of biological and/or foster parents is complicated by the fact that in most cases there is uncertainty about the life and death of the biological parents and the adoptive child has no explanation for the reasons of his abandonment. Finally, there are no relatives of the biological parents to share the child's loss, to express memories associated with the lost person(s), and to participate in the child's mourning process. A child struggling to understand abandonment does not easily accept war or poverty as explanations for the adoption. Fantasies of reunion with the lost parent deprive the child of the opportunity to address the reality of the loss and its causes. The question of how long a work of mourning is necessary remains unanswered (Stroebe et al. 1993), as mourning is done in an individual way, at various times in its own rhythm and in varying degrees of completeness.

A child needs help from meaningful adults present in a continuous relationship for his grieving. If adoptive parents are burdened by their own unprocessed losses such as the loss of their reproductive capacity or the loss of a child, it is difficult for them to help their adopted child in his mourning process. Mourning is likely to occur when the child can cognitively and emotionally recognize and accept the irreversibility of the loss. The grieving process is essential, allowing the child to continue his psychosocial development, but also to prevent, that the child repeats his traumatic experiences again and again and suffers additional traumatization.

# References

Abraham N, Torok M. The shell and the kernel: renewals of psychoanalysis. Chicago: University of Chicago Press; 1994.

Aimone JB, Li Y, Lee SW, Clemenson GD, Deng W, Gage FH. Regulation and function of adult neurogenesis: from genes to cognition. Physiol Rev. 2014;94(4):991–1026.

Andero R, Ressler KJ. Fear extinction and BDNF: translating animal models of PTSD to the clinic. Genes Brain Behav. 2012;11(5):503–12. doi:10.1111/j.1601-183X.2012.00801.x.

Anzieu D. The skin ego. New Haven: Yale University Press; 1989.

Barrois C. Les névroses traumatiques. Paris: Dunod; 1988.

Beardslee WR, Versage EM, Gladstone TRG. Children of affectively ill parents: a review of the past 10 years. J Am Acad Child Adolesc Psychiatry. 1998;37:1134–41.

Beebe B, Lachmann F, Jaffe J, Markese J, Buck KA, Chen H. Maternal postpartum depressive symptoms and 4-month mother–infant interaction. Psychoanal Psychol. 2012;29(4):383–407. doi:10.1037/a0029387.

Benoit RG, Anderson MC. Opposing mechanisms support the voluntary forgetting of unwanted memories. Neuron. 2012;76(2):450–60. doi:10.1016/j.neuron.2012.07.025.

Berrettini WH. Are schizophrenic and bipolar disorders related? A review of family and molecular studies. Biol Psychiatry. 2000;48(6):531–8.

Bleuler M. Die schizophrenen Geistesstörungen im Lichte langjähriger Kranken- und Familiengeschichten. Stuttgart: Thieme; 1972.

Bogosian A, Moss-Morris R, Bishop FL, Hadwin J. Psychosocial adjustment in children and adolescents with a parent with multiple sclerosis: a systematic review. Clin Rehabil. 2010;24:789–801.

Boszormenyi-Nagy I, Framo JL. Intensive family therapy: theoretical and practical aspects. New York: Brunner/Mazel; 1985.

Bremner JD, Elzinga B, Schmahl C, Vermetten E. Structural and functional plasticity of the human brain in posttraumatic stress disorder. Prog Brain Res. 2008;167:171–86.

Brodzinsky DM, Schechter MD. The psychology of adoption. Oxford: Oxford University Press; 1990.

Brodzinsky DM, Schechter MD, Brodzinsky AB. Children's knowledge of adoption: developmental changes and implications for adjustment. In: Ashmore RD, Brodzinsky DM, editors. Thinking about the family. Views of parents and children. Hillsdale: Erlbaum; 1986. p. 205–32.

Charmandari E, Achermann JC, Carel JC, Soder O, Chrousos GP. Stress response and child health. Sci Signal. 2012;5(248):mr1. doi:10.1126/scisignal.2003595.

Charney DS, Deutch AY, Krystal JH, Southwick SM, Davis M. Psychobiologic mechanisms of posttraumatic stress disorder. Arch Gen Psychiatry. 1993;50(4):295–305. Review.

Chwastiak L, Ehde DM, Gibbons LE, Sullivan M, Bowen JD, Kraft GH. Depressive symptoms and severity of illness in multiple sclerosis: epidemiologic study of a large community sample. Am J Psychiatry. 2002;159:1862–8.

Cirulli F, Alleva E. The NGF saga: from animal models of psychosocial stress to stress-related psychopathology. Front Neuroendocrinol. 2009;30(3):379–95. doi:10.1016/j.yfrne.2009.05.002.

Cloitre M, Stolbach BC, Herman JL, van der Kolk B, Pynoos R, Wang J. Developmental approach to complex PTSD: childhood and adult cumulative trauma as predictors of symptom complexity. J Trauma Stress. 2009;22(5):399–408. doi:10.1002/jts.20444.

Cohen MR, Pickar D, Dubois M, Bunney Jr WE. Stress-induced plasma beta-endorphin immunoreactivity may predict postoperative morphine usage. Psychiatry Res. 1982;6(1):7–12.

Coplan JD, Fathy HM, Jackowski AP, Tang CY, Perera TD, Mathew SJ, et al. Early life stress and macaque amygdala hypertrophy: preliminary evidence for a role for the serotonin transporter gene. Front Behav Neurosci. 2014;8:342. doi:10.3389/fnbeh.2014.00342.

Courtin J, Chaudun F, Rozeske RR, Karalis N, Gonzalez-Campo C, Wurtz H, et al. Prefrontal parvalbumin interneurons shape neuronal activity to drive fear expression. Nature. 2014;505(7481):92–6. doi:10.1038/nature12755.

D'Andrea W, Ford J, Stolbach B, Spinazzola J, van der Kolk BA. Understanding interpersonal trauma in children: why we need a developmentally appropriate trauma diagnosis. Am J Orthopsychiatry. 2012;82(2):187–200. doi:10.1111/j.1939-0025.2012.01154.x.

Davies PT, Windle M. Gender-specific pathways between maternal depressive symptoms, family discord, and adolescent adjustment. Dev Psychol. 1997;33:657–68.

de Kloet ER, Joëls M, Holsboer F. Stress and the brain: from adaptation to disease. Nat Rev Neurosci. 2005;6(6):463–75.

de Quervain DJ, Kolassa IT, Ackermann S, Aerni A, Boesiger P, Demougin P, et al. PKCα is genetically linked to memory capacity in healthy subjects and to risk for posttraumatic stress disorder in genocide survivors. Proc Natl Acad Sci U S A. 2012;109(22):8746–51. doi:10.1073/pnas.1200857109.

Dennison L, Moss-Morris R, Yardleya L, Kirbya S, Chalderc T. An interview study. Change and processes of change within interventions to promote adjustment to multiple sclerosis: learning from patient experiences. Psychol Health. 2013;28(9):973–92.

Do-Monte FH, Quiñones-Laracuente K, Quirk GJ. A temporal shift in the circuits mediating retrieval of fear memory. Nature. 2015. doi:10.1038/nature14030.

Donovan DM, McIntyre D. Healing the hurt child: a developmental-contextual approach. New York: Norton; 1990.

Drotar D. Impact of parental health problems on children: concepts, methods, and unanswered questions. J Pediatr Psychol. 1994;19:525–36.

Dunn B. Growing up with a psychotic mother. A retrospective study. Am J Orthopsychiatry. 1993;63/2:177–89.

Ferenczi S. The confusion of tongues between adults and children. Int J Psychoanal. 1949;30:225–30.

Field T. Infants of depressed mothers. Dev Psychopathol. 1992;4:49–66.

Field T. Postpartum depression effects on early interactions, parenting, and safety practices: a review. Infant Behav Dev. 2010;33(1):1–6. doi:10.1016/j.infbeh.2009.10.005.

Finkelhor D, Ormrod RK, Turner HA. Lifetime assessment of poly-victimization in a national sample of children and youth. Child Abuse Negl. 2009;33(7):403–11. doi:10.1016/j.chiabu.2008.09.012.

Fischer G, Riedesser P. Lehrbuch der Psychotraumatologie. München Basel: E. Reinhardt Verlag; 1999.

Flint J, Kendler KS. The genetics of major depression. Neuron. 2014;81(3):484–503. doi:10.1016/j.neuron.2014.01.027.

Franklin TB, Russig H, Weiss IC, Gräff J, Linder N, Michalon A, et al. Epigenetic transmission of the impact of early stress across generations. Biol Psychiatry. 2010;68(5):408–15. doi:10.1016/j.biopsych.2010.05.036.

Freud S. Studies on hysteria, Standard edition, vol. II. London: Hogarth Press; 1895.

Freud S. Psychoanalysis and the war neurosis, Standard edition, vol. XVII. London: Hogarth Press; 1919.

Freud S. Analysis terminable and interminable. Int J Psychoanal. 1937;18:373–405.

Freud S. Moses and monotheism. An outline of psycho-analysis and other works, Standard edition, vol. XXIII. London: Hogarth Press; 1937–1939.

Freud S. New introductory lectures on psycho-analysis and other works., Standard edition, vol. XXII. London: Hogarth Press; 1932–1936.

Gabel HW, Greenberg ME. Genetics. The maturing brain methylome. Science. 2013;341(6146):626–7. doi:10.1126/science.1242671.

Garmezy N. The study of competence in children at risk for severe psychopathology. In: Anthony EJ, Koupernik C, editors. The child in his family: children at psychiatric risk, vol. 3. New York: Wiley; 1974. p. 77–97.

Garmezy N. Stress-resistant children: the search for protective factors. In: Davids A, editor. Recent research in developmental psychopathology. Elmsford: Pergamon Press; 1985. p. 213–33.

Giusti-Rodríguez P, Sullivan PF. The genomics of schizophrenia: update and implications. J Clin Invest. 2013;123(11):4557–63. doi:10.1172/JCI66031.

Glover H. Emotional numbing: a possible endorphin-mediated phenomenon associated with post-traumatic stress disorders and other allied psychopathologic states. J Trauma Stress. 1992;5(4):643–75. doi:10.1002/jts.2490050413.

Goleman D. The New York Times. A Key to Post-Traumatic Stress Lies In Brain Chemistry, Scientists Find, 1990.

Gray JD, Milner TA, McEwen BS. Dynamic plasticity: the role of glucocorticoids, brain-derived neurotrophic factor and other trophic factors. Neuroscience. 2013;239:214–27. doi:10.1016/j.neuroscience.2012.08.034.

Green AH. Self-destructive behaviour in battered children. Am J Psychiatry. 1978;135(5):579–82.

Green AH. Dimension of psychological trauma in abused children. J Am Acad Child Psychiat. 1983;22:231–37.

Green AH. Child maltreatment and its victims. A comparison of physical and sexual abuse. Psychiatr Clin North Am. 1988;11(4):591–610.

Guyotat J. Mort, naissance et filiation: études de psychopathologie sur le lien de filiation. Paris: Masson; 1980.

Heinrichs M, Baumgartner T, Kirschbaum C, Ehlert U. Social support and oxytocin interact to suppress cortisol and subjective responses to psychosocial stress. Biol Psychiatry. 2003;54(12):1389–98.

Horner RM. Interventions for children coping with parental multiple sclerosis: a systematic review. J Am Assoc Nurse Pract. 2013;25:309–13.

Hostetler CM, Ryabinin AE. The CRF system and social behavior: a review. Front Neurosci. 2013;7:92. doi:10.3389/fnins.2013.00092.

Insel TR. Next-generation treatments for mental disorders. Sci Transl Med. 2012;4(155ps19):155. doi:10.1126/scitranslmed.3004873.

Janet P. L'automatisme psychologique: essay de la psychologie expérimentale sur les formes inférieures de l'activité humaine. Paris: Félix Alcan; 1889.

Jones E, Vermaas RH, McCartney H, Beech C, Palmer I, Hyams K, et al. Flashbacks and post-traumatic stress disorder: the genesis of a 20th-century diagnosis. Br J Psychiatry. 2003;182: 158–63.

Kendler KS, Gatz M, Gardner CO, Pedersen NL. A Swedish national twin study of lifetime major depression. Am J Psychiatry. 2006;163(1):109–14.

Khan M. The privacy of the self. London: Hogarth; 1974.

Kim-Cohen J, Caspi A, Rutter M, Tomás MP, Moffitt TE. The caregiving environments provided to children by depressed mothers with or without an antisocial history. Am J Psychiatry. 2006;163(6):1009–18. PMID: 16741201.

Kirk GS, Raven JE, Schofield M. Die vorsokratischen Philosophen. Einführung, Texte und Kommentare. Stuttgart: J.B. Metzler; 1994.

Kossowsky J, Monique PHD, Pfaltz C, Schneider S, Taeymans J, Locher C, Gaab J. The separation anxiety hypothesis of panic disorder revisited: a meta-analysis. Am J Psychiatry. 2012; AiA:1–14.

Kozhimannil KB, Kim H. Maternal mental illness. Science. 2014;345(6198):755. doi:10.1126/science.1259614.

Kroencke DG, Denney DR, Lynch SG. Depression during exacerbations in multiple sclerosis: the importance of uncertainty. Mult Scler. 2001;7:237–42.

Landolt MA, Schnyder U, Maier T, Schoenbucher V, Mohler-Kuo M. Trauma exposure and post-traumatic stress disorder in adolescents: a national survey in Switzerland. J Trauma Stress. 2013;26:209–16.

Laplanche J, Pontalis JB. The language of psychoanalysis. New York: Norton; 1973.

LeDoux J. The emotional brain. New York: Simon & Schuster; 1996.

LeDoux JE. Emotion circuits in the brain. Annu Rev Neurosci. 2000;23:155–84.

Leinonen JA, Solantaus TS, Punamaki RL. Parental mental health and children's adjustment: the quality of marital interaction and parenting as mediating factors. J Child Psychol Psychiatry. 2003;44:227–41.

Mayberg HS, Lozano AM, Voon V, McNeely HE, Seminowicz D, Hamani C, et al. Deep brain stimulation for treatment-resistant depression. Neuron. 2005;45(5):651–60.

McEwen BS. Protective and damaging effects of stress mediators. N Engl J Med. 1998;338(3):171–9. Review.

McEwen BS. Brain on stress: how the social environment gets under the skin. Proc Natl Acad Sci U S A. 2012;109 Suppl 2:17180–5. doi:10.1073/pnas.1121254109.

McEwen BS. Neuroscience. Hormones and the social brain. Science. 2013;339(6117):279–80. doi:10.1126/science.1233713.

Mehta MA, Golembo NI, Nosarti C, Colvert E, Mota A, Williams SC, et al. Amygdala, hippocampal and corpus callosum size following severe early institutional deprivation: the English and Romanian Adoptees study pilot. J Child Psychol Psychiatry. 2009;50(8):943–51. doi:10.1111/j.1469-7610.2009.02084.x.

Minuchin S, Fishman HC. Family therapy techniques. Cambridge: Harvard University Press; 2004.

Nathan T. Trauma et mémoire. In: Métamorphoses de l'identité. Nouv Rev Ethnopsychiatrie; 1986;7–18.

Nemeroff CB, Binder E. The preeminent role of childhood abuse and neglect in vulnerability to major psychiatric disorders: toward elucidating the underlying neurobiological mechanisms. J Am Acad Child Adolesc Psychiatry. 2014;53(4):395–7. doi:10.1016/j.jaac.2014.02.004.

Niwa M, Jaaro-Peled H, Tankou S, Seshadri S, Hikida T, Matsumoto Y, et al. Adolescent stress-induced epigenetic control of dopaminergic neurons via glucocorticoids. Science. 2013;339(6117):335–9. doi:10.1126/science.1226931.

O'Neill ES, Morrow LL. The symptom experience of women with chronic illness. J Adv Nurs. 2001;33:257–68.

Olfson M, Marcus SC, Druss B, Pincus HA, Weissmann MM. Parental depression, child mental health problems, and health care utilization. Med Care. 2003;41:716–21.

Pakenham KI. Development of a measure of coping with multiple sclerosis caregiving. Psychol Health. 2002;17:97–118.

Pakenham KI, Cox S. The nature of caregiving in children of a parent with multiple sclerosis from multiple sources and the associations between caregiving activities and youth adjustment over-time. Psychol Health. 2012;27(3):324–46.

Parsons R, Ressler KJ. Implications of memory modulation for post-traumatic stress and fear disorders. Nat Neurosci. 2013;16(2):146–53. doi:10.1038/nn.3296.

Plomin R. Genetics and developmental psychology. Merrill-Palmer Q. 2004;50(3):341–52.

Redondo RL, Kim J, Arons AL, Ramirez S, Liu X, Tonegawa S. Bidirectional switch of the valence associated with a hippocampal contextual memory engram. Nature. 2014;513(7518):426–30. doi:10.1038/nature13725.

Romer G, Barkmann C, Schulte-Markwort M, Thomalla G, Riedesser P. Children of somatically ill parents: a methodologic review. Clin Child Psychol Psychiatry. 2002;7:17–38.

Rutter M. Children of sick parents. An environmental and psychiatric study. London: Oxford University Press; 1966.

Rutter M. Psychosocial resilience and protective mechanism. Am J Orthopsychiatry. 1987;57(3): 316–31.

Rutter M. Pathways from childhood to adult life. J Child Psychol Psychiatry. 1989;30:23–51.

Rutter M. Resilience as a dynamic concept. Dev Psychopathol. 2012;24(2):335–44. doi:10.1017/S0954579412000028.

Rutter M, Silberg J, O'Connor TG, Simonoff E. Genetics and child psychiatry: advances in quantitative and molecular genetics. J Child Psychol Psychiat. 1999;40(1):3–18.

Rutter M, Kim-Cohen J, Maughan B. Continuities and discontinuities in psychopathology between childhood and adult life. J Child Psychol Psychiatry. 2006a;47(3-4):276–95.

Rutter M, Moffitt TE, Caspi A. Gene-environment interplay and psychopathology: multiple varieties but real effects. J Child Psychol Psychiatry. 2006b;47(3-4):226–61.

Sapolsky RM. The influence of social hierarchy on primate health. Science. 2005;308(5722): 648–52.

Shengold L. Soul murder. The effects of childhood abuse and deprivation. New Haven: Yale University Press; 1989.

Solms M. Freud returns. Sci Am. 2004;290(5):82–8.

Stams G, Juffer F, Rispens J, Hoksbergen R. The development and adjustment of 7-year-old children adopted in infancy. J Child Psychol Psychiat. 2002;41(8):1025–38.

Steck B. Multiple Sklerose und Familie—Psychosoziale Situation und Krankheitsverarbeitung. S. Karger: Basel; 2002.

Steck B. Adoption—ein lebenslanger Prozess. Freiburg Basel: S. Karger; 2007. ISBN 978-3-8055-8285-8.

Steck B, Amsler F, Dillier AS, Grether A, Kappos L, Bürgin D. Indication for psychotherapy in offspring of a parent affected by a chronic somatic disease (e.g. multiple sclerosis). Psychopathology. 2005;38:38–48.

Steck B, et al. Mental health problems in children of somatically ill parents, e.g. multiple sclerosis. Eur Child Adolesc Psychiatry. 2007a;16(3):199–207.

Steck B, et al. Disease variables and depression affecting the process of coping in families with a somatically ill parent. Psychopathology. 2007b;40:394–404.

Stierlin H, Rucker-Embden I, Wetzel N, Wirshching M. The first interview with the family. New York: Brunner/Mazel; 1980.

Stroebe MS, Stroebe W, Hanson R, editors. Handbook of bereavement: theory, research, and intervention. New York: Cambridge University Press; 1993.

Sullivan PF, Daly MJ, O'Donovan M. Genetic architectures of psychiatric disorders: the emerging picture and its implications. Nat Rev Genet. 2012;13(8):537–51. doi:10.1038/nrg3240.

Terr LC. Childhood traumas: an outline and overview. Am J Psychiatry. 1991;148(1):10–20.

Tienari P, Wynne LC, Sorri A, Lahti I, Läksy K, Moring J. Genotype-environment interaction in schizophrenia-spectrum disorder. Long-term follow-up study of Finnish adoptees. Br J Psychiatry. 2004;184:216–22.

Turner HA, Finkelhor D, Ormrod R, Sewanee SH, Leeb RT, Mercy JA. Family context, victimization, and child trauma symptoms: variations in safe, stable, and nurturing relationships during early and middle childhood. Am J Orthopsychiatry. 2012;82(2):209–19. doi:10.1111/j.1939-0025.2012.01147.x.

Udwin O. Annotation: children's reactions to traumatic events. J Child Psychol Psychiatry. 1993;34/2:115–27.

Van der Kolk BA. The compulsion to repeat the trauma: re-enactment, revictimization, and masochism. Psychiatr Clin North Am. 1989;12(2):389–411. Review.

Van der Kolk BA. Traumatic stress. London: Guilford Pres; 1996.

van der Kolk BA. Clinical implications of neuroscience research in PTSD. Ann N Y Acad Sci. 2006;1071:277–93.

Van der Kolk BA, Roth S, Pelcovitz D, Sunday S, Spinazzola J. Disorders of extreme stress: the empirical foundation of a complex adaptation to trauma. J Trauma Stress. 2005;18(5):389–99.

Van der Kolk BA, Alexander C, McFarlane AC, Weisaeth L. Traumatic stress: the effects of overwhelming experience on mind, body, and society. New York: Guilford Press; 2007.

van Ijzendoorn MH, Juffer F. The Emanuel Miller memorial lecture 2006: adoption as intervention. Meta-analytic evidence for massive catch-up and plasticity in physical, socio-emotional, and cognitive development. J Child Psychol Psychiatry. 2006;47(12):1228–45. doi:10.1111/j.1469-7610.2006.01675.x.

Wahlberg KE, Wynne LC, Hakko H, Läksy K, Moring J, Miettunen J, Tienari P. Interaction of genetic risk and adoptive parent communication deviance: longitudinal prediction of adoptee psychiatric disorders. Psychol Med. 2004;34(8):1531–41.

Wang XD, Su YA, Wagner KV, Avrabos C, Scharf SH, Hartmann J, et al. Nectin-3 links CRHR1 signaling to stress-induced memory deficits and spine loss. Nat Neurosci. 2013;16(6):706–13. doi:10.1038/nn.3395.

Weder N, Kaufman J. Critical periods revisited: implications for intervention with traumatized children. J Am Acad Child Adolesc Psychiatry. 2011;50(11):1087–9. doi:10.1016/j.jaac.2011.07.021.

Weder N, Zhang H, Jensen K, Yang BZ, Simen A, Jackowski A, et al. Child abuse, depression, and methylation in genes involved with stress, neural plasticity, and brain circuitry. J Am Acad Child Adolesc Psychiatry. 2014;53(4):417–24.e5. doi:10.1016/j.jaac.2013.12.025. Epub 2014 Jan 27.

Winnicott DW. Collected papers: through paediatrics to psycho-analysis. 1st ed. London: Tavistock; 1958.

Winnicott DW. The child, the family and the outside world. Harmondsworth: Penguin; 1964.

Winnicott DW. The family and individual development. London: Tavistock; 1965a.

Winnicott DW. The maturational processes and the facilitating environment. London: Hogarth Press; 1965b.

Winnicott DW. Fear of breakdown. Int Rev Psychoanal. 1974;1:1–2.

Young A. Our traumatic neurosis and its brain. Sci Context. 2001;14(4):661–83.

# Part VI

# Chapter 11
# Pain and Mind-Body

## Introduction

While modern neuroscience teaches us a lot about the biological mechanisms of pain, a comprehensive account of the multidimensional experience of pain is only emerging. To describe pain, we need to cover a wide spectrum of phenomena that range from the very basic experience of feeling pain, when a person, for example, burns himself, to feeling pain when we are grieving. The neurobiological machinery of the nociceptive aspect of pain is very accurately described at both molecular and physiological levels: the activation of pain receptors in the skin leads to the transmission of impulses through afferent pain fibers mapping to the sensory cortex. Physical pain from noxious stimuli, such as sensing something too hot or too cold, can be understood in a rather well-defined and limited framework. An all-inclusive conception of how these physical events are translated into the feeling of pain is not yet within reach: this quest directly points to the fundaments of the mind-body relationship.

There is no question that pain is inherently subjective, though medicine is attempting to objectively measure pain with clinical scales, while neuroscience is trying to visualize it by brain imaging techniques. Pain in neurological affections like trigeminal neuralgia can be understood in a physiological and biological framework; pain in conversion disorders seems to translate psychic conflicts into physical bodily symptoms. In this situation, physical pain functions as an indicator of complex dysfunctional mental mechanisms.

Pain itself cannot qualify as an emotion, but the expression of pain can. This was well described by Darwin (1872) in his book *The Expression of Emotions in Man and Animals*. Darwin showed that there is a continuity of pain expression across species and that pain is readable in the human physiognomy. With this analogy, Darwin demonstrated the evolutionary origin of pain expression. In this context, pain has a clear adaptive function. Facial expression and vocalization of pain are behaviors that express solicitation of help, and as such pain expression will promote prosocial behavior.

© Springer International Publishing Switzerland 2016
A. Steck, B. Steck, *Brain and Mind*, DOI 10.1007/978-3-319-21287-6_11

The emotional affective aspects of pain we experience in the context of loss of a loved one, a pain that may stay for long periods of time as part of a grieving process, will by its complex nature mobilize very large neuronal networks and thus profoundly affect our mind. Comprehending these complex interactions requires an understanding of the neural correlates of emotional states.

## Pain Mechanisms and Functions

In life we encounter a large variety of pain types that have different causes (Woolf 2010) (Table 11.1). Nociceptive pain that arises after an acute trauma is also the pain we feel when we touch something too cold or too hot. Nociceptive pain is part of the physiological early warning system essential to detect and minimize injuries to our body. It has a clear protective function. Sensory systems are designed so that a specific form of physical energy is detected by the sensors or sensory receptors in our body and converted into an electrochemical form in a process called transduction. Strong stimuli such as heat or cold activate these nociceptors.

Painful sensations such as a toothache or sore throat are variants of nociceptive pain, called inflammatory pain. This type of pain is triggered by activation of the immune system. It also has a warning function, despite inflammatory pain being part of an adaptive process of healing and repair. Clinically, nociceptive pain needs to be reduced so that suffering is alleviated while the adaptive character of inflammatory pain should be preserved. On the other hand, in patients with chronic inflammation from an autoimmune disease such as rheumatoid arthritis, pain results from a dysfunctional immune system and causal treatment is aimed at restoring normal immune function. In addition a variety of disease states affect the somatosensory system causing neuropathic pain. This pathological pain reflects different disorders such as back pain with nerve compression and neuropathies.

In all living creatures, pain's function is to protect the body from damage and wounds and ultimately serves to extend life. Evidence for genetic control of pain has been derived from familial studies with mutations in the voltage-gated sodium channel expressed in dorsal root ganglia and their axons. Gain of function mutations have been found to cause painful disorders (Faber et al. 2012), while loss of function mutations are associated with an insensitivity to pain (Cox et al. 2006). A case of insensitivity to pain was reported in a family in which the index patient was a young street performer that stabbed knives into his arms and walked on burning coals without feeling discomfort. In this patient, the loss of function mutation of the sodium channel prevented the pain fibers from being activated (Cox et al. 2006).

The protective role of pain perception is illustrated in the study of individuals with neuropathies where nociceptive perception is diminished. The affected persons often develop severe skin lesions or suffer from skeletal injuries because they do not exhibit pain avoiding behavior. Patients with diabetic neuropathy, for example, loose protective sensations and often develop skin lesions, which can lead to ulcers.

**Table 11.1** Classification of somatic pain states

| |
|---|
| Nociceptive pain: pain arising as a response to potentially body damaging stimuli |
| Inflammatory pain: pain triggered by the immune system |
| Neuropathic pain: pain caused by damage to the nervous system or by its abnormal functioning |

## The Affective Pain System

Pain contains both sensory and affective dimensions. Pain translates a multidimensional experience, including nociceptive components, as well as emotional and affective aspects. The central pathways of pain include multiple medullary and midbrain structures. This is part of the early pain response that does not necessarily involve cognition. However, the long-term and affect-related aspects of pain engage prefrontal cortical areas such as the anterior cingulate gyrus. Extensive neuroimaging studies have revealed a network of brain structures that process pain-related information (Fig. 11.1. Tracey and Mantyh 2007). This pain-processing network includes the thalamic nuclei, which have a key role in gating and processing sensory information, the somatosensory cortex, the insular cortex, and the anterior cingulate cortex. Both the insula and the anterior cingulate cortexes are important for the affective and behavioral aspects of pain (Price 2000). Prefrontal cortical areas as well as subcortical areas such as the amygdala contribute to the conscious awareness and cognitive evaluation of pain (Neugebauer et al. 2009). The amygdala is a key element in the affective component of pain and together with the prefrontal cortex forms part of the multimodal areas in the pain-processing network. Through its connection with the reward-aversion system, the amygdala plays an important role in modulating pain. This is further exemplified by the link to the periacqueductal central gray (PAG) area of the brain stem, which is known as the main endogenous opioid or endorphin-producing system of the brain. This is an essential network modulating pain by its analgesic properties. The PAG system received lay interest as the biological explanation for "the runners high," the brief and mild sense of well-being after high-intensity jogging. This mood change is due to the release of endorphins by the PAG (Boecker et al. 2008).

Sensing pain does not only mean having a nociceptive experience such as a burn, but we also feel pain when family members or friends are ill or die. One of the most interesting findings is the realization that the pain we experience when we are separated from a loved person or excluded by family or friends engages the same neural mechanisms as those when we feel physical pain. In other words, the affective and the sensory components of pain are closely related. Eisenberger et al. (2003) convincingly showed that psychological pain in humans, especially when grieving, activates the same neuronal pathways as those involved in physical pain, such as the anterior cingulate gyrus, the dorsomedial thalamus, and the PAG (Fig. 11.2, Panksepp 2003). The same neurochemicals that regulate physical pain also control

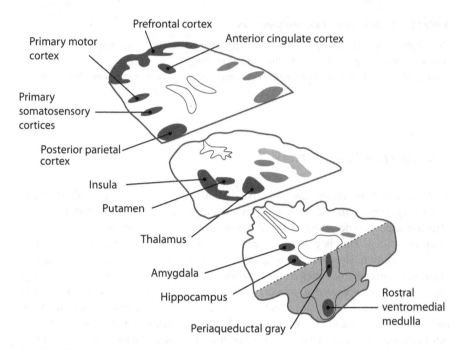

**Fig. 11.1** The pain matrix. A large distributed brain network is activated during a painful experience and is referred to as the pain matrix. This pain matrix is composed of sensory discriminatory components (laterally) and affective cognitive components (medially) (Adapted from Tracey and Mantyh 2007)

the feelings of pain in separation situations. Extensive studies in animal research demonstrated that opiates as well as endorphins but also oxytocin and prolactin are powerful regulators of separation anxiety (Panksepp 2003).

For Panksepp and Eisenberger, there are definite similarities between physical and emotional pain, explaining why it "hurts" when a person mourns a loved one.[1] Psychic pain is caused by a real or imagined loss of a loved person. Pain is caused by the fact that the significant person is indeed irreversibly lost, but the deprived subject nevertheless holds on to the loved one (Pontalis 1977).

The cingulate gyrus, in particular it's anterior part, is activated when we experience feelings such as sadness (Damasio et al. 2000). The fact that exactly the same region is activated in separation distress helps us understand why it provokes such negative feelings. On the other hand, social bonding is associated with a feeling of happiness, and in this case, the posterior part of the cingulate gyrus is activated.

---

[1] "When I lost my daughter 12 years ago in a horrendous traffic accident, among her papers I found a poem that is now carved on her tombstone. The last stanza is particularly pertinent to the question of whether love can reduce the emotional pain of loss" (Panksepp 2003, ref. 21). "When your days are full of pain, And you don't know what to do, Recall these words I tell you now—I will always care for you."

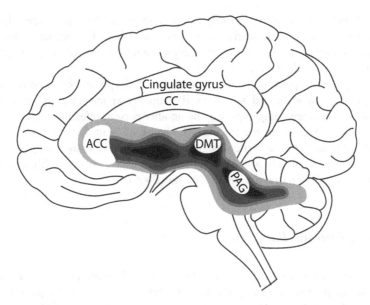

**Fig. 11.2** In subjects experiencing sadness, it is the anterior cingulate cortex (ACC) that is most responsive, but other areas that are also activated include the dorsomedial thalamus (DMT) and the periaqueductal central gray area (PAG) of the brain stem. Corpus callosum (CC) (Adapted from Panksepp 2003)

Could the fact that these core emotional experiences activate brain regions that are side by side explain why changes in mood between happiness and sadness occur so easily?[2] We have many similar examples, in particular in the brainstem, an area of the brain tightly packed with nuclei and circuits involved in different and sometimes opposing functions, where closely situated switches regulate the sleep and wake cycle or the fight and flight reaction. A minimal variation in the area where stimuli are directed can trigger opposite behavioral or affective states (Coenen et al. 2012). These closely localized opposing brain functions take on particular importance when exploring targets for deep brain stimulation to treat neurological or psychiatric disorders; exact knowledge of the detailed anatomy of these circuits is a perquisite in order to avoid stimulating the wrong area.

Recent developments shed a new perspective on the nature of human attachment bonds, including infant separation distress, as depending on the engagement of "nociceptive" mechanisms. With increasing "encephalization" of the pain system, neuronal mechanisms evolved to allow transition from pain being a purely physical phenomenon to the experience of psychic pain. In this respect, the pain system with its entire complex sensory and affective components becomes an important self-regulatory network controlling visceral and somatic functions. Tucker et al. (2005) proposed that attachment and empathic concern are directly derived from this self-

---

[2] Joyful and sorrowful; thoughtful; longing and anxious; in constant anguish; sky-high rejoicing despairing to death; happy alone is the soul that loves (Goethe 1898).

regulatory network, controlling bodily integrity, in which the pain system plays an important role. This is particularly true when one considers the fact that in humans, empathy for another's pain activates the very same region involved in physical pain experience (Bernhardt and Singer 2012).

The empathy for pain is a social emotion that is deeply rooted in all mammals and of course most developed in humans. By empathy we mean the ability to recognize emotions that are being expressed by another person, referring to the capacity to understand what others are feeling. The study of brain networks involved in empathy is bound to give us better insight into social behaviors like compassion and concern for others and will also shed light on other aspects of social life and social perception including moral reasoning (Neiman 2009).

## *Notes on Chronic Pain*

That pain is not just a pure nociceptive phenomenon is especially true for chronic pain. Chronic pain is a major health problem and one of the most frequent reasons to seek medical help. Acute pain can be considered as "hard wired," since—upon injury—pain is felt specifically at the lesion site. While some cases of chronic pain can be traced to a specific injury, other conditions have no obvious cause. Chronic low back pain, for example, can persist long after the initial nerve root compression by a herniated disk is healed and is not easily explained by a hard-wired model. Chronic pain results from changes occurring in the peripheral nerves, which become sensitized, and also from rearrangements taking place in the central nervous system. The importance of these rearrangements is best exemplified by the phenomenon of phantom limb pain.

Modern studies of phantom limb pain, considered for a long time as a curiosity, help us understand the intrinsic brain mechanisms of chronic pain. The American neurologist Weir Mitchell (1829–1914) introduced the term phantom limb in the nineteenth century (Mitchell 1871). He showed that the sensation of a phantom limb occurred in subjects who had undergone amputation of an extremity. This sensation suggests that the memory of the lost limb persists and is thus responsible for the illusion of a phantom limb. Patients frequently complain that the phantom limb is painful. We now know that after limb amputation, there is a striking and massive functional reorganization of the cortex, in particular the sensorimotor maps (Hamzei et al. 2001). This reorganization is the result of the well-known phenomenon of plasticity that allows marked changes in brain structure. As a consequence, there is a perceptual remapping of cortical representation with resulting distortion of body maps, giving rise to all kinds of illusions such as the feeling that the stump is moving. These plastic changes occur at multiple levels of the nervous system in the periphery, the spinal cord, and the central nervous system (Flor 2012). On a functional level, there is alteration of transduction molecules, especially voltage-sensitive ion channels, thus leading to painful sensations.

Instead of just feeling numbness, patients with phantom limb pain often suffer from excruciating sensations that usually do not obey somatotopic borders of the lost limb. Researchers have therefore put forward the concept that the emergence of phantom limb pain is the result of reshaping of the neurological pain pathways, such as cortical remapping, as well as changes in the dorsal horn of the spinal cord. These plastic changes depend on a multitude of factors both predetermined and acquired. The brain has been said to actively "carve" the properties of pain as it evolves from an acute to a chronic condition (Farmer et al. 2012).

The dynamic changes involved in chronic pain occur at the molecular, synaptic, cellular, and network levels (Kuner 2010). These mechanisms include classical pre- and postsynaptic potentiation, expansion of receptive fields, and structural changes such as increase in size of dendrites and even of receptive neuronal fields. Taken together the changes related to chronic pain imply learning and memory processes and are accompanied by changes in body perception.

There is good evidence that the plastic changes occurring in the nervous system of chronic pain patients are to a great extent determined by learning processes. Both implicit and explicit memory processes are involved, implicit learning processes being of particular importance. As a result, we observe that patients with chronic pain often develop avoidance activities that are associated with painful memories. Furthermore, just thinking about a given movement may trigger the pain memory and induce self-restraint.

Besides the fact that patients with chronic pain avoid certain pain-related activities, many suffer from symptoms that profoundly affect their quality of life, such as chronic fatigue, lack of motivation, and depression. Recent data show that in this context, maladaptive modifications take place in neural circuits involved in the regulation of reward and motivation. In particular, animal experiments demonstrate that chronic pain affects reward-seeking behavior (Schwartz et al. 2014). Specifically it was shown that chronic pain results in depression of the activity of the nucleus accumbens, the key dopaminergic node projecting to the prefrontal cortex. In humans, fMRI studies demonstrate connectivity changes between the nucleus accumbens and the cortex in chronic pain patients (Baliki et al. 2012). How chronic pain affects reward-seeking behavior is a subject of considerable interest if we want to better understand the relationship between pain, mood, and behavior.

# References

Baliki MN, Petre B, Torbey S, Herrmann KM, Huang L, Schnitzer TJ et al (2012) Corticostriatal functional connectivity predicts transition to chronic back pain. Nat Neurosci 15(8):1117–9. doi:10.1038/nn.3153

Bernhardt BC, Singer T (2012) The neural basis of empathy. Annu Rev Neurosci 35:1–23. doi:10.1146/annurev-neuro-062111-150536, Review

Boecker H, Sprenger T, Spilker ME, Henriksen G, Koppenhoefer M, Wagner KJ (2008) The runner's high: opioidergic mechanisms in the human brain. Cereb Cortex 18(11):2523–31. doi:10.1093/cercor/bhn013

Coenen VA, Panksepp J, Hurwitz TA, Urbach H, Mädler B (2012) Human medial forebrain bundle
    (MFB) and anterior thalamic radiation (ATR): imaging of two major subcortical pathways and
    the dynamic balance of opposite affects in understanding depression. J Neuropsychiatry Clin
    Neurosci 24(2):223–36. doi:10.1176/appi.neuropsych.11080180
Cox JJ, Reimann F, Nicholas AK, Thornton G, Roberts E, Springell K et al (2006) An SCN9A
    channelopathy causes congenital inability to experience pain. Nature 444(7121):894–8
Damasio AR, Grabowski TJ, Bechara A, Damasio H, Ponto LL, Parvizi J et al (2000) Subcortical
    and cortical brain activity during the feeling of self-generated emotions. Nat Neurosci
    3(10):1049–56
Darwin CR. The expression of the emotions in man and animals, 1st edn. London: John Murray;
    1872
Eisenberger NI, Lieberman MD, Williams KD (2003) Does rejection hurt? An FMRI study of
    social exclusion. Science 302(5643):290–2
Faber CG, Lauria G, Merkies IS, Cheng X, Han C, Ahn HS et al (2012) Gain-of-function Nav1.8
    mutations in painful neuropathy. Proc Natl Acad Sci U S A 109(47):19444–9. doi:10.1073/
    pnas.1216080109
Farmer MA, Baliki MN, Apkarian AV (2012) A dynamic network perspective of chronic pain.
    Neurosci Lett 520(2):197–203. doi:10.1016/j.neulet.2012.05.001
Flor H (2012) New developments in the understanding and management of persistent pain. Curr
    Opin Psychiatry 25(2):109–13. doi:10.1097/YCO.0b013e3283503510
Goethe JW (1898) 1749–1832 from Egmont. Act III, Clärchen's song
Hamzei F, Liepert J, Dettmers C, Adler T, Kiebel S, Rijntjes M et al (2001) Structural and func-
    tional cortical abnormalities after upper limb amputation during childhood. Neuroreport
    12(5):957–62
Kuner R (2010) Central mechanisms of pathological pain. Nat Med 16(11):1258–66. doi:10.1038/
    nm.2231
Mitchell SW (1871) Phantom limbs. Lippincott's Magazine Popular Literature and Science
    8:563–9
Neiman S (2009) Moral clarity: a guide for grown-up idealists. Random House, New York
Neugebauer V, Galhardo V, Maione S, Mackey SC (2009) Forebrain pain mechanisms. Brain Res
    Rev 60(1):226–42. doi:10.1016/j.brainresrev.2008.12.014
Panksepp J (2003) Neuroscience. Feeling the pain of social loss. Science 302(5643):237–9
Pontalis JB (1977) Entre le rêve et la douleur. Editions Gallimard, Paris
Price DD (2000) Psychological and neural mechanisms of the affective dimension of pain. Science
    288(5472):1769–72, Review
Schwartz N, Temkin P, Jurado S, Lim BK, Heifets BD, Polepalli JS et al (2014) Chronic pain.
    Decreased motivation during chronic pain requires long-term depression in the nucleus accum-
    bens. Science 345(6196):535–42. doi:10.1126/science.1253994
Tracey I, Mantyh PW (2007) The cerebral signature for pain perception and its modulation.
    Neuron 55(3):377–91, Review
Tucker DM, Luu P, Derryberry D (2005) Love hurts: the evolution of empathic concern through
    the encephalization of nociceptive capacity. Dev Psychopathol 17(3):699–713
Woolf CJ (2010) What is this thing called pain? J Clin Invest 120(11):3742–4. doi:10.1172/
    JCI45178

# Chapter 12
# Somatization-Psychosomatics

*The human body is the best picture of the human soul.*

(Ludwig Wittgenstein, 1889–1951)

## The Mind-Body Dilemma

As we turn our attention to what clinicians call psychosomatic disorders, in other words, disorders in which symptoms are not explained by an organic condition, we are directly confronted with the thorny issue of the mind–body relationship. The mind–body interaction is an important topic in contemporary neuroscientific literature and pertains to the complex problem of how the body is represented in the brain.

Consciousness is not only a state of cognition but is inherently affective (Solms and Panksepp 2012). In other words the cortex, the seat of cognition, can never be conscious without the subcortical structures, the seats of affects. Being conscious is not only being able to think but also being capable to feel one's own body. In this sense, consciousness consists of a "binding state" where cognition and feelings are "merged." The body, with its sense of touch, takes a special place. Tactility is not only sensorial but cognitive too. The tactile sense makes us human by "keeping in touch" with things or responding to people's feelings. Compassion and concern require the ability to feel and to be felt in turn (Kearney 2014).

An infant's desire for pleasurable exchange is initially aimed at bodily touch with the mother, searching to bring as much as possible large body areas into physical contact. The erogenous zones of the infant are awakened by the care of the primary caregivers. According to Anzieu (1989), the primary contact between mother and baby is tactile in nature.[1] The development of desire and lust is not exclusively tied to the erogenous zones but can be carried out by any skin or mucous membrane that is by the whole skin as an envelope of the self.[2] The communication between infant and mother are first rooted in bodily sensorimotor experiences.

---

[1] Tactile stimulation by massage (moderate pressure stroking) and kinesthetic stimulation by exercise (passively moving the limbs into flexion and extension) increase weight gain in preterm infants, as studies by Field (2014) demonstrate.

[2] According to Anzieu the "skin-ego" is a containing envelope, built up by proprioperception and epidermal sensations. Anzieu enlarged this concept to psychic envelopes.

© Springer International Publishing Switzerland 2016
A. Steck, B. Steck, *Brain and Mind*, DOI 10.1007/978-3-319-21287-6_12

The infant's searching for and finding pleasure is therefore dependent on the bodily and emotional availability of the mother.

> "If the child who cries hears sympathetic sounds and sees a particular facial expression, along with feeling a soothing touch, the child's schemas of pain or fear will develop to incorporate responses of turning to others and expectations that others can help. If the caregivers typically respond to the child's cries with annoyance or withdrawal, schemas of negative expectations and associated responses will develop" (Bucci 2011: p. 49).

Understanding psychosomatic disorders implies on one side the information processing abilities of the brain and on the other the affective dimensions of a subject. The word psychosomatic is derived from the Greek terminology psyche ψυχή[3] (mind) and soma σῶμα (body). The whole issue of psychosomatics resolves around the relationship between mind and body and between brain and mind. A distinction between psyche or mind and soma or body is no longer relevant today in neuroscientific literature but still remains an issue in some psychoanalytical literature.

For Winnicott (1988) the mind must be considered "as a special case of the functioning psyche-soma" (p. 11). "The basis of psyche is soma and in evolution the soma came first. The psyche begins as an imaginative elaboration of physical functioning, having as its most important duty to bind together past experiences, potentialities and present moment awareness, and expectancy for the future. Thus the self comes into existence" (p. 19). "Human nature is not a matter of mind and body—it is a matter of interrelated psyche and soma. Disorders of the psyche-soma are alterations of the body or of the body functioning associated with psychic states" (p. 26). "The psychic part of the person is concerned with relationships, relationship within, relationship to the body, to the external world. Arising out of what may be called the imaginative elaboration of body functioning of all kinds and the accumulation of memories, the psyche (specifically dependent on brain functioning) … makes sense of the person's sense of self …" (p. 28).

## Psychosomatics

According to Franz Alexander, every disease can be regarded as psychosomatic as there is always interaction between mind and body (Alexander 1950). He and Georg Groddeck are generally considered as the founders of psychosomatic medicine (Groddeck 1923).[4]

"Somatization" refers to a variety of phenomena and has different definitions. For some authors, patients with somatization have psychiatric disorders but present with somatic symptoms (Goldberg and Bridges 1988); others such as Barsky (1992) emphasize the influence of psychological distress on the perception or reporting of somatic symptoms as "somatosensory amplification"; finally for some authors,

---

[3] The Greek word ψυχή = psyche from the verb ψύχω = blowing, breathing, meaning soul, life, and spirit

[4] For the history of psychoanalytic psychosomatics, see Smadja (2011).

there is denial of psychological distress and its substitution with somatic symptoms. From this perspective, somatization is a psychological defense against the awareness or expression of psychological distress (Simon et al. 1992, 1999). Somatization is considered as the presence of physical symptoms out of proportion to any demonstrable physical disease (Livingston 1992; Livingston et al. 1995). These symptoms are associated with substantial anxiety, sorrow, pain, and impairment.

The importance to distinguish between organic pain and a psychosomatic disorder can be exemplified by patients presenting with facial pain. In neurological practice, it is customary to differentiate typical facial neuralgia from atypical facial neuralgias. In the former, pain is related to dysfunction of the trigeminal nerve, while in the latter, trigeminal dysfunction cannot be found. Patients with typical facial neuralgia present with physical pain symptoms in the distribution of the trigeminal nerve and report their pain with words that fit a neuropathic pain description. In contrast, in atypical facial neuralgia, the pain narrative takes on a more emotional than physical meaning. Pain is not restricted to the area innervated by the trigeminal nerve. These patients do not respond to typical neuropathic pain drugs and similarly should not be submitted to surgical treatment.

Pain-processing circuits can be visualized by neuroimaging techniques (Tracey and Mantyh 2007). The neuromatrix of pain that we described in the previous chapter involves not only the sensory but also the affective and cognitive components of pain. Recent studies in patients with psychosomatic disorders demonstrate a critical activation of "affective areas" such as the anterior cingulate and prefrontal cortex (Derbyshire 2014). In these patients, the connectivity between cortical and subcortical structures is modified. Whether these functional changes are causal or secondary remains to be shown.

Pierre Marty (1918–1933) the founder of the Psychosomatic School in Paris[5] considered psychosomatic symptoms as expressions of intrapsychic conflicts (Marty et al. 1963; Marty 1980). Patients with psychosomatic disorders have great difficulties to fantasy and symbolize, perceive and express feelings; they resort to "une pensée opératoire, operational thinking," being unable to move from concrete to abstract thinking. In 1973 Sifneos (1995) introduced the term alexithymia[6] to describe patients with psychosomatic disorders who have difficulty in identifying and expressing their emotions as well as appreciating and responding to the emotions of others. They lack fantasy and display a utilitarian way of thinking.

Fischbein (2011) distinguishes patients who suffer from acute and transient psychosomatic episodes from patients whose identity is organized by illness. "They 'are' the illness...." In the former, "the body is responding to an inability to process conflict adequately at a mental level," while in the latter, patients "are

---

[5] The Paris School of Psychosomatics was founded in 1963 by Pierre Marty. Today it is referred to as the Paris Psychosomatic Institute (IPSO = Institut de Psychosomatique).

[6] Alexithymia: in Greek λέξις (lexis = word) and θυμός (thumos = soul), and α = alpha-privative, meaning deprived of words of the soul.

For a psychoanalytical conception of alexithymia and operational thinking, see Pirlot and Corcos (2012).

unable to go through the experiences of mourning, disintegration and emptiness involved in moving towards an identity organized outside their pathology" (pp. 197–198). If psychic pain is attached to a significant person (through overidentification in a fusional relationship), pain cannot be given up, as this would represent not only disloyalty with respect to the loved person but above all risking to lose a part of one's self, leading to feelings of unbearable loss of love with immense sadness and narcissistic void.

According to the attachment theory, somatization is the failure to build up a secure attachment in infancy; in early development, the integration of sensory, visceral, and motor excitations with images and words does not take place. "A fundamental aspect of this learning is dependent on the parents' ability to mirror and regulate the infant's emotional states and in this way help the infant to convert emotional arousal into psychic elements that can then be thought about, named and communicated"(Fonagy et al. 2004, cited in Gubb 2013: p. 122).

## Speaking Body, Speechless Mind

According to the attachment theory, if a mother fails to regulate the infant's emotional states, the child does not develop sufficient mentalization abilities to reflect on his experiences. He then expresses his emotional states through his "speaking body." According to the Paris School of Psychosomatics, the origin of psychosomatic illness is considered as an excessive drive and physical sensation that cannot be thought about and made sense of, the so-called speechless mind. "…an excess of excitation and the resulting displeasure causes the individual to have difficulties in the development of mentalizing abilities" (Gubb 2013: p. 115). Both theories contain the idea that psychosomatic illness results from disturbances in early development. Both schools suggest that the aim of therapy is for bodies and minds to express themselves in conjunction, but in the right registers, in the right locations, and with the right emphases. This will allow the patient to "speak" his or her mind and not his or her "body" (Gubb 2013: p. 139).

According to Stuart and Noyes (1999), somatizing patients display anxious attachment behavior that derives from adverse childhood experiences with caregivers. Early exposure to illness increases the likelihood that distress will be manifested somatically. Patients with somatization disorders seem to be unable to engage in a mourning process of their lived traumatic events; their feelings of distress such as anger, frustration, pain, and despair are expressed through their bodily complaints. Somatoform disorders may also have their roots in childhood through processes that involve enhanced parental focus on health, leading to transmission of somatoform disorders between mother and child (Craig 2002; Craig et al. 2004). Somatizing behavior is then a unique form of interpersonal behavior that is driven by an anxious and maladaptive attachment style and is fostered by real or perceived rejecting responses from significant others. The attachment to psychic pain favors the past over the present and future. The experience of pain maintains a loyalty to a painful relationship.

Patients with psychosomatic disorders show regressive behavior to preverbal somatosensory states; their lack of internal representations renders them dependent on external relationships, yet establishing bonding in order to build up significant relationships often remains extremely difficult. The ability to refer and rely on one's own mental internal world seems to have protective features against psychosomatic illnesses, whereas psychosomatic complaints have mainly the function to sooth psychic pain.

## Somatization in Children and Adolescents

According to Leon Kreisler (1912–2008), considered as the founder of psychosomatics in children, psychosomatic diseases are manifestations of essentially somatic expression, their development being strongly influenced by psychological or psychopathological factors (Kreisler 1983). Kreisler mentions insomnia, infant anorexia, psychogenic vomiting, rumination, idiopathic colic, spasms of sob, early asthmatic events, eczema, and headache, as well as some type of enuresis and encopresis and psychogenic dwarfism as frequent examples of psychosomatic manifestations or psychosomatic participation in infancy and early childhood.

The human being is a unity: soma and psyche are closely related, affect each other, and are indissociable (Aisenstein 2006). Psychological distress may have a visible or sometimes more hidden impact on the body; conversely, somatic illness or physical dysfunction often has an immediate impact on the child's affectivity. When overwhelming emotions cannot be psychologically digested, they are unconsciously redirected to the body and manifested physically. This is especially true for children; they do not have—before a certain age—the tools to perceive and represent emotions and distress to themselves, neither to express them with words to others. However, they may feel strong tensions, struggling to attribute meaning and finding themselves helpless to cope. Psychosomatic manifestations are common in children (e.g., vomiting before going to school) and are very often accessible to psychotherapeutic intervention.

The infant's and child's somatic manifestations are closely linked to interaction with his surroundings and to early psychic disorders. Somatization in children and adolescents (e.g., abdominal pain) is often an expression of psychological concerns on a physical level and tends to decrease during development. Psychosomatic symptoms are relatively frequent in children, as they are not yet as able as adults to separate psychic conflicts from somatic sensations. The process of somatization in small children can be a preferred way to communicate, sometimes imitating somatic expressions of their caregiver; they can also be understood as resulting from lack of symbolization. For assessment of psychosomatic symptoms in infants and young children, it is essential to consider developmental aspects. Since the infant is in constant interaction with the mother or primary caregivers, one has to pay attention to the caregiver–child dyad, a kind of psychophysical unity.

Somatic dysfunction with no detectable somatic substrate may show up in motor, sensory, somatic, visceral, and other functional areas. Early relationship disturbances between infant and caregiver may be expressed pre-symbolically, e.g., in the form of nutritional problems. Nutrition is closely linked to the construction of the earliest relationship with primary caregivers as the exchange around food, and feeding contains a wide range of tactile, visual, auditory, and emotional perceptions and explorations.

Unbearable feelings in children and adolescents due to early childhood traumatic events, lack of holding and containment experience, and affect regulation difficulties are expressed in the form of psychosomatic reactions. Intolerable emotions, which cannot be named with words, nor mentally integrated, will be inscribed in the body and appear in the form of psychosomatic symptoms.

The attempt to solve conflicts can be expressed at the somatic level and often leads to conversion disorders. Conversion is an active process of symptom formation: contradictory impulses are mentally symbolized and—by means of corresponding phantasms—expressed in a kind of body language. Conversion symptoms are often transient and grafted onto different psychopathological structures. The conversion—an unconscious mechanism—corresponds to unconscious needs and desires of a subject and his defensive strategies. Conversion phenomena are most often observed during puberty. Any part of the body can be chosen for the conversion-localization. There may be a genetic predisposition or a current stress situation for the organ choice. Familial constellations may create symptom traditions, e.g., headache families. But also emotional and relationship problems, narcissistic conflicts, or development difficulties may lead to conversion symptoms—often representing an attempt to find a solution.

It is of great importance for the child to know how his parents react to his somatic symptoms and how they verbalize their emotional state or express their feelings in somatic manifestations. Complex family factors are often involved in the development of serious psychophysical disorders in childhood or adolescence. There is also a risk that a functional disorder may have physical consequences (e.g., persistent vomiting).

Hypochondria is a differential diagnosis to psychosomatic symptoms, which should only be made if a child is preoccupied with the idea that he has a serious illness over a long period of time. Children and adolescents of severe physical-diseased parents as well as siblings of somatically ill children often complain of hypochondrial fears.


### Clinical Vignette Manuel

A first child psychiatric consultation is required for 5-year-old Manuel by his pediatrician, who has known Manuel since birth. Manuel's development was within normal range. Since age 2 and until now, however, he has been vomiting. All somatic investigations were negative.

In the initial consultation (with Manuel and his parents), the mother brings plastic bags, so that Manuel, who is accustomed to vomit into bags, does not soil the consulting floor, yet Manuel never vomits in the sessions with the psychotherapist. The parents let their son explain why they asked for help. Manuel immediately begins to draw, "I draw what scares me," and explains his drawings. He describes one nightmare after another. Despite his acute anxiety state, Manuel draws and explains with amazing speed and agility for his age. He comments the first drawing as follows: "A flower, she is very old. She will be killed by a truck. The truck has a tire that has no air; a rose has burst this tire with its thorns. The truck is very upset about the flower; he inflates the tire again. A new flower will come and stay forever young."

The issues of youth, age, violence, death, revenge, and reparation with the hope of eternal life are introduced. Manuel tells more stories of survival struggles of flowers with machines and says: "The story repeats itself again and again." He also speaks of his fear of trucks, tractors, machinery, and their never-ending noise.

In other nightmares, witches and monsters with pointy teeth, ugly eyes, and broken legs eat, bite, and kill various animals. Manuel's oral destructive fantasies are pronounced. He verbalizes his fears that old people could die; his paternal grandmother is very old. He is afraid that his mother could be run over by a truck and that his father could be caught by the police and taken to jail. "I would have no one left; I'd be all alone." Manuel does not want to leave his drawings on the blackboard because he thinks that they could scare other children. He forbids his parents to look at his drawings, as they would be shocked by their ugliness, and he does not want his parents to be sad or worry about him. He is afraid that the child psychiatrist might be killed by these monsters and says to her: "I will save you." Manuel—at the end of the first hour—leaves his drawing of a "fairy with a star" on the blackboard. The fairy has a magic stick she uses to make Pinocchio's body come alive.

In this first interview, the parents report their son's separation anxiety and vomiting. These symptoms have been going on for 3 years and increase with each new situation or novel event. Currently, Manuel refuses to be separated from his mother. He vomits, often refuses food, and runs continuously to the toilet. He does not want to sleep in his own bed, suffers from nightmares, and is frightened by any noise. He resists leaving the house and reacts with panic when he meets disabled people.

At age 2, Manuel's parents left him with his paternal grandparents for 3 weeks while they went abroad. The grandparents at this time were occupied with constructions around their house. Manuel saw how the flower garden was destroyed by construction equipment and trucks. In the last 3 years, he witnessed the death of two cats and a dog. The mother also mentioned the death of her own father, whom Manuel did not know, and the fact that she could not speak about her father's death. Manuel has always been too great a burden for her; therefore, she did not wish to have a second child. The father remains silent most of the time during the first consultation.

In the following individual meetings (Manuel is now able to be separated from his mother), he tells the psychotherapist his dreams of big machines, into which he falls and which annihilate him so that he no longer exists—nightmares from which he wakes up in terror. In another nightmare, there is a castle with a ghost and a frightened boy like himself. The ghost eats 5-year-old boys. Then the boy comes out the mouth of the ghost, but the ghost kills him.

Manuel draws and simultaneously talks about horrible skeletons, ghastly ghosts, which have bad teeth and possess swords, appearing in his dreams. Evil snakes and lions threaten Manuel; a spider-man eats him so that he has only one leg left. He draws a lion that has no body and says that the body has been taken away because the lion did not obey. "If you have no body, then you die. Everything you see is evil." Subsequently Manuel wishes to be a very lucky and very kind lion that does not hurt anybody and loves to be petted. "Nobody has ever seen such a lion." If he were a lion, he would never be afraid again. Later, he wants to be a dinosaur, so that he could scratch and bite, but the evil dinosaur that has come in the consulting room has to die and disappear. "All my bad dreams have to remain here" (in the consulting room).

### *Discussion*

Manuel's development at intellectual and cognitive levels is precocious. He has an excellent capacity of graphic- and verbal expressions and representations. On an emotional level, Manuel is overwhelmed with existential and archaic fears such as separation, death, and annihilation anxieties and fears of fragmentation and mutilation, physical disintegration, and loss. He experiences his aggressiveness as destructive and turns it mainly against himself.

The separation from his parents and placement with his grandparents, living—in Manuel's subjective perception—in a threatening environment, was experienced as a traumatic event. Manuel apparently felt exposed and completely helpless and powerless. He was not able to integrate these experiences and the associated overwhelming anxiety and threat feelings. For the last 3 years, Manuel manifests his traumatic experience in constant repetition of anxiety states, nightmares, and phobic behavior.

Manuel is permanently dependent on the presence of an adult because of his persistent intensive fear state. But his mother fails to reassure him. The mother's depression, probably partly due to the unprocessed loss of her father, prevented her from being emotionally available for Manuel and to provide adequate security, protection, and support. Manuel suppressed his rage against his vulnerable mother. He expresses his aggressive impulses mainly in vomiting and anorexia symptoms: Manuel refuses what his mother gives him to eat or gives it back in vomiting.

Manuel's separation anxiety originates partly from his own feelings of helplessness and powerlessness, partly from his fear that his aggressive impulses toward his mother could harm her and he could lose her. The refusal to be separated from his mother allows Manuel also to care for and control his depressed and vulnerable mother. Manuel is highly parentified; he takes over an adult role with regard to his parents. This is already the case at the beginning of the first interview when the parents leave it up to Manuel to explain the reason for their consultation-request. Manuel's concern, not to burden his parents with sadness or worry about him, demonstrates his parentification, as well as his caring attitude to protect his parents, a behavior Manuel also showed toward the child psychiatrist.

Manuel's symptomatology quickly disappeared after a few psychotherapeutic interventions. Manuel integrated rapidly into kindergarten and according to his teacher even attended with great joy. The parents unfortunately prematurely stopped the treatment.

### Follow-Up

One and a half years later, the mother called to ask again for professional help for Manuel who showed the same symptomatology of vomiting, anorexia, and school phobia, with additional breathing disorders and fears of suffocation.

In the interview with Manuel and his mother, she reported her car accident and the sudden deaths of Manuel's maternal grandmother and paternal grandfather. Manuel also underwent adenoidectomy surgery. All these events took place in the last 6 months. Manuel told the following dream: "The two dead persons, grandmother and grandfather, descend from the sky, every night; they are glad to see me and glad to see that I am not in heaven."

Manuel was integrated into a psychoanalytically oriented psychotherapy group with children of the same age. Again his symptomatology disappeared quickly. This time it was possible to obtain parental consent to conduct Manuel's therapeutic process to the end.

Manuel's mother—in accompanying interviews with her—was able to begin a grieving process. Her helplessness in the face of death was already one of her preoccupations in the first interview. Up to now, she had never been able to speak about death to her son. She felt it was far too terrible for Manuel to learn that the body of a person was forever lost.

Manuel already expressed in words and drawings in the first consultation the unspeakable fear of his mother: "If you have no body, then you die." At the end of the first hour, Manuel presented his desire to rebuild the body—a kind of physical resurrection—when he drew on the blackboard a fairy, which with her magic stick made Pinocchio's body alive.

Manuel's symptomatology is complex, marked not only by his own traumatic experiences but also by his mother's pathological mourning state and the self-exclusion of the father. Manuel's anxiety symptoms, accompanied by terrible representations of monsters, ghosts, and skeletons, refer to an early psychic intergenerational transmission from his mother, incapable of mourning (Abraham and Torok 1987) (see Chap. 14). This form of communication is unconscious and preverbal.

Manuel expressed unprocessed psychological conflicts with an eating disorder. The dialogue between mother and child about nutrition represents a manifold range of tactile, visual, auditory, and emotional perceptions. The developmental history of nourishment is closely connected to the construction of the earliest relationships with primary caregivers. Therefore, nutritional problems in infancy and early childhood reveal symbolically interactive communication features in the mother–child relationship. Manuel's symptoms drew attention to the psychological problem of his mother and its impact on the mother–child relationship.

# References

Abraham N, Torok M (1987) L'écorce et le noyau. Flammarion, Paris

Aisenstein M (2006) The indissociable unity of psyche and soma: a view from the Paris psychosomatic school, Jaron S, translator. Int J Psychoanal 87(Pt 3):667–80

Alexander F (1950) Psychosomatic medicine: its principles and applications. Norton, New York

Anzieu D (1989) The skin ego. Yale University Press, New Haven. ISBN 0300037473

Barsky AJ (1992) Amplification, somatization, and the somatoform disorders. Psychosomatics 33:28–34

Bucci W (2011) The interplay of subsymbolic and symbolic processes in psychoanalytic treatment: it takes two to tango—but who knows the steps, who's the leader? The choreography of the psychoanalytic interchange, psychoanalytic dialogues. Int J Relat Perspect 21(1):45–54. doi:10.1080/10481885.2011.545326

Craig TKJ, Cox AD, Klein K (2002) Intergenerational transmission of somatization behaviour: a study of chronic somatizers and their children. Psychol Med 32:805–816

Craig TKJ, Bialas I, Hodson S, Cox AD (2004) Intergenerational transmission of somatization behaviour. Observations of joint attention and bids for attention. Psychol Med 34:199–209

Derbyshire SW (2014) The use of neuroimaging to advance the understanding of chronic pain: from description to mechanism. Psychosom Med 76(6):402–3. doi:10.1097/PSY. 0000000000000092

Field T. Massage therapy research review. Complement Ther Clin Pract. 2014;20(4):224–9. doi:http://dx.doi.org/10.1016/j.ctcp.2014.07.002

Fischbein JE (2011) Psychosomatics: a current overview. Int J Psychoanal 92(1):197–219

Fonagy P, Gergley G, Jurist EL, Target M. Affect regulation, mentalization and the development of the self. London: Karnak; 2004. Cited In: Gubb K. 2013; p. 122.

Goldberg DP, Bridges K (1988) Somatic presentations of psychiatric illness in primary care setting. J Psychosom Res 32:137–44

Groddeck G (1923) The book of the it. New York, International Universities Press

Gubb K (2013) Psychosomatics today: a review of contemporary theory and practice. Psychoanal Rev 100(1):103–42. doi:10.1521/prev.2013.100.1.103

Kearney R. Losing our touch. New York Times; 2014, 31:8.

Kreisler L (1983) The bases of clinical psychosomatics in childhood. Springer, New York

Livingston R (1992) Children of people with somatization disorder. J Am Acad Child Adolesc Psychiatry 32:536–44

Livingston R, Witt A, Smith GR (1995) Families who somatize. J Dev Behav Pediatr 16:42–6

Marty P (1980) L'ordre psychosomatique: les mouvements individuels de vie et de mort, vol. 2. Desorganisation et regression [The psychosomatic order: Individual life and death motions, vol. 2. Disorganization and regression]. Payot, Paris

Marty P, de M'Uzan M, David C (1963) L'investigation psychosomatique: sept observations cliniques [Psychosomatic investigations: seven clinical observations]. PUF, Paris

Pirlot G, Corcos M (2012) Understanding alexithymia within a psychoanalytical framework. Int J Psychoanal 93:1403–25

Sifneos PE (1995) Psychosomatic, alexithymie et neurosciences [Psychosomatics, alexithymia, and neurosciences]. Rev Fr Psychosom 7:27–35

Simon GE, Gater R, Kisely S, Piccinelli M (1992) Somatic symptoms of distress: an international primary care study. Psychosom Med 58:481–8

Simon GE, Von Korff M, Piccinelli M, Fullerton C, Ormel J (1999) An international study of the relation between somatic symptoms and depression. N Engl J Med 341:1329–35

Smadja C (2011) Psychoanalytic psychosomatics. Int J Psychoanal 92(1):221–30. doi:10.1111/ j.1745-8315.2010.00390.x

Solms M, Panksepp J (2012) The "Id" knows more than the "ego" admits: neuropsychoanalytic and primal consciousness perspectives on the interface between affective and cognitive neuroscience. Brain Sci 2(2):147–75. doi:10.3390/brainsci2020147

Stuart S, Noyes R Jr (1999) Attachment and interpersonal communication in somatization. Psychosomatics 40:34–43

Tracey I, Mantyh PW (2007) The cerebral signature for pain perception and its modulation. Neuron 55(3):377–91

Winnicott DW (1988) Human nature. Free Association Books, London

# Part VII

# Chapter 13
# Resilience

## A Dynamic Concept

Resilience[1] is an interactive concept and refers to the relative resistance of a subject to environmental risk experiences or to his overcoming of stress or adversity. Underlying psychosocial and biological processes, risk, and vulnerability as well as gene–environment interactions are all factors contributing to resilience. The current interest in resilience in childhood and adolescence is based on the findings that critical life events in early childhood can be followed by severe and long-lasting psychopathological disorders. Resilience research arose from an effort to better protect children, adolescents, and young adults from the impact of adverse life experiences, such as traumatic events, unfavorable burdens, or the management of stress. Longitudinal studies concerning the effects of psychosocial constraints on the development of resilience demonstrate that indicators of child resilience such as adequate behavioral and emotional self-regulation contribute to later competence. However severe environmental adversities prevail over the individual resilience resources.

Stress exerts a double toll on physical or emotional health and on well-being. As a consequence of chronic load, stress not only contributes to diseases but disrupts functions responsible for coping and self-regulation. Good intellectual functioning and parenting resources are associated with good outcomes across competence domains, even in the context of severe, chronic adversity. Children having different temperament styles seek out environments that may increase risk or promote resilience. The quality of interpersonal relationships between the infant and his caregivers, parental attachment models, and the child's binding security play an essential role in the development of resilience and in intergenerational transmission. Preventive and therapeutic interventions at both individual and family levels are important measures promoting resilience (Bürgin and Steck 2008).

---

[1] "Act of rebounding" from Latin resilire "rebound, recoil."

© Springer International Publishing Switzerland 2016
A. Steck, B. Steck, *Brain and Mind*, DOI 10.1007/978-3-319-21287-6_13

Resilience is responsible for the individual variation in the response of children and adolescents to similar experiences. The exposure to stress and not its avoidance may in certain circumstances strengthen the resistance to later stress, the so-called "steeling" effect, in other words when risk experiences have been mastered by successful coping. "… resilience can be defined as reduced vulnerability to environmental risk experiences, the overcoming of a stress or adversity, or a relatively good outcome despite risk experiences" (Rutter 2012: p. 336). Resilience leads to successful adaptation and integration despite high risks, chronic stress, and psychosocial adverse conditions (Welter-Enderlin and Hildenbrand 2008). Protective mechanisms against psychosocial risks associated with adversity are reducing risk impact and negative chain reactions, establishing and maintaining self-esteem and self-efficiency, and opening up of opportunities.

A major prospective study in resilience (Werner 1989, 1992), known as the Kauai longitudinal study, was carried out on a large population born in 1955 on the island of Kauai, the oldest of the main Hawaiian Islands.[2] The author describes each individual life—from birth to age 40—of children who grew up in poverty or other adverse conditions (parental divorce, alcoholism, mental illness). Two thirds of the children, who were exposed to four or more risk factors up to the age of 2 years, developed learning or behavioral problems by age 10 or by age 18 committed offenses and/or had mental health problems. However, one third of the children developed into competent, caring adults. The resilience of these children seemed to be related to the fact that they displayed a temperament to which most family members reacted in a positive way. The caregiving environment described them as active, balanced, and easy to handle regarding nutrition, sleep, and other behaviors. In cases of separations or other failures of the parents, they were able to quickly use adults from the surrounding environment as substitutes. They integrated rapidly into school and entered professional, familial, or other social relationships.

Resilience is not constant, but can fluctuate in the course of life, depending on situations and context. Ungar stresses the importance of taking into account protective as well as harmful factors of the environment with respect to resilience, which he defines as follows: "In the context of exposure to significant adversity, resilience is both the capacity of individuals to navigate their way to the psychological, social, cultural and physical resources that sustain their well-being, and their capacity individually and collectively to negotiate for these resources to be provided and experienced in culturally meaningful ways"(Ungar 2010: p. 425). He emphasizes the need to consider children's context and culture, as well as the environmental role of social and physical contributions, challenging or fostering resilience (Ungar 2011).

In spite of experiencing significant discriminatory conditions or trauma, resilient children, adolescents, and young adults show positive adaptation (Luthar and Cicchetti 2000). Positive adaptation is usually defined as social skills or as successful passage through distinctive phases of specific developmental tasks. Traumatic life experiences can trigger maturation processes, particularly in three areas: self-awareness, interpersonal relationships, and attitude toward life (Tedeschi et al. 1998).

---

[2] According to legend, a Polynesian navigator named the island after his favorite son.

Resilient children are generally very early in a position to establish relationships with surrogate persons and use them for their development, having a high interactive capacity.

## Gene–Environment Interactions

The risk of developing psychopathological conditions is best understood through studies investigating gene–environment interactions. It is increasingly realized that changes in the environment influence gene expression. Genes and environmental features affect almost every psychopathological traits and associated disorders (Eley et al. 2004a). Environmental events can modify the expression of genes through epigenetic mechanisms (Bird 2007). These mechanisms consist of DNA methylation and histone modifications and do not directly alter the nucleotide sequence of the gene. The epigenetic changes are not as stable as genetic alterations caused by mutations and are usually not transmitted more than one or two generations.

A paradigmatic example of epigenetic-mediated changes includes the negative effect of early adverse rearing on the regulation of the hypothalamic–pituitary–adrenal (HPA) axis (Bagot and Meaney 2010). Following exposure to stress glucocorticoids stimulate the glucocorticoid receptor in the hippocampus and eventually inhibit the HPA axis. In abused children, this negative feedback loop is blunted through epigenetic change of the glucocorticoid receptor in the hippocampus, so that there is an increase in the HPA response to stress. What is particularly interesting is the fact that this negative effect of adverse rearing can be reversed. Studies in animals show that through subsequent ideal fostering, the HPA axis response to stress is again normalized (Weder and Kaufman 2011).

The contribution of single genes to the development of resilience has also been intensively investigated. The serotonin transporter gene, the oxytocin receptor gene, the dopamine receptor D4 gene, and the corticotropin-releasing hormone receptor gene are among these genes, and each has been linked to some aspects of resilient functioning (Cicchetti and Rogosch 2012). In addition recent genetic findings demonstrate that the risk conferred by these genes is implicated in a range of neurodevelopmental disorders such as schizophrenia, autism, attention-deficit hyperactivity disorder, and forms of intellectual disability (Owen 2012). This overlap reveals the complexity of the combination of genes and environmental factors affecting individual development and psychological processes.

Changes in manifestations of resilience take place especially during developmental transitions, such as adolescence (Silk et al. 2007), in which new risk factors arise and protective factors will be challenged. It is well known that the individual answers to being exposed to adverse conditions are heterogeneous. The majority of persons are able to cope with stressful situations and do not develop psychopathology. Yet in a significant minority, severe symptomatology may result from traumatic experiences, even in later life. Multiple genetic and environmental factors are involved in developmental processes and therefore in the outcome of resilience or vulnerability differences. Epigenetic changes in various regions of the brain—during critical periods of development—seem to be responsible for the emergence of vulnerability or resilience to stress-related psychiatric disorders (Dudley et al. 2011).

## *Adoption*

Adoption research allows a unique insight into the malleability of child development demonstrating children's recuperation from adversities in infancy. Long-term studies of severely deprived children in Romanian institutions, who were adopted by well-functioning British families, did not show persistent effects of deprivation if adopted before the age of 6 months; however children who were adopted at 6–12 months showed multiple impairments, which persisted for many children up to age 11. Some children were able to improve their cognitive functions between the ages 6 and 11. The findings show great heterogeneity in outcomes (Rutter 2006; Beckett et al. 2006). The quality of the adoptive mother–child relationship plays an essential role (Stams et al. 2002).

Research on adults, who were internationally adopted around 2 years of age, showed that early severe or multiple adverse experiences increased their risk of psychiatric disorders in adulthood. However children having suffered from less severe early adversity seemed to be resilient (van der Vegt et al. 2009).

Studies on the development of specific executive functions demonstrate their contribution to adaptive and maladaptive socio-emotional outcomes among children having experienced early psychosocial deprivation (McDermott et al. 2013). Data are still inconclusive with regard to the moderating factors that promote resilience in children who have experienced extraordinarily severe deprivation. Research on deprivation-specific psychological patterns demonstrates their persisting influence up to the age of 15 years (Rutter and Sonuga-Barke 2010; Rutter et al. 2010). Genetic contributions are responsible for only part of the variance seen in psychopathology (Kendler and Prescott 2006; Rutter 2006). Further explorations of long-term impacts following early deprivation experiences on underlying neurobiological systems are required (Rutter and Sonuga-Barke 2010; Rutter et al. 2010).

## Development

Resilience processes are dynamically influenced during developmental phases, in which the social and biological adaptation systems are reorganized. The resilience process thus changes in the adolescence period. Long-term studies on development in children and adolescents from birth to 18 years show that the characteristics of the social context represent better predictors of resilience than the individual characteristics of a child (Sameroff and Rosenbaum 2006). The quality of parental functions, the parent–child relationships, and the family milieu constitute effective mediators and moderators in unfavorable stress situations.

Indicators of childhood resilience such as behavioral and emotional self-regulation—a characteristic for mental health—and cognitive processes contribute to later competence of children and youths. But the effects of such individual features of resilience do not overcome the impacts of high environment challenges, such as poor parental relationships and functions, antisocial peers, low community resources, and financial hardship. The effects of single environmental burden become quite strong when accumulated into multiple risk scores. They may even affect the development of offspring in the next generation. These longitudinal studies of children from birth to 18 years also examined the relative contribution of early childhood resilience and the environmental challenges to mental health and school performance. The results demonstrate that the groups of children with high individual resilience properties in high-risk environments later show poorer mental health and cognitive competence than the groups of children with low individual resilience properties in a low-risk environment (Sameroff and Rosenbaum 2006).

# Temperament

Temperament refers to the biologically rooted individual differences in behavioral characteristics. These predisposing characteristics may change during the child's development, both qualitatively and quantitatively, and manifest themselves differently depending on the nature of the context in which the child is placed (Wachs 2006). Temperamental differences rooted in infancy are important for understanding individual discrepancies in vulnerability and resilience (Schwartz et al. 2012).

Temperament is to nature what personality is to nurture; in other words temperament can be viewed as a biological property by which we react in a characteristic way to experiences, while personality reflects our constructed self. Of course in everyday life, temperament and personality have traits that are exchangeable. Kagan (2003) proposed that temperament reflects behavioral features that are inherited. He described two primary temperamental types which he termed high reactive and low reactive. Kagan postulated that the amygdala is the primary brain structure that determines the affective reactivity of the infant. Longitudinal studies showed however that the assessment between low and high reactivity in infancy did not necessarily correspond to the behavioral profile of older children, which emphasizes the role of environmental influences in the development of temperament and in particular the enormous importance of parenting. Parental responses to innate temperamental profiles should be considered as a significant factor in the development of a child. Neurobiological traits and temperamental dispositions are clearly shaped by environmental factors. Temperament as well as personality should never be reduced to biological characteristics. As noted by Blandin (2013), it is important to consider the layers between biology and the environment. Subjectivity is often missing in neuroscience, even though a hallmark of our personality and, by extension, of the culture in which we live.

Individual variations in temperament reflect underlying differences in reactivity and self-regulation. As for the biological roots, temperament characteristics reflect individual brain functions and structures. The amygdala plays a central role in shaping behavioral patterns to adverse events. Individual variations are not only due to genetic traits and neurobiological features but also to ecological factors, like diet, environment, and familial characteristics, such as parental–child relatedness and family functioning. Particular temperament patterns may heighten vulnerability or facilitate resilience. Children with different temperament styles seek out environments that may increase risk or promote resilience; caregivers or teachers will respond to children according to their temperaments in distinctive ways. Between child temperament characteristics and environmental demands, there can be a goodness or poorness of fit. Temperamental differences influence coping strategies of children in dealing with stressful situations. These will further contribute to vulnerability or resilience.

## Stress

Genetic and epigenetic factors interact in shaping brain structure and function and lead to multiple individual variants. Therefore the response to stress is always influenced by the personal genetic makeup (nature) and the environmental context (nurture). Studies demonstrate how the epigenetic regulation of neuronal gene transcription may contribute to either subjective vulnerability or resilience in challenging stressful environmental situations (Zannas and West 2014). Gene–environment interaction research shows that the genetic influence is only expressed through interaction with the environmental risk. The genetic variability per se neither constitutes a risk nor a protective factor. There is no single generally applicable resilience trait. As François Jacob[3](1970) said, the human being is not prisoner of its genome.

Children who have high levels of positive emotionality, emotional access and activity, are more likely to use active coping mechanisms to deal with stress, while children with low scores in these items tend to use avoidance strategies. Children who use active and flexible coping and adaptive mechanisms are more successful in dealing with stressful situations, and in this sense more resilient, than children who apply avoidance strategies. The effects of psychosocial stress and the related nature of coping strategies are of great importance for the understanding and management of resilience in childhood and adolescence (Compas 2006).

The psychological and biological processes of reactivity to psychosocial stress and the related nature of confrontation and coping, as well as the recovery from stress, are fundamental to the understanding of the extent of the emotional and physical consequences of long-lasting chronic stress. Stress not only contributes to somatic illnesses

---

[3] François Jacob (1920–2013) was a French biologist and geneticist who received the Nobel Prize in Medicine in 1965 for his work on DNA transcription.

and emotional and behavioral problems but also interrupts the functions in the brain that are primarily responsible for effective coping and self-regulation; stress impairs hippocampal integrity resulting in diminished cognitive functioning and affects the development of frontal regions implicated in emotional regulation (Bremner et al. 2008). The direct effect of chronic stress is thus reinforced by the impairment of the ability to effectively cope with stress (see Chap. 10).

## Depression

Silk et al. (2007) investigated the resilience of children and young persons at risk for depression. They reviewed the interaction of the social environment with brain functions involved in emotional reactivity and emotional regulation. They discuss the influence of the social context on resilience processes at the neurobiological level, such as the dysfunction in the serotoninergic system as well as the dopaminergic reward system. The interaction of genetic factors, stress reactivity, positive emotions, and sleep was investigated as possible processes contributing to resilience in children and young persons with depression. Insufficient ability to adaptively regulate negative emotions is associated with anxiety and depressive disorders in children and adolescents. Research in the field of depression considers disturbances in emotional reactivity and regulation as risk factors. Forbes and Dahl (2005) define the regulation of emotion as internal (by the self) and external (by others) processes which are involved in the initiation, maintenance, and modification of the quality, intensity, and timing of emotional responses. Emotional reactivity relates to the subject's variance in the intensity of his response to an emotional stimulus. The ability to effectively regulate emotions contributes to resilience of children at risk for depression (Masten 2004). The social context of supportive parental care also protects children with genetic risk factors against the onset of a depression (Eley et al. 2004a, b; Kaufman et al. 2006).

## Attachment

Current research toward understanding the brain systems influencing parenting demonstrates the presence of universal networks that are highly conserved between animals and humans. The neurohormone of the hypothalamus, oxytocin, has been known for a long time to be important for reproductive behavior and has been studied for its role in enhancing mother–infant bonding (Pedersen and Prange 1979). Interest in the role of oxytocin as a "resilience hormone" is derived from its broad effects on behavior, such as fostering attachment, improving social memory, and reducing fear. Oxytocin depresses amygdala activity and HPA stress response and thus "serves to inhibit defensive behaviors associated with stress, anxiety or fear, and allows positive social interactions and the development of bonds" (Carter 1998: p. 782).

Functional imaging studies showed that—when parents view videos of their children—there is activation of the mesolimbic dopaminergic system including the ventral tegmental area (VTA), the nucleus accumbens, and the orbitofrontal cortex. The activation of these brain regions is thought to be related to positive parental engagement and interaction with their children (Rilling 2013; Rilling and Young 2014). Animal studies have demonstrated that oxytocin stimulates the dopaminergic VTA, increasing maternal motivation. Oxytocin modulates the prefrontal cortex and the anterior cingulate gyrus through the VTA, fostering empathy. In addition oxytocin is known to inhibit components of the fear system in the amygdala.

Given the importance of a secure attachment in infancy for normal psychological development, the role of oxytocin goes well beyond its primary role in fostering early child–parent relationships and is at the root of the development of good quality in social relationships in adulthood. There is interest today in the use of oxytocin as a treatment for psychiatric disorders such as autism or schizophrenia, because oxytocin is thought to improve social functioning. It is however unlikely that this drug may help address the principal deficits at the core of these diseases. A secure attachment represents part of the mediation process, in which resilience is observed (Fonagy et al. 1994). Parental attachment and relationship models affect the binding safety of the child, i.e., each parent transmits his internal attachment and relationship patterns, regardless of the other parent. Eventually the child is able to integrate the two separate internalized relationship models of his primary caregivers. One assumes that one secure internal relationship model represents a sufficiently protective factor and contributes to the resilience of the child in a situation of deprivation.

Uncertain representation of maternal attachment figures not only influences the mother's affective and cognitive properties but also leads to distortions in the perception of her child and interferes with her ability to build a secure relationship with her child. Psychotherapies with young children and their parents proved to be an effective intervention to promote secure attachment organization in children of depressed mothers (Lieberman 1992; Cicchetti 2013).

## Resilience Promotion

Resilience research clearly shows that children and adolescents growing up in stressful situations or exposed to critical life events do not necessarily develop psychopathological symptoms. Children's and adolescents' vulnerability can be compensated by mediating early, protective, and long-lasting interventions.

A longitudinal study conducted in Jamaica showed that psychosocial intervention for disadvantaged children in early childhood compensates for developmental delays. For 2 years community health workers visited growth-retarded toddlers and their mothers living in poverty once a week to teach parental skills and favor mother–child interactions, which stimulated cognitive and emotional development. Twenty years after the intervention, the stimulated group of children had increased their earnings by 25 %, thus catching up the earnings of a non-growth-retarded comparison group (Gertler et al. 2014).

Interventions at all phases of development are of highest value (Rutter 2000); longer interventions are more efficient than shorter ones (Luthar et al. 2006). Interventions for children at risk prove to be particularly advantageous at the time of developmental transitions, such as starting school, adolescence, or entering the world of work. Reduction of risk impact, promoting self-reliance and self-efficacy, and opening new opportunities and prospects through available stable and supportive relationships or successful task accomplishment are crucial measures to foster resilience as the following investigation demonstrates: in a longitudinal study of adolescent development, Hauser et al. (2006) led annual interviews with 150 young persons over a period of 4 years; they were previously hospitalized because they presented a serious danger to themselves or others. Interviews were conducted to investigate the contribution of narratives to resilience promotion. Storytelling initiates a symbolic process and attributes meaning to adverse or traumatic life events, which have interrupted the continuity of a subject's personal life history. The narrative coherence reflects the ability to deal with stress and integrate personal painful events. The authors wondered how resilience develops through new life experiences. The results show that—in the process of resilience in adolescents—their personal responsibility and commitment to overcome adverse living conditions are essential. Adolescents have to be actively engaged in their own development and their reflectivity competence in order to enhance their commitment to relationships and master emotional and social interactions in relationships.

Resilient families often have strong value systems; reliable relationships; clear forms of communication based on trust, empathy, and tolerance; flexible social and economic resources; and the ability to find solutions and to adapt to new challenges (Welter-Enderlin and Hildenbrand 2008).

Today adversity or stressful environmental conditions are not less frequent, although they are better perceived and their long-term effects are better known. Resilience tries to grasp the variance that cannot be explained by risk-and protective factors. Resilience can be described as an adaptive and developmental process of a child or young person in a stressful context in which multiple risk and protective factors take place in highly complex interactive ways. To successfully deal with a challenge, physiological adaptation and psychological habituation are required, as well as the acquisition of effective adaptive and coping skills. In addition a sense of self-efficacy and a self-reflecting ability are involved to redefine the lived experience.

# References

Bagot RC, Meaney MJ. Epigenetics and the biological basis of gene×environment interactions. J Am Acad Child Adolesc Psychiatry. 2010;49(8):752–71. doi:10.1016/j.jaac.2010.06.001.

Beckett C, Maughan B, Rutter M, Castle J, Colvert E, Groothues C, Kreppner J, et al. Do the effects of early severe deprivation on cognition persist into early adolescence? Findings from the English and Romanian adoptees study. Child Dev. 2006;77(3):696–711.

Bird A. Perceptions of epigenetics. Nature. 2007;447(7143):396–8.

Blandin K. Temperament and typology. J Anal Psychol. 2013;58(1):118–36. doi:10.1111/j.1468-5922.2013.02020.x.

Bremner JD, Elzinga B, Schmahl C, Vermetten E. Structural and functional plasticity of the human brain in posttraumatic stress disorder. Prog Brain Res. 2008;167:171–86.

Bürgin D, Steck B. Resilienz im Kindes- und Jugendalter [Resiliency in childhood and adolescence]. Schweiz. Arch Neurol Psychiatry. 2008;159:480–9.

Carter CS. Neuroendocrine perspectives on social attachment and love. Psychoneuroendocrinology. 1998;23(8):779–818. Review. p. 782.

Cicchetti D. Annual research review: resilient functioning in maltreated children—past, present, and future perspectives. J Child Psychol Psychiatry. 2013;54(4):402–22. doi:10.1111/j.1469-7610.2012.02608.x.

Cicchetti D, Rogosch FA. Gene×environment interaction and resilience: effects of child maltreatment and serotonin, corticotropin releasing hormone, dopamine, and oxytocin genes. Dev Psychopathol. 2012;24(2):411–27. doi:10.1017/S0954579412000077.

Compas BE. Psychobiological processes of stress and coping. Implications for resilience in children and adolescents—Comments on the papers of Romeo & McEwen and Fisher et al. Ann N Y Acad Sci. 2006;1094:226–34.

Dudley KJ, Li X, Kobor MS, Kippin TE, Bredy TW. Epigenetic mechanisms mediating vulnerability and resilience to psychiatric disorders. Neurosci Biobehav Rev. 2011;35(7):1544–51. doi:10.1016/j.neubiorev.2010.12.016. Epub 2011 Jan 18. Review.

Eley TC, Sugden K, Corsico A, Gregory AM, Sham P, McGuffin P, et al. Gene-environment interaction analysis of serotonin system markers with adolescent depression. Mol Psychiatry. 2004a;9:908–15.

Eley TC, Liang H, Plomin R, Sham P, Sterne A, Williamson R, et al. Parental familial vulnerability, family environment, and their interactions as predictors of depressive symptoms in adolescents. J Am Acad Child Adolesc Psychiatry. 2004b;43(3):298–306.

Fonagy P, Steele M, Steele H, Higgitt A, Target M. The Emanuel Miller Memorial Lecture 1992. The theory and practice of resilience. Review. J Child Psychol Psychiatry. 1994;35(2):231–57.

Forbes EE, Dahl RE. Neural systems of positive affect: relevance to understanding child and adolescent depression? Dev Psychopathol. 2005;17(3):827–50. Review.

Gertler P, Heckman J, Pinto R, Zanolini A, Vermeersch C, Walker S, Chang SM, Grantham-McGregor S. Labor market returns to an early childhood stimulation intervention in Jamaica. Science. 2014;344(6187):998–1001. doi:10.1126/science.1251178.

Hauser S, Allen JP, Golden E. Out of the Woods. Tales of resilient teens. Cambridge: Harvard University Press; 2006.

Jacob F. La logique du vivant. Une histoire de l'hérédité. Paris: Gallimard; 1970. «Bibliothèque des sciences humaines».

Kagan J. Biology, context, and developmental inquiry. Annu Rev Psychol. 2003;54:1–23.

Kaufman J, Yang BZ, Douglas-Palumberi H, Grasso D, Lipschitz D, Houshyar S, Krystal JH, Gelernter J. Brain-derived neurotrophic factor-5-HTTLPR gene interactions and environmental modifiers of depression in children. Biol Psychiatry. 2006;59(8):673–80.

Kendler KS, Prescott CA. Genes, environment, and psychopathology : understanding the causes of psychiatric and substance Use disorders. New York: Guilford Press; 2006.

Lieberman AF. Infant–parent psychotherapy with toddlers. Dev Psychopathol. 1992;4:559–74.

Luthar SS, Cicchetti D. The construct of resilience: implications for interventions and social policies. Dev Psychopathol. 2000;12(4):857–85. Review.

Luthar SS, Sawyer JA, Brown PJ. Conceptual issues in studies of resilience. Past, present, and future research. Ann N Y Acad Sci. 2006;1094:105–15.

Masten AS. Regulatory processes, risk and resilience in adolescent development. Ann N Y Acad Sci. 2004;1021:310–9.

McDermott JM, Troller-Renfree S, Vanderwert R, Nelson CA, Zeanah CH, Fox NA. Psychosocial deprivation, executive functions, and the emergence of socio-emotional behavior problems. Front Hum Neurosci. 2013;7:167. doi:10.3389/fnhum.2013.00167. eCollection 2013.

Owen JM. Implications of genetic findings for understanding schizophrenia. Schizophr Bull. 2012;38(5):904–7.

Pedersen CA, Prange Jr AJ. Induction of maternal behavior in virgin rats after intracerebroventricular administration of oxytocin. Proc Natl Acad Sci U S A. 1979;76(12):6661–5.

Rilling JK. The neural and hormonal bases of human parental care. Neuropsychologia. 2013;51(4):731–47. doi:10.1016/j.neuropsychologia.2012.12.017. Epub 2013 Jan 16. Review.

Rilling JK, Young LJ. The biology of mammalian parenting and its effect on offspring social development. Science. 2014;345(6198):771–6. doi:10.1126/science.1252723. Epub 2014 Aug 14. Review.

Rutter M. Resilience reconsidered: conceptual considerations, empirical findings, and policy implications. In: Shonkoff JP, Meisels SJ, editors. Handbook of early childhood intervention, vol. 2. New York: Cambridge University Press; 2000. p. 651–82.

Rutter M. Implications of resilience concepts for scientific understanding. Ann N Y Acad Sci. 2006;1094:1–12.

Rutter M. Resilience as a dynamic concept. Dev Psychopathol. 2012;24(2):335–44. doi:10.1017/S0954579412000028.

Rutter M, Sonuga-Barke EJ. X. Conclusions: overview of findings from the era study, inferences, and research implications. Monogr Soc Res Child Dev. 2010;75(1):212–29. doi:10.1111/j.1540-5834.2010.00557.x.

Rutter M, Sonuga-Barke EJ, Castle J. I. Investigating the impact of early institutional deprivation on development: background and research strategy of the English and Romanian Adoptees (ERA) study. Monogr Soc Res Child Dev. 2010;75(1):1–20. doi:10.1111/j.1540-5834.2010.00548.x.

Sameroff AJ, Rosenbaum KL. Psychosocial constraints on the development of resilience. Ann N Y Acad Sci. 2006;1094:116–24.

Schwartz CE, Kunwar PS, Greve DN, Kagan J, Snidman NC, Bloch RB. A phenotype of early infancy predicts reactivity of the amygdala in male adults. Mol Psychiatry. 2012;17(10):1042–50. doi:10.1038/mp.2011.96.

Silk JS, Vanderbilt-Adriance E, Shaw DS, Forbes EE, Whalen DJ, Ryan ND, Dahl RE. Resilience among children and adolescents at risk for depression: mediation and moderation across social and neurobiological contexts. Review Dev Psychopathol. 2007;19(3):841–65.

Stams GJM, Juffer F, van IJzendoorn MH. Maternal sensitivity, infant attachment, and temperament in early childhood predict adjustment in middle childhood: the case of adopted children and their biologically unrelated parents. Dev Psychol. 2002;38(5):806–21. doi:10.1037/0012-1649.38.5.806.

Tedeschi RG, Park CI, Calhoun LG. Posttraumatic growth: conceptual issues. In: Tedesci RG, Park CI, Calhoun LG, editors. Posttraumatic growth: positive changes in the aftermath of crisis. Mahwah: Lawrence Erlenbaum; 1998.

Ungar M. Families as navigators and negotiators: facilitating culturally and contextually specific expressions of resilience. Fam Process. 2010;49(3):421–35. doi:10.1111/j.1545-5300.2010.01331.x.

Ungar M. The social ecology of resilience: addressing contextual and cultural ambiguity of a nascent construct. Am J Orthopsychiatry. 2011;81(1):1–17.

van der Vegt EJ, Tieman W, van der Ende J, Ferdinand RF, Verhulst FC, Tiemeier H. Impact of early childhood adversities on adult psychiatric disorders: a study of international adoptees. Soc Psychiatry Psychiatr Epidemiol. 2009;44:724–31. doi:10.1007/s00127-009-0494-6.

Wachs TD. Contributions of temperament to buffering and sensitization processes in children's development. Ann N Y Acad Sci. 2006;1094:28–39.

Weder N, Kaufman J. Critical periods revisited: implications for intervention with traumatized children. J Am Acad Child Adolesc Psychiatry. 2011;50(11):1087–9. doi:10.1016/j.jaac.2011.07.021.

Welter-Enderlin R, Hildenbrand B (Hrsg.) Resilienz—Gedeihen trotz widriger Umstände. Heidelberg: Carl-Auer; 2008.

Werner EE. Children of the garden island. Sci Am. 1989;260(4):106–11.

Werner EE. The children of Kauai: resiliency and recovery in adolescence and adulthood. J Adolesc Health. 1992;13(4):262–8.

Zannas AS, West AE. Epigenetics and the regulation of stress vulnerability and resilience. Neuroscience. 2014;264:157–70. doi:10.1016/j.neuroscience.2013.12.003.

# Part VIII

# Chapter 14
# Grief

*Give sorrow words; the grief that does not speak,*
*Whispers the o'erfraught heart and bids it break.*

(William Shakespeare (1564–1616), Macbeth, Act 4, Scene 3)

## Introduction

Grief is an internal process—following experiences of loss and/or psychic injuries—that involves an active engagement of the subject. The grieving person recalls all his experiences with the loved one and must recognize the loss as permanent and irrevocable. Remembering is thus a process of continuous disruption of the bonds with the beloved person. Mourning is known since ancient times and among all nations. Religion, literature, philosophy, and art relay expressions of traumatic experiences and associated grief.

Freud (1917) wrote:

"... although mourning involves grave departures from the normal attitude toward life, it never occurs to us to regard it as a pathological condition and to refer it to a medical treatment. We rely on its being overcome after a certain lapse of time, and we look upon any interference with it as useless or even harmful". (p. 243)

Kubler-Ross (1969) described five stages of mourning: denial and isolation, anger, bargaining, depression, and acceptance of loss. After an initial shock state, the loss is denied, followed by a state of protest in an attempt to undo what has happened, accompanied by aggressive feelings (anger, hate, etc.). A state of depression and grief arises only after, which eventually leads to acceptance of the loss. These stages do not usually proceed sequentially, but in parallel. Individuals who suffer repeated losses often remain in a stage of aggression, with anger, hatred, and revenge, and are unable to perform the grieving process.

The traumatic loss of a significant person may reactivate all the painful emotions of the previous losses an individual has experienced. For Kernberg (2010) one way to handle the pain of loss lies in engaging to achieve the aspirations of the deceased person. "It is as if the most effective way to deal with the pain of loss were the commitment to carry out that mandate, a commitment that has an ethical quality" (p. 616). It contains the wish of restitution and maintains—as part of the identification process—the internalized relationship with the beloved person. Yet one of the most

© Springer International Publishing Switzerland 2016
A. Steck, B. Steck, *Brain and Mind*, DOI 10.1007/978-3-319-21287-6_14

difficult aspects of mourning is enduring the continuous internal presence of the loved one and at the same time being confronted with his external absence. In special situations such as the disappearance of a loved person, the grieving process is hindered and takes the form of an "enigmatic mourning." The survivor may idealize the lost person and identify with the disappeared loved one. His mind is haunted by the lost person. "…like the ghost of Hamlet's father,[1] 'who knows a secret to be revealed or a wrongdoer to be apprehended', the disappeared body is now inside the mind of those who knew him, as well as roaming the outside world rather than resting in a silent grave…" (Taiana 2014: p. 1095).

## Prolonged Grief Disorder or Complicated Grief

To live is to suffer; to survive is to find some meaning in the suffering.

Friedrich Nietzsche (1844–1900) (1967)

Acute grief and associated symptoms such as pain, sadness, and anger are considered normal processes after bereavement, not generally needing mental health intervention. Symptoms of grief may reappear at anniversaries of the lost person or in stressful situations. The stress caused by bereavement, like other stressors, can increase the likelihood of onset or worsening of other physical or mental disorders. According to various studies, prolonged grief disorder (PGD) occurs in about 10 % of bereaved persons, the rates being higher among parents who have lost a child (Shear et al. 2011).

PGD is diagnosed following a period of 6 months to 1 year after the loss of a significant loved one. There is a symptomatology of persistent and intense yearning for the lost one with feelings of loneliness, emptiness, bitterness, and great difficulty to detach from and accept the loss of the significant person. The surviving person is affected by images, hallucinations, and nightmares of the deceased person and preoccupied with questions of why, accompanied by feelings of worthlessness and loss of meaning of one's own life. Complicated grief (CG)

> "… also leads to dysfunctional thoughts, maladaptive behaviors and emotion dysregulation such as troubling ruminations about circumstances or consequences of the death, persistent feelings of shock, disbelief or anger about the death, feelings of estrangement from other people and changes in behavior focused on excessive avoidance of reminders of the loss or the opposite, excessive proximity seeking to try to feel closer to the deceased, sometimes focused on wishes to die or suicidal behavior" (Shear et al. 2011: p. 105).

Risk factors or increased vulnerability of developing PGD include among others a history of mood disorder, low perceived social support, insecure attachment style, and increased stress. Vanderwerker et al. (2006) show that childhood separation anxiety was associated with complicated grief in adults. In their research, Lichtenthal et al. (2010) found that almost half the parents who lost a child expressed—in their written narratives—that they could not make sense of the loss of their child. These parents

---

[1] Hamlet, Act I, Scene 5, by William Shakespeare.

suffered greater levels of grief and were at a higher risk for PGD. Most helpful and relevant for attributing meaning to the loss were religious beliefs. The idea that their child was relieved from suffering was a way to make sense of the loss.

"The most common benefit-finding themes centered around a desire to help others and an enhancement in compassion and understanding of deep pain. ... it seemed that the unique and profound anguish that followed the loss of their child for the majority of the parents heightened their sensitivity to the distress of others also contending with emotional pain. In fact, parents who reported helping other bereaved individuals were less likely to meet potential criteria for PGD" (Lichtenthal et al. 2010: p. 12).

The importance of being able to attribute meaning to the loss of a significant person was demonstrated by investigations of the relation between meaning reconstruction following the death of a loved one and complicated grief symptomatology in young adults in the first two years of bereavement (Neimeyer et al. 2006). The results show that strong continuing attachment to the deceased person predicted higher levels of separation distress, if the survivor was unable to make sense of the loss in personal, practical, existential, or spiritual terms.

According to Neimeyer (2011), the loss of a significant loved one interrupts the self-narrative of the surviving person. In his research dealing with the consequences of bereavement, he shows the relation between the incapacity to make sense of the loss and complicated grief. A crisis of meaning in the context of bereavement is more challenging after traumatic losses in situations of a fatal accident, suicide or homicide, than after loss by natural death. The search for signification and sense making is found in religious beliefs and in the desire to help others in their suffering. Psychotherapeutic interventions play a key role in fostering the process to "reconstruct" the life narrative of the bereaved.

Numerous studies on complicated grief have elaborated risk factors and diagnostic criteria to identify—if possible early on in the mourning process—the symptomatology of grief complications and to differentiate CG from depression, anxiety disorder, or post-traumatic stress disorder (PTSD). The period of acute grief is of course individually variable; a mourning process of 6–12 months is considered necessary to cope with the loss of a significant person. In the so-called integrated grief, the loss of the beloved one is accepted as definitive and accompanied by return to daily life activities and relationships. Grief emotions may be reactivated at crucial times such as anniversaries or other reminders of the lost person. Guidelines for counseling and therapy come to the conclusion that interventions are efficient for individuals who ask for help and present several risk factors (Shear 2012; Simon 2013; Stroebe et al. 2005, 2007).

# Grief in Children and Adolescents

And when your sorrow is comforted (time soothes all sorrows) you will be content that you have known me. You will always be my friend.

Antoine de Saint-Exupéry (1900–1944) in: The little Prince 1943 (1945)

Mourning in children is different from that in adults. The child has to mourn his loss at each new developmental phase. Only at the age of latency (6 years to puberty) can a child understand at the cognitive level that death is a loss forever. Often the child imagines that death is reversible as his desire for reunion with a lost parent is so strong that even if the child knows the truth, his fantasies have a greater impact. A child is not able to accomplish a grieving process alone; he needs the help of a meaningful adult person to fulfill a process of mourning.

According to Freud (1925–1926), the construction of the human personality is shaped by ongoing losses; at birth the infant experiences its first loss, namely, the warmth and well-being in utero. Infant and early childhood development is accompanied by loss and gain, i.e., growing up goes hand in hand with losing. However one always tries to compensate for loss and instead of loss to obtain a gain. During the growth process, the child gains an ever-greater autonomy. This simultaneous gain may allow in parallel a grieving process of experienced losses.

Infants and toddlers have no memories when everything goes well but do remember if the continuity in their lives has been interrupted, which leads to distrust (Winnicott 1965). Holding[2] creates a feeling of trust in the environment, of stability that allows the continuity of personal experience; a "silent" communication takes place long before speech develops.

Children's mourning can be described as a mental process that a child goes through after a loss and allows him to continue his development in the normal range. A child's grief cannot be compared to that of an adult because mourning as such occurs only after adolescence. For his mourning process, the child needs an emotionally significant adult, available in a continuous relationship. The child understands a loss only according to his psychological development. The loss of a significant relationship arouses existential fears and needs for security, protection, and narcissistic gratification. The child has not yet developed the maturity to cope with the intense feelings of sadness, fear, anger, and longing; therefore he denies the loss. Very often the child maintains—on a fantasy level—his bond to the lost caregiver, i.e., he continues an inner relationship with the lost person. Such fantasy occupations and internal dialogues may be—if not excessive—temporarily helpful. In this way feelings of loss can be fended off until a level of development is reached at which the child can endure his psychic pain.

### Clinical Vignette Jacqueline and Samuel

Jacqueline, living in the United States, lost her father at the age of 2 years and 9 months. The mother left the United States after the death of her husband and lived with her two children in Switzerland. For half a year after her father's death,

---

[2] Winnicott's concept of holding means safeguarding and maintaining the continuity of the infant's or child's experience of being and being alive over time.

Jacqueline continued to call him (in her play) every night, just as she had previously phoned him while he was in hospital. Her brother Samuel who is 5 years older than her told at school that his father worked in America. Two years after the father's death, the mother returned with her two children to the United States. At the father's grave, Jacqueline broke down and cried for hours as she had expected to find her father again.

Both children had denied their father's death and maintained in their phantasms the hope of seeing him again. Phantasms have an omnipotent character and are also expressed by playing over and over again the same scene, such as being reunited with the lost person. These are symbolic repetitions of preserving and losing, of being present and absent, in order to better cope with the traumatic experience of the loss. Children try to understand and cope with traumatic experiences by building an imaginary world "explaining" what has happened to them. A child can tell his phantasms in the form of stories. He needs to share his trauma-associated memories, fantasies, and feelings with a relevant adult person in a continuous relationship. If parents are burdened with their own unprocessed losses, they are not available to help their child with his grief. The meaning of the lived experience is revised again and again by the child during the course of his development.

A grieving process proves necessary, not only for the child to continue his developmental process but also to prevent him from reproducing his traumatic experience and undergoing additional traumatization.

A child, to a much greater extent than an adult, needs outside help to meet the psychophysical needs (e.g., food, shelter), to limit his fears and not to be left alone with his feelings and fantasies. Various identification-, individuation-, and separation processes can be disturbed through losses, which aggravate the grieving process in children.

Without the presence of a significant relationship, children have trouble mourning the loss of relevant related persons. Developing a relationship with a new person meeting the needs of the child is no guarantee that the child is able to disengage from the lost, beloved person. Often it is simply an attempt to shift the old love for a new person—a defensive measure against the longing pain. Processes of undoing and reversing, aggressiveness, and idealization of a lost parent may be used in order to prevent perception of ambivalence toward the deceased person and to avoid feelings of guilt. The construction of a new relationship is a difficult task since children must mourn their bonding-losses and in parallel build up new relationships. The ability to accept the reality of an irretrievable loss is indispensable for mourning. Triggered by internal development phases or by external experiences, the child has to take over again and again the grieving process.

The working through of loss by a child is particularly difficult when the specific circumstances of the death lend apparent reality to the child's developmental problems (e.g., oedipal situation, rivalry). Fantasies over the cause of death or preconscious fantasies that contain aggressive impulses (e.g., death wishes) and guilt feelings can complicate the mourning process, thereby affecting a fresh mental start.

### Grief in Children Who Do Not Live with Their Biological Parents

Children growing up in institutions or with foster or adoptive parents can cleave their feelings by maintaining a love relationship and a longing for their biological parents, and building up aggressive relationships with the actual care persons; grieving of the separation or loss of loved, still-living persons cannot take place. These children have a tendency to repeatedly form relationships in the hope of being relieved from the internalized relationship with a non-deceased but absent parent, mainly the biological mother.

Often children deny the loss and hold on to the bonds with their biological parents or primary caregivers (Manzano 1989). Their life happens in the past, in a hidden way. They maintain a dialogue with the lost parent, or they imagine before falling asleep that their most meaningful person is present, holding them in his or her arms, telling them all their misfortunes, praying to God for them. They fantasy a reunion with the lost parent, to whom all their love is devoted. This helps the child to alleviate the painful loss of parental love and to maintain a much-needed narcissistic gratification. The emotional significance of the internal parental representation does not diminish, but on the contrary is idealized and overinvested. The denial of the loss of a parent exists simultaneously with the conscious and correct knowledge of the reality of the loss (Freud 1927–1931). If these children allow themselves to begin mourning, they have to give up the hope of again finding the parent and being able to (re)establish a relationship with him or her. From the absent or dead parent, information or knowledge is not available and there are no witnesses or testimony from family members with memories of the lost parent, no funeral, and no grave. Therefore mourning for these children is impaired as the loss cannot be perceived and recognized as permanent and irrevocable.

*PATRICE,* 9 years old, living with foster parents, wants to return to the past to see his mother again. "I cannot accept that my (biological) mother died; I do not want to admit that she no longer lives; there is no reason why she should have died; therefore I have no explanation and God, I can ask only when I am dead."

Children who do not have contact with biological parents are unable to explain why they were abandoned, felt as being rejected. They often ask the same question: why have I been abandoned and why me, what is my otherness, my fault that my mother did not want to take care of me? The child is not satisfied with answers that explain the context, e.g., situations of war or poverty. The idea of having been rejected, given away, is associated with very painful, even unbearable feelings.

### Grief After the Loss of a Parent or a Significant Caregiver

The death of a parent is considered as one of the most stressful life events that a child can experience. It may be anticipated (e.g., cancer); the parent may die unexpectedly (e.g., myocardial infarction, cerebral hemorrhage) or traumatically by accident, suicide or homicide. A child may also lose his single parent.

Offspring who lose a parent by suicide, accident, or sudden natural death have a higher risk for psychic illness, such as depression or PTSD. This may be explained in part by a higher incidence of psychiatric disorders in the deceased and/or surviving parent, compared to controls (Melhem et al. 2008).

Feelings of grief are often suppressed or expressed through somatic complaints. The desperate sadness may suddenly be revealed through weeping crises, when, for example, a beloved pet dies or when the child suffers a minor physical injury. Children also rely on pets or animated objects, such as stuffed animals with which they engage a dialogue. The animal serves as a kind of binding to the lost caregiver and provides comfort and represents a support-giving companion.

(Un)conscious aggressive emotions toward the lost caregiver are caused by feelings of having been abandoned and rejected and are expressed in aggressive and destructive behavior toward present caregivers who are blamed for the loss, as they cannot be directed against the lost parent/caregiver. Anger and rage are revealed in play and by destructive activity. The loss or death of a parent "confirms" a child's mainly unconscious aggressive wishes and feelings toward his parent. Children deny the often strong feelings of guilt. Their presumed fault is to have caused the death or loss, and therefore they deserve punishment or even death.

Thoughts of death or even suicide attempts arise from fantasied wishes to be reunited with the lost parent. The desire to die also expresses the need to be punished. Severe illness, injury, and separation are equivalent to death or loss, and in all these situations, the child is afraid of dying or wishes to die.

*PETER,* a 10-year-old boy who lost his father at the age of 4, was found by his mother on the window sill, wanting to jump out of the window. To the child psychotherapist, he explained: "Now I know that a dead person does not come back. This would be a miracle. I have to kill myself to be reunited again with my father."

Upon the death of a parent, a child is deprived of his fundamental identificatory references. A child may fight against identification with a sick or dead mother; if it is a girl, she may behave like a boy and express her wish to become a father. Smaller children, contrariwise, may identify with the lost loved person and become ill like their mother or father. Some children identify with the death (personification) and not with the deceased person. They develop fears that death will call upon them or that the dead parent may come back for revenge (fantasies of retaliation).

Eight-year-old *MAURICE,* who lost his father through suicide, suffered from panic anxiety and sleep disorders: he believed that his father would come back to kill him. In his play he repetitively built ladders and telephone connections, which—as he said—reach up to heaven, so that he could establish contact with his father and be reunited with him.


## Mourning of a Sibling

The adaptation processes of parents and siblings of a dying child are described as "anticipatory grief." The more the healthy siblings sense that their parents can endure their feelings of sadness and anger, the more likely they are able to tolerate their own emotions. The siblings of dying children are considered as one of the most neglected group in bereaved families. Studies show that siblings benefit the most from counseling sessions with bereaved families, while the parent's mourning difficulties do not fundamentally change.

Children and young adults intensively mourn a sibling lost during childhood. A close emotional relationship with a sibling before his death increases the grief reaction. Feelings of rivalry among siblings may turn over to guilt feelings after the death of the sibling. "Because of the mixed feelings that accompany any relationship, as well as a myriad of unconscious fantasies, a death of a sibling is likely to bring with it a range of reactions, including grief, relief, guilt, shame, anger, blame, and remorse" (Christian 2007: p. 51).

After losing a sibling, a child always loses his "former" parents; thus children and adolescents who lose a sibling have to cope with multiple losses. Parents face a threefold task: besides their own grief, they have to help their dying child and the surviving siblings with their grief processes. Siblings' angry feelings toward the parents unable to mourn the loss of their child and therefore unable to help the surviving brothers and sisters are an additional source of guilt. The enhanced and generalized anxiety of losing someone dominates and modifies social interactions. For each child or adolescent, mourning a deceased sibling will be an individual process, sometimes carried out only years later. As adults, they consider the loss of a sibling during childhood as one of the most important life events that has left traces and will persist throughout their life.

Grief work after the loss of a child or a sibling is in about half the parents only partially or not at all achieved.[3] Fathers seem to have more difficulties to grieve and often take refuge in work. Mothers succeed better—even during the period of their child's illness—to allow and express their sad and painful feelings. Guilt feelings arise from the idea of having transferred illness and death to their child, instead of health and life. For many years after the loss of a child, parents are occupied with maintaining their relation to the deceased child.

## Pathological Grief and Secret

The delineation of normal and pathological grief is difficult and controversial. There is pathological grief when mourning is delayed, particularly long, unusually grave, suppressed, or even nonexistent. The assessment of pathological grief in children must consider the circumstances of the loss, the grieving process, subsequent events,

---

[3] "One knows that the acute mourning after such a loss will run its course, but one will remain unconsoled and never find a substitute. Everything that takes its place, even if it should fill that place entirely, remains something else. And actually, it's good that way. It is the only way to continue the love, which after all one does not want to give up" (Freud in a letter to Binswanger, April 11, 1929. 1960: p. 386).

and the personal developmental changes. Generally, one can speak of pathological mourning when the child expresses sadness in behavior and symptoms that—according to his level of development—can no longer be considered as an appropriate response to the loss. For a small child, this is the case when there is loss of already acquired functions, such as walking or talking, and/or the loss of affects or when a persistent regression (a return to earlier behavior and modes of experience) takes place. The preschool child and the child in latency may present a behavior of retreat, depression, or the abandonment of pleasurable functions or skills. In adolescence, the inability to perform the mourning process can also seriously affect the engagement of relationships or learning processes (Bürgin and Steck 2013).

Studies on prolonged grief disorders in children and adolescents demonstrate the necessity for investigation and treatment (Spuij et al. 2012; Melhem et al. 2007, 2013). Ten percent of children and adolescents confronted with sudden death of a parent suffer extended and persistent grief reactions up to 3 years after the parental death. Following the death of a parent, a sibling, or another close relative, children and adolescents may present with a symptomatology similar to PTSD, anxiety, or depression disorders but also with additional manifestations including shock and refusal to acknowledge the death, feelings of intense longing for the lost person, suicidal ideas, and loss of the sense of meaning of one's life and of one's Weltanschauung (worldview).

Traumatic experience of loss in a family, which could not be dealt with and overcome, often represents the starting point for the development of family secrets. The formation of a family secret seems to be comparable to the creation of a "void," a hidden space in the mind of the individual, which is subsequently often filled with bizarre intrapsychic fantasies (Khan 1976). A secret always arises in a meaningful relationship and is a shared experience (Abraham and Torok 1987). In painful loss situations, such as ruptures of relationships or origins, the child records and "integrates" a "picture" of the moment of the event and the persons involved, along with associated feelings of shock, fear, pain, anger, guilt, and shame. A child or adolescent may, under certain circumstances, later identify with these stored memories or express associated or fantasied affects and feelings again (Tisseron 1992).

The child has no organized representation of traumatic experiences occurring in early childhood—not even in the form of images—but they leave sensorimotor traces. Repression capacity or mental processing in infancy is still insufficiently formed. Under certain circumstances, especially in adolescence, the traces of these events "wake up" and are expressed as somatic or motor manifestations or experienced as intense feeling states or acted out as emotional outbursts. Events that cannot be mentally adequately represented risk merging with archaic fantasies and fears of the subject (Tisseron 1992). The presence of a secret involves any meaningful relationship, for example, in a relationship where an individual depends on the other person—as in the case of a child on his parents—or in a love relationship. The affective experience in the personal history of an individual is in such cases reactualized. The reactivation harbors the hope that the meaningful person, for example, a parent, will open the secret, explain its meaning, and help the child to understand its importance.

When painful or violent situations of loss such as relationship-ruptures are silenced in the family and the child receives no help to cope with such an event, then his emotional resonance is partly cleaved or encapsulated so that the child does not perceive the feelings of shock, fear, pain, anger, and shame associated with the event. At a later point in his life, the child may again feel and sometimes express these emotions which have been changed by the process of retrospective attribution.[4] They are first felt as strange, sometimes even as a foreign body. "Enigmatic message" is "a perplexing and impenetrable implicit communication that is overloaded with significance. Such messages implant themselves as foreign bodies, haunting questions in the child's psyche" (Laplanche 1999: p. 242, fn.17).

## Transgenerational Transmission of Traumatic Events

The consequences of severely psychic traumata can—under certain circumstances—be transmitted from one generation to another like a cultural heritage. The history of the parents blends into the personal history of their child and is inseparable. The past of the parents becomes the present for their child. An individual psychic traumatic event of the child can lead to the discovery of a transgenerationally transmitted trauma that represents a traumatic event in the life of a subject's parent.

Numerous authors studied the transmission of traumata and losses through the process of identification including—to mention a few—Abraham and Torok (1987) who speak of "endocryptic identification," Faimberg (2005) of "telescoping," Kestenberg (1993) of "transposition," Kogan (1995) of "concretization," and Oliner (1995) of "hysterical identification."

Abraham and Torok (1987) contrast "introjection," a process that enriches the self, endowing it with certain features of the lost person, and "incorporation," a mechanism that merely transfers the lost person within the self without acknowledging the loss. There is incorporation whenever loss is denied. As a result, the lost person attaches itself to the subject as a "ghost" would, and this inclusion of another being through the process of "incorporation" turns the subject into a "crypt carrier".

Communication from unconscious to unconscious[5] (Abraham and Torok 1987; Nachin 1993) takes place in the earliest preverbal interactions (whose variables are of tactile, visual, auditory, or sensorimotor nature) between infant/toddler and the primary caregiver. Nonintegrated, unprocessed traumatic experiences of a parent can be passively transmitted by unconscious, nonverbal forms of communication to the child (Nachin 1993). Through identification with life experiences of persons from

---

[4] Retrospective attribution (Modell 2006) or deferred action (in German Nachträglichkeit) implies a complex and reciprocal relationship between a significant event and its later reinvestment with meaning, a reinvestment that lends it a new psychic efficacy.

[5] As part of intersubjective processes, two minds can transmit and receive unconscious "messages."

the previous generations, the child actively assumes unconsciously intrapsychic, transgenerational conflict configurations (Faimberg 2005). These identifications are often alienating.

In transgenerational mandates by a parent (or sometimes both), with which a child is overidentified in an intrapsychic archaic–fusional relationship, the child makes himself available to take over the mourning that the parent was unable to accomplish. In these cases the mourning process involves the differentiation and detachment from mental representations, the working through of multiple, often strange feelings associated with the past of the mourning ill parent, and finally the abandonment of the fantasied narcissistic omnipotence, such as to heal the parent(s). In this process—often very difficult to understand—the individual (un)consciously fears to live an intolerable loss of love and a narcissistic emptiness.

If mourning cannot be fulfilled, secret intrapsychic crypts or enclaves, a form of pathological grief, are formed. These are set up by incorporation fantasies. They preserve an irreplaceable representation of a highly significant person whose sudden loss must be radically denied. However the child of a parent, bearer of a crypt, is at risk to unconsciously "import" the crypt—through identificatory processes—into his own mind. The child thus becomes a "phantom carrier" (Abraham and Torok 1987). The phantom corresponds to the unconscious processing of a non-confessable secret of another significant person. The child's play represents not only the symbolic production of his own instinctual impulses but also unconscious facts, hidden suffering, and concealed fears of his parents. The child symbolizes what it does not understand and what cannot be named. Sometimes a child acts out scenes that are intended to represent a kind of fantasied solution to the parent's problem, but sometimes the child suffers serious mental and intellectual inhibition. The clinical manifestations result from the psychic stress and the coping attempts of the child, coupled with his hope to understand his parents and, in turn, to be better understood and loved by his parents. At the same time, the child seeks to fill gaps in his own representations. According to Diatkine (1986), a family secret leads to intellectual inhibition when a child incorporates the crypt of a parent who denies the loss of the loved person. Under these conditions, the child is not stimulated by the secret. On the contrary such inherited mental representations oblige the child not to know and forbid him even to think.

### Clinical Vignette Sandra and Andrew

Incorporation fantasies keep the lost person intrapsychically in a state of dead–alive or dead–dying person. An adopted 9-year-old girl (with severe learning difficulties, but good intelligence) and her 11-year-old brother (with behavioral and psychosomatic symptoms) were abandoned by their mother and their father was murdered. The children are integrated into two different psychoanalytical oriented psychodrama therapy groups.

Sandra suggests playing the story of a boy who is always hungry and wants to eat. During the play, Sandra, who assigned the role of the boy to someone else, tells what happened to the boy. "He was so very hungry that he ate his mother, killed, and lost her. Therefore he's an orphan; he is always hungry and has to eat." Sandra's fantasies show that she has incorporated her mother and has to feed her, but stays forever insatiable. Sandra maintains a loyal, vampire-like fantasy-bond with her biological mother.

Her symptom points to an encapsulated sadness (Steck and Bürgin 1996). Incorporation fantasies assume that thoughts, feelings, ideas, or persons can be incorporated like objects into the body in a magical way. Incorporation fantasies tend to maintain—inside the subject—the lost loved person in a strange state between dead and alive. The actual fate of the person and the reality of the loss are denied.

Sandra's brother Andrew constantly proposes stories of violence-related death and chooses the role of the dying or the dead. Sick with influenza, he cries and screams in the arms of his adoptive father for hours, telling him that he is going to be killed and that he wants to die.

The examples show that Sandra maintains her loyal bond to the lost person, her biological mother, in a state of an alive person, feeding her, while Andrew maintains his fantasy bond to his murdered father in a state of an ever-again dying person. Both incorporation fantasies allow a continuity binding to a loved person of whom the subject does not need to separate. The pain of the missing person is in this way alleviated. The subject does not have to admit the real pain of the "wound".

## Neurobiology of Grief and Depression

Grief, pain, and depression are states of mind that remain subjective, not truly measurable because they contain a major personal and cultural dimension. The neurobiological strategy proposed to apprehend these affects and emotions is to relate them to neuronal structures and specific brain systems. This approach is based on the general concept that emotions are primarily understood as a response to biologically important life challenging situations. Emotions represent primary affective processes that serve adaptive evolutionary purposes. Positive affects tell us that we can go on, while negative affects inform us that we might be in a threatening situation.

These basic emotional elements have been classically studied in a behavioral perspective of reward and punishment in animals. There is a growing body of evidence demonstrating that similar emotional systems are found in humans. Therefore, researchers today are looking intensively at the subcortical structures uncovered in nonhuman mammals to explain, at least in part, the emotional reactions occurring in grief and related psychic stress situations. Attempts are being made to study primary emotional processes according to their affective quality (Zellner et al. 2011).

Panksepp tried to clarify the functional neuroanatomical processes involved in the generation of grief (Panksepp 2011). Especially in its intensive form, grief activates the panic–loss system, resulting in feelings of distress and helplessness.

This panic–loss system includes the periacqueductal gray (PAG) in the midbrain and ascends through the dorsomedial thalamus to various basal forebrain nuclei and cingulate forebrain regions. It is under the control of brain opioids. We previously described (see Chap. 11) this system as an important center for modulating pain, and as we noticed, there are similarities between the brain pathways involved in physical and social pain (Eisenberger et al. 2003), suggesting that the separation distress system evolved from the more ancient and basic physical pain system.

In the grieving process, very often feelings of anger and rage arise. This can be part of the very early response, the so-called fight-or-flight reaction. In its acute form, the fight-or-flight reaction in mammals is typically associated with a motor response such as grimacing, a defensive body posture, and is sometimes accompanied by aggressive sounding noises. The limbic brain, especially the medial part of the amygdala, processes this emotional reaction. Rage or uncontrollable anger should not only be understood as depicting violent behavior but can also express despair and hopelessness. Rage represents a final and innate path of an emotion with multifaceted traits. In the end separation and loss—if sustained—is followed by chronic despair and a depressive mood.

Rage or anger is very often a symptom of depression: it is as if a depressive state impairs our emotional control. Impulsive and aggressive behavior has been linked to dysfunction of the neurotransmitter serotonin. Of interest is the fact that serotonin reuptake inhibitors are useful to treat patients with depression but are also used in the treatment of aggressive personality disorders (Owens and Nemeroff 1994; Lesch et al. 2012). Patients with brain injuries, particularly of the basal forebrain, have difficulties regulating their emotions and often suffer from violent rage outbursts. Many research findings point to the fact that deficits in emotional regulation resulting in aggressive and violent behavior can be attributed to dysfunction of the serotonergic system (Lesch et al. 2012). Serotoninergic neurons are found in the raphe nucleus of the brain stem, and these neurons project to the amygdala, hippocampus, basal ganglia, thalamus, hypothalamus, and cortex, thus mediating multiple functions such as perception, cognition, emotion, and visceral functions like circadian rhythm and food intake. This multiplicity of functions exemplifies a well-known problem in brain research. On the one hand, we have the rather well-defined subcortical networks proposed by Panksepp (2011)[6] based on animal experiments, to explain basic emotional subtypes. On the other hand, we have the much more complex organizational networks revealed by imaging studies in humans. For example, multiple cortical regions such as somatosensory areas are activated when we feel emotions (Damasio et al. 2000). To get a coherent view and to understand grief and associated emotions and behaviors in humans, we need to integrate the topology of small brain networks to the larger-scale representations present at any moment in the brain of the grieving subject.

---

[6] Panksepp describes seven basic primary emotional subtypes consisting of *SEEKING* (reward), *RAGE*, *FEAR*, sexual *LUST*, maternal *CARE*, separation distress *PANIC–GRIEF* (simply *PANIC*), and joyful *PLAY*.

The networks generating negative affects, activated during grieving, such as the panic–loss system, will ultimately impair the brain reward system leading to further emotional imbalance and depression. The seeking or reward system in rodents classically connects the brain stem and the hypothalamus with the olfactory and frontocortical apparatus and is only part of the much more complex system found in humans (Ikemoto and Panksepp 1999).

The importance of the reward-seeking circuitry in emotional processing has been the subject of intense interest with respect to depression and its treatment. It started with the observation of hypomania in Parkinsonian patients treated with deep brain stimulation of the subthalamic nuclei. Coenen et al. (2009) were the first to point out that hypomania was the consequence of the inadvertent stimulation of the seeking system or, as it is now also called, the medial forebrain bundle (MFB). The complex functional neuroanatomy of the MFB has been dissected. It is composed of multiple distinct circuits containing the ascending monoamine system, the mesolimbic dopamine system, and interneurons producing different neuropeptides such as orexin. The MFB should be conceived as an important and complex system with multiple subcomponents (Coenen et al. 2012).

Anatomical and imaging studies have shown that the anterior thalamic radiation system or ATR, thought to be the anatomical correlate of the panic system in humans, runs so closely to the MFB that it has often been mistaken for it (see Fig. 5.2 in Chap 5). Fibers from the ATR system are directed to the orbitofrontal cortex and the anterior cingulate gyrus (CG), in particular CG25,[7] an area that is overactive in depressed patients (Mayberg et al. 2005). Another area that is overactive in the depressive state is the lateral habenula, a brain region activated by negative emotional cues such as fear or stress (Li et al. 2013).

## New Treatments for Depression

The current thinking is to view depression as a multimodal system-level disorder affecting discrete and specific pathways that are altered in response to negative external stimuli. Under certain circumstances this leads to maladaptive changes at both cellular and molecular levels, in which individual susceptibility plays a role.

Based on these findings, focal neuromodulation has been advocated to treat depression. Researchers are using deep brain stimulation (DBS) in areas such as the subcallosal cingulate gyrus to deactivate the ATR or panic systems (Coenen

---

[7] Area 25 of Brodmann is located under the anterior part of the corpus callosum and has extensive connections to the nucleus accumbens, the amygdala, the frontal cortex, the thalamus, and the periacqueductal gray. Dysfunction of this area can therefore result in an imbalance of many functional circuits.

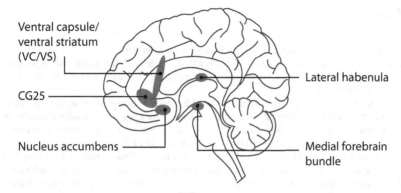

**Fig. 14.1** The different target areas currently explored in studies of deep brain stimulation to treat depression. CG (cingulate gyrus) 25 corresponds to Brodmann area 25 (Adapted from Underwood 2013)

et al. 2012), but other putative affect regulating systems, such as the nucleus accumbens, the lateral habenula, or the MFB, have also been targeted (Fig. 14.1).[8]

A far less invasive approach to treat depression is pharmacological modulation. It is widely accepted that serotonin reuptake inhibitors are effective in the treatment of depression (Gibbons et al. 2012). Many patients will however relapse. There is also a need to predict the therapeutic responses to specific classes of antidepressants since the response to drug treatment is highly individual. The identification of novel molecular targets such as neuronal-specific protein kinases (Li et al. 2013) may help to find new antidepressant drugs for treating core symptoms of depression.

Neuroimaging techniques have shown that psychotherapeutic treatment of depression is accompanied by considerable changes in large brain networks. Neuroimaging remains however very much a research tool because of the tremendous heterogeneity of psychiatric disorders (Mayberg 2014). Currently much research is devoted to a better understanding of the neural correlates of psychotherapy. The induced changes are complex, but fit with the general model of a limbic-cortical dysregulation that psychotherapy helps to reset (Messina et al. 2013). In longer therapies, psychotherapeutic treatment combined with antidepressants is associated with greater improvement compared to drug treatment alone (Nemeroff et al. 2003).

---

[8] The many different targets that are stimulated in depression reflect the conflicting views on the pathogenesis of this condition. For example, if depression is viewed as a consequence of anhedonia, the medial forebrain bundle, part of the reward system, is stimulated. Not all patients undergoing DBS will improve and there is a lack of controlled studies, so that the method remains experimental. How DBS "resets" a circuit or corrects a chemical imbalance remains to be shown (Underwood 2013).

# References

Abraham N, Torok M. L'ecorce et le noyau. Paris: Flammarion; 1987.

Bürgin D, Steck B. Indikation psychoanalytischer Psychotherapie bei Kindern und Jugendlichen, Diagnostisch-therapeutisches Vorgehen und Fallbeispiele. Stuttgart: Klett-Cotta; 2013. ISBN 978-3-608-94829-5.

Coenen VA, Honey CR, Hurwitz T, Rahman AA, McMaster J, Bürgel U, et al. Medial forebrain bundle stimulation as a pathophysiological mechanism for hypomania in subthalamic nucleus deep brain stimulation for Parkinson's disease. Neurosurgery. 2009;64(6):1106–14. doi:10.1227/01.NEU.0000345631.54446.06; discussion 1114-5.

Coenen VA, Panksepp J, Hurwitz TA, Urbach H, Mädler B. Human medial forebrain bundle (MFB) and anterior thalamic radiation (ATR): imaging of two major subcortical pathways and the dynamic balance of opposite affects in understanding depression. J Neuropsychiatry Clin Neurosci. 2012 Spring;24(2):223–36. doi:10.1176/appi.neuropsych.11080180.

Christian C. Sibling loss, guilt and reparation: a case study. Int J Psychoanal. 2007;88:41–54.

Damasio AR, Grabowski TJ, Bechara A, Damasio H, Ponto LL, Parvizi J, et al. Subcortical and cortical brain activity during the feeling of self-generated emotions. Nat Neurosci. 2000;3(10): 1049–56.

Diatkine G. Chasseurs de fantômes, dans: le secret sur les origines; problèmes psychologiques, légaux, administratifs. Paris: Editions ESF; 1986. p. 71–90.

De Saint-Exupéry A. Le Petit Prince. Paris: Gallimard; 1945.

Eisenberger NI, Lieberman MD, Williams KD. Does rejection hurt? An FMRI study of social exclusion. Science. 2003;302(5643):290–2.

Faimberg H. The telescoping of generations. London: Routledge; 2005.

Freud S. Mourning and melancholia, Standard edition, vol. XVII. London: Hogarth Press; 1917. p. 237–60.

Freud S. An autobiographical study, inhibitions, symptoms and anxiety, the question of lay analysis and other works, Standard edition, vol. XX. London: Hogarth Press; 1925–1926.

Freud S. The future of an illusion, civilization and its discontents, and other works, Standard edition, vol. XXI. London: Hogarth Press; 1927–1931.

Freud S. Letter to Binswanger. Letter 239, 1929. In: Freud EL, editor. The letters of Sigmund Freud. New York: Basic Books; 1960.

Gibbons RD, Hur K, Brown CH, Davis JM, Mann JJ. Benefits from antidepressants: synthesis of 6-week patient-level outcomes from double-blind placebo-controlled randomized trials of fluoxetine and venlafaxine. Arch Gen Psychiatry. 2012;69(6):572–9. doi:10.1001/archgenpsychiatry.2011.2044.

Ikemoto S, Panksepp J. The role of nucleus accumbens dopamine in motivated behavior: a unifying interpretation with special reference to reward-seeking. Brain Res Brain Res Rev. 1999;31(1):6–41. Review.

Kernberg O. Some observations on the process of mourning. Int J Psychoanal. 2010;91:601–19.

Kestenberg J. What a psychoanalyst learned from the holocaust and genocide. Int J Psychoanal. 1993;74:1117–29.

Khan M. The privacy of the self. London: Hogarth; 1976.

Kogan I. The cry of mute children. London: Free Association Books; 1995.

Kubler-Ross E. On death and dying. New York: Macmillan; 1969.

Laplanche J. Essays on otherness. London: Routledge; 1999.

Lesch KP, Araragi N, Waider J, van den Hove D, Gutknecht L. Targeting brain serotonin synthesis: insights into neurodevelopmental disorders with long-term outcomes related to negative emotionality, aggression and antisocial behaviour. Philos Trans R Soc Lond B Biol Sci. 2012;367(1601):2426–43. doi:10.1098/rstb.2012.0039. Review.

Li K, Zhou T, Liao L, Yang Z, Wong C, Henn F, et al. βCaMKII in lateral habenula mediates core symptoms of depression. Science. 2013;341(6149):1016–20. doi:10.1126/science.1240729.

Lichtenthal WG, Currier JM, Neimeyer RA, Keesee NJ. Sense and significance: a mixed methods examination of meaning making after the loss of one's child. J Clin Psychol. 2010;66(7): 791–812. doi:10.1002/jclp.20700.

Manzano J. La séparation et la perte d'objet chez l'enfant. Un point de vue sur le processus analytique. Rev Franç Psychanal. 1989;1:241–72.

Mayberg HS, Lozano AM, Voon V, McNeely HE, Seminowicz D, Hamani C, et al. Deep brain stimulation for treatment-resistant depression. Neuron. 2005;45(5):651–60.

Mayberg HS. Neuroimaging and psychiatry: the long road from bench to bedside. Hastings Cent Rep. 2014;Spec No:S31-6. doi:10.1002/hast.296.

Melhem NM, Moritz MPH, Walker MSW, Shear MK, Brent D. Phenomenology and correlates of complicated grief in children and adolescents. J Am Acad Child Adolesc Psychiatry. 2007; 46:493–9.

Melhem NM, Walker M, Moritz G, Brent DA. Antecedents and sequelae of sudden parental death in offspring and surviving caregivers. Arch Pediatr Adolesc Med. 2008;162(5):403–10.

Melhem NM, Porta G, Walker Payne M, Brent DA. Identifying prolonged grief reactions in children: dimensional and diagnostic approaches. J Am Acad Child Adolesc Psychiatry. 2013;52(6): 599–607.e7. doi:10.1016/j.jaac.2013.02.015.

Messina I, Sambin M, Palmieri A, Viviani R. Neural correlates of psychotherapy in anxiety and depression: a meta-analysis. PLoS One. 2013;8(9), e74657. doi:10.1371/journal.pone.0074657. eCollection 2013.

Modell AH. Imagination and the meaningful brain. Cambridge: MIT Press; 2006.

Nachin C. Les fantômes de l'âme. Paris: L'Harmattan; 1993.

Neimeyer RA, Baldwin SA, Gillies J. Continuing bonds and reconstructing meaning: mitigating complications in bereavement. Death Stud. 2006;30(8):715–38.

Neimeyer RA. Reconstructing meaning in bereavement. Riv Psichiatr. 2011;46(5-6):332–6.

Nemeroff CB, Heim CM, Thase ME, Klein DN, Rush AJ, Schatzberg AF, et al. Differential responses to psychotherapy versus pharmacotherapy in patients with chronic forms of major depression and childhood trauma. Proc Natl Acad Sci U S A. 2003;100(24):14293–6.

Nietzsche F. The will to power. In: Kaufman W, editor. (Kaufman W, Hollingdale RJ, trans.). New York: Vintage Books; 1967.

Oliner M. Hysterische Persönlichkeitsmerkmale bei Kindern Überlebender. In: Bergmann M, Jucovy M, Kestenberg J, Hrsg. Kinder der Opfer Kinder der Täter S. . Fischer Verlag GmbH: Frankfurt am Main; 1995.

Owens MJ, Nemeroff CB. Role of serotonin in the pathophysiology of depression: focus on the serotonin transporter. Clin Chem. 1994;40(2):288–95.

Panksepp J. Cross-species affective neuroscience decoding of the primal affective experiences of humans and related animals. PLoS One. 2011;6(9), e21236. doi:10.1371/journal.pone.0021236. Review.

Shakespeare W. Macbeth, Act 4, Scene 3 (1564–1616)

Shear MK, Simon N, Wall M, Zisook S, Neimeyer R, Duan N, et al. Complicated grief and related bereavement issues for DSM-5. Depress Anxiety. 2011;28(2):103–17, p. 105.

Shear MK. Grief and mourning gone awry: pathway and course of complicated grief. Dialogues Clin Neurosci. 2012;14:119–28.

Simon NM. Treating complicated grief. JAMA. 2013;310(4):416–23.

Spuij M, Reitz E, Prinzie P, Stikkelbroek Y, de Roos C, Boelen PA. Distinctiveness of symptoms of prolonged grief, depression, and post-traumatic stress in bereaved children and adolescents. Eur Child Adolesc Psychiatry. 2012;21(12):673–9. doi:10.1007/s00787-012-0307-4.

Stroebe WT, Schut H, Stroebe MS. Grief work, disclosure and counseling: do they help the bereaved? Clin Psychol Rev. 2005;25:395–414.

Stroebe M, Schut H, Stroebe W. Health outcomes of bereavement. Lancet. 2007;370:1960–73.

Steck B, Bürgin D. Über die Unmöglichkeit zu trauern bei Kindern trauerkranker Eltern. Kinderanalyse. 1996;4:351–61.

Taiana C. Mourning the dead, mourning the disappeared: the enigma of the absent–presence. Int J Psychoanal. 2014;95:1087–107. doi:10.1111/1745-8315.12237.

Tisseron S. Tintin et les secrets de famille. Paris: Aubier; 1992.

Underwood E. Short-circuiting depression. Science. 2013;342(6158):548–51. doi:10.1126/science.342.6158.548.

Vanderwerker LC, Jacobs SC, Parkes CM, Prigerson HG. An exploration of associations between separation anxiety in childhood and complicated grief in later life. J Nerv Ment Dis. 2006;194(2):121–3.

Winnicott DW. The maturational processes and the facilitating environment: studies in the theory of emotional development. London: Hogarth; 1965.

Zellner MR, Watt DF, Solms M, Panksepp J. Affective neuroscientific and neuropsychoanalytic approaches to two intractable psychiatric problems: why depression feels so bad and what addicts really want. Neurosci Biobehav Rev. 2011;35(9):2000–8. doi:10.1016/j.neubiorev.2011.01.003.

# Part IX

# Chapter 15
# Dreams and the Dreaming Brain

## History

Dreams have been regarded as messengers since antiquity. In Mesopotamia, dreams were written on clay tablets. For the Egyptians and Greeks dreams were considered as oracles from the gods,[1] predicting the future. For the ancient Hebrews dreams were the voice of their unique god, Yahweh. Ancient priests or shamans[2] could "read" the wisdom of dreams. In the Melanesian Kanak population, the elders slept on "dream boards," to be given prophetic dreams.[3]

In order to receive divine revelation—in ancient Greece—dreams were induced or incubated by performing a symbolic operation, for example, by sleeping in a dream temple. According to Hippocrates and Aristotle—in the Hellenistic period—dreams predicted on the one hand illnesses and on the other suggested how to heal a person from disease. In indigenous tribes and Mexican culture dreams allowed contact with the ancestors. As the Old Testament tells stories of dreams, Christians believed that God was speaking to them through their dreams. For St. Augustine and St. Jerome dreams had an important influence on the course of their lives. In the Middle Ages dreams were seen as evil temptations.

---

[1] "The lord who owns the Oracle of Delphi neither reveals ούτε λέγει (oute legei) nor hides ούτε κρύπτει (oute kruptei) but gives a sign αλλά σημαίνει (alla saemainei)" (Kirk et al. 1994).

[2] A shaman is a true practitioner of the dream; his task is to exceed the limits of this world in order to receive sacred power (Perrin 1992).

[3] These dream boards, located at an intermediate distance between the ground and the ceiling of the hut, formed an ideal space where the elder communicated with the world of the ancestors or the divine power.

© Springer International Publishing Switzerland 2016
A. Steck, B. Steck, *Brain and Mind*, DOI 10.1007/978-3-319-21287-6_15

## The 24-Hour Brain

The brain is very active when it is "doing nothing." This is at first glance a paradoxical statement, but the fact is that our brain is never inactive. There is considerable brain activity that goes by quietly in the background when the brain isn't "doing much of anything"; this "resting activity" may even constitute the bulk of brain activity. Indeed, it has been pointed out that the total energy consumption supporting neuronal firing in the conscious awake brain is orders of magnitude larger than that from specific brain activity during mental processes (Shulman et al. 2009). When performing a focused mental task, brain energy consumption is increased by less than 5 %. While in anesthesia there is a large decrease in the energy consumption of the brain, this is not the case in sleep. During rapid eye movement (REM) sleep, the brain's oxygen consumption is as high as in the awake state. Modern research suggests that sleep is a well-organized activity with dreams going on every night. This shows that the brain, even when disconnected from environmental stimulation, can itself generate an entire world of "conscious experience" (Nir and Tononi 2010).

## Neurophysiology of Dreams

As we fall asleep and consciousness is fading, a change in brain activity and brain chemistry occurs and in parallel a dreamlike mental activity appears. The sleeping brain remains active: we know that dreaming occurs in REM sleep periods, but it also occurs in non-REM sleep.[4] During REM sleep, brain activity is quite similar to that in the waking period: the brain awakes, while the subject remains asleep. The association of an activated cortical EEG, reminiscent of waking, along with muscle paralysis, led Jouvet (1967), a French neurophysiologist, to term the REM state "le sommeil paradoxal," paradoxical sleep. Brain imaging studies can explain this curious phenomenon. Indeed, some regions of the brain are awake, while others are sleeping. Cerebral areas responsible for image production are turned on, which explains the visual nature of dreams. Areas remaining dormant, however, include those responsible for placing objects in their physical context, such as parietal brain areas. This explains why proportions are often distorted in dreams and we see, for example, giant objects or on the contrary large objects appear as miniature. These distortions or scale anomalies, not unusual in dreams, may also be explained by the fact that frontal cortical areas involved in critical thinking are turned off in dreaming. During REM sleep the attentional network, a frontoparietal function, is turned down, so that external stimuli are ignored.

---

[4] Sleep architecture comprises non-REM sleep, further subdivided into four stages corresponding to increasing depth of sleep and REM sleep. In man a non-REM –REM sleep cycle lasts about 90 min.

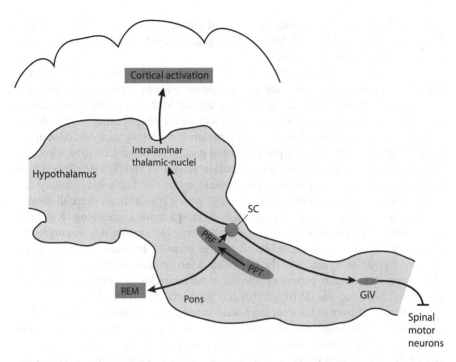

**Fig. 15.1** The pontine generator of REM sleep is constituted by the glutamatergic pontine reticular formation (PRF) and the cholinergic pedunculopontine tegmental nuclei (PPT). They induce ascending activation of the cortex and generation of rapid eye movement (REM) in the pons. They trigger also a descending activation of the noradrenergic subcoeruleus (SC) nuclei, which in turn activates the glycinergic/gabaergic ventral gigantocellular nucleus (GiV), promoting muscle atonia (Adapted from Brown et al. 2012)

The main excitatory sources for REM sleep are located within the reticular formation of the brain stem and project to the thalamus to activate the cortex, forming an extended thalamocortical system. This main generator is found in the mesopontine tegmentum (Fig. 15.1). Lesions in this region suppress REM sleep (Lin 2000). As we know REM and non-REM sleep alternate during the night as the activity of the sleeping brain switches from a cholinergic state, driven by the acetylcholine-producing neurons in the mesopontine tegmentum, to another set of neurons in the dorsal raphe nucleus and the locus coeruleus, which produce monoamines such as noradrenaline, serotonin, or dopamine.[5] Dreams occur preferentially in REM sleep, but a fair proportion of our dreams take place in non-REM sleep, especially when falling asleep and during the awakening period, but dreaming is possible at any time during the night. In a night's sleep, we usually experience about four or five periods

[5] The brain mechanisms controlling sleep and wakefulness and REM and non-REM sleep, especially the neurotransmitters responsible for the switch between these states, have been identified. Readers interested in a more in-depth description will find up-to-date information in Brown et al. (2012) and Ramaligam et al (2013).

of REM sleep. The relative amount of REM sleep varies considerably with age. A newborn baby spends about 80 % of sleep time in REM, while there is an overall decline of REM sleep in the elderly.

Considerable research has been devoted to understanding the "driving forces" behind the dreaming process. They are thought to reside in a functional system that includes parts of the limbic, occipital, and temporal lobe regions, but that excludes two critical cortical regions involved in memory and self-representation. The first is the dorsal lateral prefrontal cortex, a key region for working memory (Goldman-Rakic 1988). The second is the posteromedial portion of the parietal lobe, a cortical region involved in internal self-representation (Cavanna and Trimble 2006). The exclusion of these two important cortical areas explains the break in continuity that we experience during dreaming and especially why it is so difficult to recall dreams and why we are unaware of our physical body in space when dreaming (Kahn and Gover 2010). In view of the many functions attributed to dreams, it is no surprise to find that the "dreaming machine" involves large areas of the brain. fMRI investigations have given us a picture of the functional neuroanatomy of REM sleep. These studies reveal a complex pattern of activation and inhibition of multiple cortical and subcortical brain regions (Perogamvros and Schwartz 2012, Fig. 15.2).

Anything that arouses the sleeping brain can trigger the dreaming process. Solms and Turnbull (2002) state that in order to dream, arousal of the inner source of consciousness—an activation of the basic mechanisms of core consciousness—has to take place. The arousal trigger can be waking thoughts before falling asleep or the REM state, the latter being the most reliable trigger. Even though most dreams

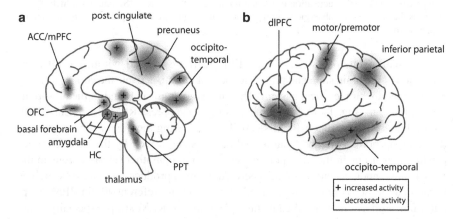

**Fig. 15.2** The complex pattern of activation and inhibition of multiple cortical and subcortical brain regions during REM sleep as visualized with fMRI. (**a**) medial view and (**b**) lateral view. The main activated regions are the pedunculopontine tegmental nuclei (PPT), the thalamus, the hippocampus (HC), the amygdala, the basal forebrain, the anterior cingulate cortex (ACC), the medial prefrontal cortex (mPFC), the motor and premotor cortex, and the occipitotemporal cortex. Downregulated areas include the dorsolateral prefrontal cortex (dlPFC), the orbitofrontal cortex (OFC), the precuneus and the inferior parietal cortex (Adapted from Perogamvros and Schwartz 2012)

occur during REM sleep, a state triggered by brain stem generators, dreaming is dependent on the integrity of cortical structures. For example, the ventromesial frontal region, an area involved in motivational behavior, is essential for dreaming suggesting that dreaming is a "motivated" process (Kaplan-Solms and Solms 2000). In other words dreaming only occurs when arousal stimuli during sleep attract motivational interest, so in a way dreams occur as a kind of a motivated action. Because the motor system is inhibited in REM sleep, voluntary motor activity does not take place during dreaming. The frontal lobes in general are inhibited or underactivated during sleep. "In the absence of the ability of the frontal lobes to program, regulate and verify our cognition, affect and perception, subjective experience becomes bizarre, delusional and hallucinated" (Solms and Turnbull 2002: p. 212).This explains the backsliding or "regressive" nature of the dreaming process.

The claim that dreams also occur during non-REM sleep is supported by many studies. For example, patients with damage to specific parts of the REM-generating structure still dream. Furthermore, epilepsy patients having seizures during non-REM sleep frequently report dreams or nightmares, reflecting the involvement of the emotional part of the brain, the limbic system (Solms and Turnbull 2002). The physiological mechanisms of dreams are similar to those for the basic emotions; the dreaming brain and the emotional brain overlap quite a bit. The fact that the hippocampus and amygdala, both parts of the limbic system, affect the emotional quality of dreaming has been confirmed by studies in patients with hippocampus damage. These patients report dreams that are short, stereotyped, and unemotional (De Gennaro et al. 2011; Torda 1969).

Of particular interest is the fact that forebrain lesions that completely spare the brain stem eliminate dreaming. Patients with focal lesions in the parieto-temporo-occipital association area experience a dramatic loss of dreaming. A complete loss of dreaming has been reported in patients with prefrontal leucotomies, where the orbito-mesial prefrontal cortex is damaged (Kaplan-Solms and Solms 2000). Based on these clinical examples, Solms and Turnbull (2002) consider that the "primary driving forces of dreaming" are to be found in an activation involving the mesocortical, mesolimbic dopaminergic system. This meso-cortico-limbic system is implicated in motivated behaviors, in emotional processing, and most importantly in reward processing. The reward-seeking property is key to the generation of an intentional goal, leading to anticipatory actions. From animal experiments it is known that lesions in this system lead to amotivational states with a marked reduced reward-seeking behavior (Ikemoto and Panksepp 1999).

Obviously not only the reward system is turned on in dreaming. The fear system, part of a defense mechanism in which the amygdala plays a key role (LeDoux 1996), is also activated most evidently in nightmares. These two systems are in fact widely interconnected, both heavily relying on limbic structures and exerting a mutually inhibitory influence. One assumes that these systems constitute an essential chain of behavioral control that is central to the dreaming state. Although it is generally admitted (Malcolm-Smith et al. 2012; Perogamvros and Schwartz 2012) that dreaming is essentially generated by the reward-seeking system, the high incidence of threatening dreams would argue for an important role of the fear system in coloring the content of dreams.

Pharmacological and clinical studies have shown that dopaminergic modulation plays an important function in dreaming. Administration of dopaminergic agonists such as L-dopa or amphetamine increases dreaming (Perogamvros and Schwartz 2012). Prefrontal leucotomy causes a diminution of dreams (Jus et al. 1973) as a result of damage to the orbito-mesial prefrontal cortex. Overall these data point to an important role of the dopaminergic reward-seeking system in the generation of dreams. By contrast dopaminergic blocking agents like neuroleptics are associated with a reduction in vivid dreaming.

## Transition States of Sleep

In falling asleep or in awakening, we often find ourselves in a unique state of consciousness, somewhere between sleep and wakefulness. The transitional state to sleep is called hypnagogia,[6] while the onset of wakefulness is called hypnopompia. In these transition states a variety of sensory experiences from vague sensations to full-blown hallucinations can occur. They include lucid dreaming and sleep paralysis. Hypnagogic experiences are often characterized by visual features but also by elaborate imagery, as if the visual cortex was fully active. It seems that the brain in default or idling modes engages the occipital cortex to play with every permutation possible, giving rise to unlimited varieties of visual phenomena. While in hypnagogic states visual imagery is often prominent, other phenomena such as sounds, voices, and smells are sensed. Hypnagogic sensory experiences are different from dreams. The formers come in flashes, while the latter have more continuity and a narrative character. Sacks (2012) suggested that in a dream one is a participant, while in the hypnagogic state one is merely a spectator of a "creation" by the visual or auditory content.

A fascinating and at the same time very frightening phenomenon is sleep paralysis or an inability to move. This is a rather rare event in the normal population but occurs frequently in neurological disorders such as narcolepsy (Ohayon et al. 1999; see Chap. 2). Instead of going gradually into the different stages of deep sleep, the person falls directly into REM sleep, his body paralyzed at the onset of sleep. Alternatively as the subject wakes up, the REM sleep state persists so that the person is unable to move. Sleep paralysis is often accompanied by hallucinatory experiences that have a vivid multimodal and terrifying character. These hallucinations not only have visual characteristics but are also often accompanied by sensory feelings such as suffocation and pressure on the chest together with a sense of total helplessness. People find themselves in a quasi-state of terror, akin to a nightmare. Nightmare is a term often utilized to mean a bad dream, but a "real" nightmare brings about an extreme sense of terror. These extraordinarily terrifying feelings are vividly expressed by Heinrich Füssli in his painting "the Nightmare," showing a

---

[6] Hypnagogia (υπναγωγία) is the experience of the transitional state from wakefulness to sleep, the hypnagogic state of consciousness. Hypnopompia is the onset of wakefulness. The related words from the Greek are Ὕπνος, "sleep"; αγωγός, "leading, inducing"; and, πομπή "act of sending."

sleeping woman with a demon sitting on her body.[7] This strong feeling of terror is the consequence of a "misinterpretation" of the dreamer who feels horribly threatened by a menacing person or animal, present in very close vicinity or an equally frightening situation. This threatening situation originates from amygdala activation, resulting in a sense of deep fear and a feeling of suffocation.

## Functions of Dreams

The study of the function of dreams cannot be dissociated from that of sleep. While many aspects remain mysterious, considerable advances have been made. At the neurobiological level it has been proposed that sleep promotes brain plasticity and stabilizes memory (Vyazovskiy et al. 2008). More specifically sleep has a key role in synapse formation and learning (Yang et al. 2014). According to this perspective dreams reflect a biological process of memory consolidation, serving to maintain and store memory representations. But there is more to it than that. Dreams may—through their hyper-associative character—not only help us organize internal memories but through unexpected associations may also lead to fresh ideas. Creativity, in the domain of scientific or artistic activities, often comes from the inspiration of dreams.

According to Modell (2006) the dream is an example of the autonomy of imagination and "bears the imprint of an individual self" (p. 58). At the same time it is a product of a neurophysiological process. The biological function of dreaming is still controversial and one cannot generalize about the function of dreams. There are probably multiple functions of dreaming. Some dreams may reflect an unconscious intentionality or may process memories of the previous day. The brain is a self-activating system and so is dreaming, which expresses the autonomy and uniqueness of an individual's imagination. "…There remains the problem of explaining the dreams self-generated content as the product of a neurophysiological process that is presumably uniform and universal" (p. 49).

The unconscious intentionality of dreams may include an inner psychic state of the previous day, may anticipate a task of the following day, or may illustrate a problem-solving process. There is no standard interpretation of dream images. Solms and Turnbull (2002) suggest that dreams occur instead of a motivated action. Because dreaming is so much linked to the seeking rewarding system, we are not far from the idea that Freud (1900, 1900–1901) proposed, namely, that dreams are a form of "wish fulfillment." Dreams can be viewed as an attempt to solve a conflict or problem.

Hartmann (2010a) makes the point that dreams reported in clinical literature (dreams in psychotherapy or psychoanalysis) and dreams reported in research literature are quite different in their content: the first are vivid and rich in images, and the latter are often dull. The dreams reported from awakening in a laboratory situation are also less interesting than those reported at home. This reflects the importance of the context and the intersubjectivity in the reporting of dreams. Working with dreams is an important tool in psychotherapy.

---

[7] The nightmare is a 1781 oil painting conserved at the Detroit Institute of Arts.

Dreaming is a form of mental functioning, representing one end of the spectrum, which goes from dreaming in sleep, through daydreaming to focused thinking in the waking state. Contemporary theories of dreaming emphasize that a major functional role of dreaming consists of creating links. These links are usually broader and looser than in the waking mind, reflecting REM sleep, with inactivation of parts of the prefrontal cortex. When dreaming we are able to connect recently experienced events to old memories in a kind of hyper-connective way or, as Freud (1900) expressed it, in a process of condensation. Hartmann (2010a) emphasizes the fact that these connections are not made randomly but are guided by the emotions of the dreamer, positive or negative, which are a major driving force in the generation of dreams. He suggests also that dreams have an adaptive function, by weaving in new material—in other words taking up new experiences and gradually connecting them into existing memory systems. It is considered as an evolutionary advantage to be able not only to think clearly and logically but also to associate thoughts more loosely, for example, in the process of creative thinking, which happens in daydreaming and dreaming. In making connections, dreams help us to condense or contextualize the dominant emotions.

After any kind of traumatic event, dreams do not necessarily picture the traumatic experience but record the intense feelings of the dreamer. The images corresponding to the underlying emotions may represent the overwhelming or terrifying feelings as, for example, flooding from a torrent or falling into void, emotions expressing helplessness and hopelessness. The dreamer's vulnerability may be revealed by an injured, bleeding, or dying animal. The nightmares may also show the emotions of being exposed, abandoned, or feelings of guilt, especially survival guilt and of mourning (Hartmann 2010b), as the following dream shows.

*RUTH*, a young female patient, musician, tells her psychotherapist the dream she had at the anniversary of her father's death: "My father, in his wheelchair, is assisting at a graduation ceremony at which I should sing…Then the scenery changes: My dad is on stage, plays the piano, and sings joyfully an English Gospel song and I start to cry…." Ruth, overwhelmed by sadness, weeps.

Maggiolini et al. (2010) analyzed typical dream contents (e.g., characters, actions, and situations) and compared them with waking life events. They explored the coherence and continuity between dream content and waking life episodes. They consider that dreams are not just thoughts represented by images but more akin to "emotional thoughts," representing affective symbolization and expressing affective consciousness. The results of their analysis demonstrate that there is no difference with regard to characters and social interactions between dream and waking life narratives, except for physical aggression, which is more frequent in dreams. From an evolutionary perspective the representation of threats in dreams may prepare the person for situations in real life and serve the survival of the species (Revonsuo 2000). Situations, where dreams appear to be most in discontinuity with waking life, are those in which the subject is trying to perform a physical action but has difficulties in mastering it, particularly when the dreamer is unable to situate himself in space and loses the control of his body. "Such sensations—sensations of falling, for instance, or floating, or being inhibited—provide a material which is accessible at any time and of which the dream-work makes use, whenever it has need of it, for expressing the dream-thoughts" (Freud 1900: p. 590). Cognitive activities such as writing, reading, or calculating are rarely present in dream and waking event narratives.

According to psychoanalytical theories (Blum 2011), the functions of dreams are multiple. For Freud (1900) dreams generally represent fulfillment of unconscious infantile wishes and are "the guardian of sleep." Dreams are always a form of communication and are probably influenced by the interest of the listener, in psychotherapy the psychoanalyst. The verbalization of a dream can hardly ever exactly report the subjective dream experience with all its somatosensory, emotional, and visual contents. "All aspects of the dream are significant for the understanding of the dreamer and the dream, including the sequence of associations before as well as after the dream report" (Blum 2011: p. 276). According to Freud "Even the unintelligible dream must be a valid psychical act ... which we can use in analysis" (Freud 1933: p. 9 in Blum 2011: p 276).

For da Rocha Barros (2011) "Dreams function as a form of unconscious thinking"... which "transforms affects into memories and mental structures" (p. 270). The mind in a dream attempts "to deal with conflicts by giving expressive pictorial representation to the emotions involved in a conflict: it is a first step to thinkability" (p. 270). According to Martin Cabre (2011) the function of dreams is a source of information on a patient's current affects and may be his preferred approach in the analytic relationship. A second function is the reactivation and symbolizing of earlier emotions, dating from past (traumatic) experiences, e.g., from early childhood, stored in implicit memory.

Ferenczi (1931) called the function of dreams, which express emotions of traumatic events, "traumatolysis." He postulated that some dreams had a recovery function when patients expressed their bodily or sensory suffering, especially in dreams where images, psychic contents, and language were missing, but represented affective memories. Winnicott (1949) attributed a healing function to the dream.

## Clinical Vignette Elisa

This vignette demonstrates different dream functions of *Elisa*, a female middle-aged patient in analysis. In her dreams she lives extensively terrifying and overwhelming feelings, yet without the corresponding images of the multiple separations, she has suffered in early childhood. These emotions dating from past traumatic experiences, stored in implicit memory, are reactivated and appear in her dream.

"I am standing alone on a bare mountain, on the uttermost peak; thousand meters underneath I hear the roaring sea. I am wearing only a straw bag over breasts and hips. There is an endless vastness, no horizon to be seen, only a power pylon rising high up into the sky. Suddenly I tumble and I fall, fall, fall and wake up screaming, with horror, panic fear, my heart racing and my body freezing."

The dream demonstrates the vivid emotions of threat, despair, and fears of annihilation and death and shows how lonely, desolate, abandoned, and helpless the patient felt in her dream. On telling her dream in the analytical session, it gains consciousness and its presence demonstrates its actuality.

Elisa then associates, telling her analyst: "I am exposed, abandoned to the bare and roaring archaic elements, almost naked, without any orientation or references; there is no hold except a dangerous high power pylon: death is certain if I grasp the pylon, but I fall. Everything hurts me, my soul but also my whole body. All my strength is gone; I can only cry. I feel like a leaf in the wind, wherever I fall, death is certain; it is only a question of when and where. Threatened in my existence, I am without orientation, confused, bewildered. What is outside, what is inside in me? What happens inside me is mirrored in the outer reality. Is there any way to distinguish inside from outside? The outer reality feels as if it takes place within me. My fear is terrifying. It is as if I would be threatened from inside and from outside. Without any protection I am at the mercy of death."

The patient is no longer able to distinguish between outer and inner reality, a confusional state she must have lived in her childhood when she was not able to integrate the traumatic events she had experienced.

The analysand's and analyst's shared understanding of the unconscious emotional experiences was helpful in (re)constructing these implicit memories. Identifying connections between past lived experiences and the present allows the elaboration for gradual emotional understanding and significant meaning. The verbalization of "emotional thoughts" and bodily sensations and the ensuing associations helped the patient to conscious awareness of her feelings, to symbolization of her affects, and to attribute meanings to her experiences. Implicit memories of her past history gained over the course of time conscious representations, alleviated her fears, and reduced her confusion.

Interestingly, sensation of pain in dreams is rarely reported and seems to be associated to pain in sleep or in waking life; in other words pain in dreams is seldom perceived, without any pain experience in the waking life of the dreamer (Schredl 2011). The lack of pain in dreams may be related to inhibitory processes in sensory transmission during REM sleep (Nielsen et al. 1993).

## Lucid Dreaming

When we dream, we have no voluntary control over the imaginary, the visual pictures, or the emotional feelings of our dreams. In dreams there may be no continuity in time and space with the waking state. In lucid dreaming the subject is aware that the ongoing dream is only a dream and not reality (Voss et al. 2012). This suggests that one has the ability to watch the dream from "outside" as the dream unfolds. Lucid dreaming may not be very frequent but is experienced by most persons. It can be considered as a specific state of consciousness, a so-called proto-consciousness where part of the brain remains asleep, while other parts display a waking level of functioning (Hobson and Voss 2011). Interestingly lucid dreaming occurs essentially during REM sleep, a stage of sleep where there is a strong physiological dissociation, part of the brain being very active and others remaining inactive, as sensory informations from the outside world are shut off.

Lucid dreaming is a process of conscious awakening, in which the person knows that he is dreaming. He is engaged in dreaming and at the same time has access to the awaken consciousness. There are different degrees in lucid dreaming: e.g., to know that one is dreaming up to directing the narrative of the dream, for example, trying to find a better solution to a problematic content in the dream (Kahn and Gover 2010).

*NICOLE*, a female patient, dreams repetitively of her beloved dog, which is lost or abandoned, paralyzed, or in danger of being killed, always threatened by death. In her dreams Nicole tries to do everything and anything to save her dog. She is desperate, overwhelmed by fear and then—knowing it is a dream—directs the content of her dream to a happy ending: the dog is alive and safe and the patient is overjoyed. "Finally I could not be happier; it is as if I am participating in the dream—from the outside—to protect my dog from menacing situations over and over again."

## Daydreaming

Daydreaming or mind wandering takes up a large part of our waking life. fMRI studies demonstrate that with decreasing external task demands, certain regions of the brain are increasingly activated. Regions that are activated during daydreaming are the medial prefrontal cortex, the posterior cingulate cortex, and the posterior temporoparietal cortex, areas that are part of the default network. Surprisingly the dorsolateral prefrontal cortex (DLPFC), a main region of the executive network, may also be recruited in daydreaming. While it was assumed from behavioral investigations that mind wandering interferes with cognitively demanding tasks, studies show that mind wandering may actually be a unique mental state associating reflective subjective states to executive resources, thus combining two brain networks that are usually viewed as working in opposing directions (Christoff et al. 2009).[8]

In support of the hypothesis that there is a continuum of mental functioning between the awake and dreaming states, several authors consider that dreaming is in many ways continuous with waking fantasies, reveries, and daydreams (Hartmann 2012). This does not mean that dreaming is like thinking, but suggests that there is a gradual change between waking thoughts and dreaming. It is interesting to consider these arguments on a neurobiological level. Brain imaging studies show a progressive shift in cortical brain regions with a strong activation of the dorsolateral prefrontal cortex (DLPFC) in focused waking thought. In daydreaming there is reduced activity in the DLPFC, but increased activity in the ventromesial portion of the prefrontal area (Perogamvros and Schwartz 2012). Eventually in REM sleep the

---

[8] Our brain operates classically in two modes: a task-focused network, the so-called cognitive control network (CCN), also referred to as the central executive network, and the default mode network (DMN) that is active when our mind is wandering. The shift between these two modes involves the insula, a region of the brain constituted by the parietotemporal junction.

DLPFC is completely inactivated (Fig.15.2), which explains the lack of cognitive control. It appears therefore that different cortical activity patterns underlie wakeful thoughts and dreaming, including daydreaming. The fact that cortical regions play such a paramount role in dreaming is supported by clinical studies reviewed by Solms (1997). For example, patients with brain damage following a stroke showed either a global cessation or a reduction of dreaming.

Freud (1908) and other psychoanalysts were particularly interested in daydreaming or what they call interior monologue (Singer 2003). Freud (1908) focused on the link between the child's early play and future creative activities. Pretend play in childhood, the occurrence of imaginary playmates, and various forms of as-if or make-believe plays are essential parts of an infant and small child's life and development. The content of these plays shows many different and individual aspects: the child presents himself with his desires and how he perceives the context in which he lives; very often the child's play presents his attempt to deal with a situation, to master problems, and to playfully search for solutions and has therefore an adaptive and healthy function. As children enter school, their playing activities continue above all at home; the contents of their play are internalized as fantasies, thus allowing a continuity of their inner world. Whereas small children verbalize their thoughts loudly while playing, latency stage children tend to keep their thoughts private.

Daydreaming consists mainly of pictures and emotions. In daydreaming we can imagine what we wish for or what we fear—which can turn into daymares—but also how we may deal with a difficult situation or find a solution to a problem. Dreaming, daydreaming, fantasies, and reveries can also be considered as some kind of art or creation. Artists and scientists confirm this view when they emphasize that their ideas, discoveries, and creative work are directly related to or came from their night- or daydreaming. Creativity, in scientific or artistic domains, often comes from the inspiration of dreams or daydreams. In his autobiography *The Statue Within,* François Jacob (1920–2013) describes how—while watching a boring movie—his mind started wandering (Jacob 1988). Suddenly, as he daydreamed, he came upon an association that gave him the long-missing link he was looking for to establish a novel theory on DNA replication in bacteria. He was then able to finalize his new concept in a seminal paper for which he eventually received the Nobel Prize in Medicine.

Daydreaming allows dissociation from an intolerable reality into a scene in which we are omnipotent actors, providing a flight into our own wished fantasied world. Imaginative fantasy and fantasizing are different psychological processes (Colombi 2010). Fantasy is part of the individual's effort to deal with *inner* reality out of creative imagination, which provides meaning and is inscribed in a developmental process (Winnicott 1958). On the opposite side, *fantasizing* is—contrary to creative imagination—leading to omnipotent manipulations of *external* reality. Colombi (2010) considers fantasizing as a defense mechanism, a withdrawal or detachment from reality, which is characterized by dissociation. Children live then in a different world that is not chaotic, nor filled with unbearable thoughts, feelings, or memories. Fantasizing furnishes such an omnipotent pleasurable situation that it may be preferred to the emotional experience in a relationship with another person. Fantasizing may isolate the subject, who then remains inaccessible in his dissociated world. The emotional development essential for the formation of the sense of self may be impaired.

A common daydream of children in the latency period is the fantasy of having a twin, a companion who shares all difficulties, disappointments, and understands and loves the child unconditionally, never leaving it to his solitude and loneliness. According to Winnicott (1958) personalization of an imaginary companion is an important part of the development of the self. "...this very primitive and magical creation of imaginary companions is easily used as a defense, as it magically bypasses all the anxieties ..." (p. 151).

Fourteen-year-old *LEA* is sent to a psychotherapist because she is unable to pay attention in school, preoccupied with constant and intensive daydreaming. She fantasies a companion who dictates her to act. The content of these fantasies is potentially dangerous and reveals instructions of auto- and hetero-aggressive behaviors. She herself has no responsibility for her actions: it is not her who is executing dangerous acts; she only obeys the commands she is told.

Lea's other fantasies express her wish to be protected and saved: she imagines herself as a princess in danger and there is a knight, a chevalier, who protects and saves her. "For me," says Lea, "my father is dead; he was never interested in me, he left me when I was 3 years old and never contacted me for 9 years. When I went to see him, I discovered that he is married and has two children; he never even told me that I have a half-brother and a half-sister." Lea displaces her emotions of rage, hatred, and retaliation—associated with being abandoned by her father—onto the companion, allowing her to maintain wishful fantasies that her father, a knight, protects her.

# Nightmares

Dreams reflect not only the images of the waking life but also the emotions and even exaggerate them. Nightmares are ubiquitous in the general population. They are common following a traumatic experience. They have been defined as a disturbing mental experience that generally occurs during REM sleep and often results in awakening. One differentiates between bad dreams that are low in distress and nightmares that are high in distress (Levin and Nielsen 2007). Schredl and Wittmann (2005) define nightmares as distressing dreams with awakening. Night terrors, more frequent in children than in adults, occur in deep, slow-wave sleep.

Posttraumatic nightmares may depict traumatic-related content and sometimes even replicate the traumatic experience with great distress. Not only is fear present in nightmares but also other negative emotions, like anger, embarrassment, and sadness. Nightmares may often be so emotionally vivid that they are accompanied by autonomic activation such as tachycardia, sweating, and difficulty in breathing. Nightmares are more prevalent in women than in men. Studies of the sociodemographic variables show that only gender was significantly associated with nightmare frequency, i.e., women reported higher nightmare frequencies than men. While there are many possibilities to explain this gender difference, one factor could be the variance in coping strategies. With regard to the content, the most common themes were falling, being chased, being paralyzed, being late, and the death of a close person. Whereas the nightmare frequency is related to the existence of actual stressors in daily life, the nightmare topics such as falling, being chased, or being paralyzed did not directly correspond to waking life experiences (Schredl 2010).

Nightmares can occur when there is an increase in daytime affective load, especially of negative emotions. This is the case for occasional nightmares that express a response to short-term stressors. Posttraumatic persistent nightmares often directly incorporate trauma-related experiences and are an example of lack of extinction of fear memories. It is well known that the amygdala modulates emotional memory and enhances memory for emotionally intense stimuli. Nightmares are associated with hyperactivation of the amygdala. This hyperactivation may follow a similar pattern to that in post-traumatic stress disorder (PTSD), namely, lack of inhibition of fear-related memory elements by the hippocampus and the anterior cingulate cortex (Pitman et al. 2012). Nightmares are among the most distressing symptoms of PTSD. There is an increase in recurrent nightmares in patients with lesions in the anterior cingulate cortex (Solms 2000).

In their evaluation of nightmares in adults (investigating behavioral effects of nightmares and their relation to personality traits), Köthe and Pietrowsky (2001) come to the conclusion that nightmares influence the waking behavior of the dreamer and his mood, activity, social contact, and coping strategies. Anxiety and physical complaints were frequent after nightmares. Behavior patterns were related to the dreamer's personality with, for example, symptoms such as guilt and anxiety. The authors postulate that the occurrence of nightmares may have an impact on the interest of a subject to seek psychotherapy.

In his quantitative studies regarding the recurrence of nightmares in children over a period of 2 years, Schredl et al. (2009) found that children with chronic nightmares showed more psychopathological symptoms such as emotional disturbances, hyperactivity and inattention, and conduct- and peer problems.

Numerous studies (Wittmann et al. 2007) show a close association between troubled dreaming and PTSD. Up to 70 % of patients with PTSD report nightmares. Whereas recovery—after a traumatic event—takes place in many patients within a year, others continue to be affected by recurrent episodes or chronic nightmares. The content of the nightmares may have no relation to the traumatic event or may be more or less a replication of the trauma. According to Terr (1979, 1983), children reported—immediately after the traumatic event—dreams that replicated the traumatic experience. Four years later, there were still repetitive, but no more replicative dreams. Fifty percent of the children told disguised dreams and dreams were less frequent.

Eight-and-a-half-year-old *MATTHIEU* draws and comments his repetitive nightmare waking him up: A man of his country of origin kidnaps him, wanting to bring him back to where he lived (before his immigration). He is so afraid of this man and of the darkness at night that he cannot fall asleep again. The man carries a weapon, a pistol, has a dreadful look, and intends to kill him. Matthieu erases—in his drawing—the person who represents himself and resumes his story: The police try to put the man in prison, but the man kills the police officer. Matthieu continues his drawing: "I have grown up, I have a sword and I defend myself. I kill this man; he is dead, he can no longer move and I can calmly sleep."

This nightmare shows the fantasies of infanticide and parricide according to the law: "either me or the other," a kind of fundamental violence (Bergeret 1984). It expresses the boy's overwhelming emotions of fear, rage, and vengeance of having been abandoned and rejected.

With children one has always to keep in mind that their nightmares may reflect a parent's never-grieved traumatic experience, transmitted to the child through unconscious nonverbal communication. The child identifies with the split-off parts of the parental representations, which he internalizes in his own self-representation.

Nine-year-old *NATHALIE* suffers since early childhood from sleep problems and nightmares. She dreams again and again that an obscure phantom with a mask intends to kidnap her. The psychotherapy of the girl's mother reveals that she lost her father, a war invalid, at the age of 3. She has never been able to mourn this loss, not knowing if he was still alive or if he was confined to a psychiatric institution. It is her daughter's symptomatology that led the mother to accept psychotherapeutic help.

To sum up, nightmares are marked by high emotional distress, accompanied by sleep disturbances, and can be associated with mental disorders such as PTSD, depression, and schizoaffective diseases, as well as neurodegenerative conditions such as Parkinson's disease and dementias. The frequency of nightmares after a traumatic event is extremely high and nightmares may persist for a lifetime. "This inseparable association between nightmares and PTSD is one of the clearest illustrations of our suggestion that affect distress mediates nightmare production" (Levin and Nielsen 2007: p. 494).

## Music in Dreams

In Greek Mythology the power of music is represented by Orpheus, who—thanks to his singing voice and playing the lyre—was able to charm wild animals, uproot trees, and convince Hades to return his wife Eurydice.

It is not astonishing that music is more frequent in dreams of professional musicians, especially those who were instructed in music at a very early age (Uga et al. 2006). Musicians create musical themes in their dreams and play or listen to music. According to Walker (1979) "the background level of musical structure [is] truly unconscious." (p. 1643). Many composers tell that music first appeared to them in a dream, initiating the creation of their musical composition. Music like other arts has its roots in unconscious motivation. There is not necessarily a direct correspondence between the content of a dream and the musical partition that may arise from it, but it emphasizes the importance of unconscious processes leading to creative activity like musical composition.

For Carta (2009), music is "the most fundamental human symbolic experience" (p. 85). He considers music in dreams as "the most direct representation of the emerging self" (p. 85), the core affect, previous to visual pictures or verbal meaning. Music contains an expression of sense and of time and holds the subject in an emotional sphere. Images and words arise afterward, from the source of music.

On a developmental level we know that the infant needs to mirror himself in the mother's face, a face in motion and in emotion, with the sounds and "singing" of mother's voice.

In his book *Musicophilia* Sacks (2007) tells his own musical dreams, which continued into the waking state. "I found something deeply disturbing and unpleasant about the music, and longed for it to stop." (p. 280). His attempts to expel the music failed as he kept on hearing hallucinatory German music. Finally after the interpretation of a friend who revealed to him "your mind is playing Mahler's Kindertotenlieder" [9] (p. 280), the music disappeared and never recurred. The dream symbolically expressed an event of the previous day: Oliver Sacks had resigned his position at the Children's unit at the hospital where he had been working and had burnt a book of essays he had written. In the intermediate states between waking and sleep, "free-floating reverie and dreamlike or hallucinatory apparitions are particularly common" (p. 281).

## Dreamwork in Psychotherapy

A dream consists of "layer upon layer of meaning related to past, present, and future, and to inner and outer, and [is] always fundamentally about" [the dreamer] (Winnicott 1971: p. 35).

The narrative analysis of nightmares and dreams offers multiple possibilities in dreamwork: it allows the dreamer to appreciate the culmination or greatest intensity of the dream, to complete the story of the dream, and to search for solutions of a problem presented in the dream. Dreams in psychotherapy—embedded in a continuing narrative—enable the dreamer to perceive and understand the content of the dream in a different light and may thus have an impact on the dreamer's waking life (Jenkins 2012).

Based on the assumption that dreams are useful for helping persons to understand themselves more deeply, Hill and Knox (2010) developed a "cognitive–experiential dream model," in which they analyze the cognitive, emotional, and behavioral components of dreams. For therapists it is important to explore connections of dream images to waking life and to collaborate with patients to construct dream interpretations in relation to past experiences. Conflicts represented in dreams can be elaborated and dream images used as metaphors in therapy (Crook and Hill 2003).

According to Ogden (2003), one has, in psychoanalytical therapy, "access to psychological "structures" only in so far as they are experienced in the medium of unconscious, preconscious and conscious dreaming, thinking, feeling and behaving". In the end, "it is emotional response—what feels true—that has the final word in psychoanalysis: thinking frames the questions to be answered in terms of feelings" (p. 596).

The experience of dreaming has a direct connection to the unconscious and is not inscribed in temporality. In *telling* a dream, timelessness is abolished; the dream is

---

[9] Songs on the Death of Children.

inscribed in time and reaches consciousness (Parsons 2007). For Bollas (2011) dreams allow us to gain wisdom of unconscious features of our life and to experience new creative meaning, thus enhancing our self-knowledge. "…Dreaming, together with the experience of recollecting, recounting and exploring dreams in analysis, increases and deepens communication between conscious and unconscious selves" (Bollas 2011: p. xxii). Bollas distinguishes two aspects of the self and a form of intrasubjective relationship between the two. "… Two subjective positions—the night self and the day self—that are continuously interdependent throughout the lifespan and seem to recognize their relative positions". He considers the lucid dream as "a rendezvous of two parts of a self" (pp. 252, 254). The narration of a dream relates to the subjective emotional experience of past events of a patient but does not necessarily represent the historical truth. Identifying connections between the infant's past and the present history allows the elaboration for gradual emotional understanding and significant meaning. Implicit memories of the past history with their impact on the present of the patient gain—over time—conscious representations and relieve the patient of his confusion and anxiety states (Giustino 2009).

Dreams are the expression of mental processes that differ qualitatively from waking thoughts. The dream occurs outside the dreamer's consciousness. On telling the dream in the analytical session, it gains consciousness and its presence demonstrates its actuality. There is transformation of timeless unconscious elements into conscious experience. "Consciousness is inseparable from existential time and chronology". "Those processes that (are) not yet inscribed in a time sequence (past-present-future) tend to repeat themselves—that is, to occur in an ever-present form" (Scarfone 2006: pp. 810, 827). Working through the patient's nightmare's unconscious fantasy system includes retrieval of painful memories and "re"construction of a tormented childhood. In the process of a psychoanalytical therapy through the narration of dreams, meaning is discovered, enlarged, and transformed. The accompanying emotions are revealed, understood, and framed in a time sequence.

A patient who is unable to dream or wakes up from night terrors or suffers from nightmares needs the analyst's wording his emotional experiences, thus—with conscious reflecting—engaging the patient to (un)conscious psychological work and enabling him to sense and differentiate his feelings. "Coming to life emotionally is … synonymous with becoming increasingly able to dream one's experience, which is to dream oneself into existence" (Ogden 2004: p. 864).

Emotional arousal makes memory stronger; when the memory is of traumatic experience, persistence can be debilitating. Sometimes only the affects, emotions, and feelings of lived (traumatic) experiences are memorized. Associations to a dream may show how a childhood event or impression is revived and how recollections belonging to different periods of life become apparent. As affective memories from infancy and early childhood are retained in the unconscious as implicit memories, they cannot be remembered (LeDoux 1996). Infantile amnesia persists until about age two and a half. Infants remember affective interactions with their caregivers but they remain implicit (Beebe et al. 1997).

**Clinical Vignette Rebecca**

Toward the end of analysis, Rebecca, a patient in her middle age, tells her analyst the following nightmare: "A woman, about 30 years old, her eyes are covered by a thick white bandage, which she takes off; her eyes are red and swollen. She looks horrible. I am this woman but also myself, much younger. I am asking her what happened. She answers that she has been crying so much that she cannot see anymore; she is blind. I tell her to see a doctor; she replies that she has consulted a lot of doctors; nobody is able to help her. We walk together on an asphalt road. Then I see a naked baby, much bigger than a normal baby; I do not know if he is alive, to whom he belongs, to this woman, to me, or to another person? Finally someone wants to care for the baby; I think that this is not the right person".

Rebecca continues: "Then there is a new scene, where I have my age and I am on the same asphalt road as before and meet an old gray, wrinkled woman, the one who took the baby with her. The baby has not changed: he is exactly the same as he was years ago: he looks giant, naked, pink, but this time he is dead. The old woman looks at me and throws the baby in the river. I am terrified, overwhelmed by sobbing; I see how the baby is going to drown in the cold water and to be eaten up by fishes. The old woman, she appears to me like a witch, turns away from me, disappears into the forest, while I am returning on the asphalt street, still looking backwards. I wake up fearful, feeling miserable, my heart beating, and I cannot fall asleep again."

The work-up during her analysis showed the fusional relationship of the patient with her mother: "I am this woman, but also myself." Rebecca always identified with her mother, wishing to understand and to help her. Her mother never answered her questions concerning the death of her father, Rebecca's grandfather. Her mother's sadness had been so overwhelming that she could not see anymore. Her only possible survival was to blind herself, a defense mechanism against the unbearable reality, an inner and outer reality she had never been able to grieve for, remaining with feelings of helplessness: "Nobody is able to help her."

Rebecca further associates: "The baby is me—far too big a burden for my mother to take care of—and expresses my feelings of not-belonging and my everlasting longing for a "right person to take care of me." I always—since I can remember— fantasied in my daydreaming to be loved and appreciated by a significant person. The baby represents also my mother's inner abandoned child (she lost her father at the age of 2) and at the same time her dead first-born baby she was never able to mourn. My mother is the old grey women, who could not take care of her inner child, whose development had come to a standstill."

The patient weeps: she has not been able in all these years to help her mother mourn her losses. Even though she knows—rationally—that her mother's depression was not her fault, she still feels guilty toward her. But what is worse is that she feels guilty in any meaningful relationship, as soon as she perceives that the other person is not content. Even if she tries to think that she is not at all so powerful to be responsible for the emotional state of another person, she has to ask herself if anything in her behavior or words could have hurt this person. Her depressed mother could not take care of her. Rebecca's mother has never been able to mourn the loss of her father at age 2 and her childhood situation of extreme poverty (she suffered hunger), with an ill brother. She and her older sister had no possibility to undertake universities studies. Married, Rebecca's mother lost her first two children.

The history of this patient reminds us of the famous concept of Green (1997) *"the dead mother"*. He describes an infant or young child's response to a chronically depressed, emotionally absent mother. The mother is physically present, but psychically "dead" for her young child, which is terrified and confused. This interaction has been observed by Stern (1994) who states: "Compared to the infant's expectations and wishes, the depressed mother's face is flat and expressionless. She breaks eye contact and does not seek to reestablish it". "After the infant's attempts to invite and solicit the mother to come to life, to be there emotionally, to play, have failed, the infant, it appears, tries to be with her by way of identification and imitation" (pp. 12, 13). For Rebecca this nightmare is like a summary of her life, beginning with her childhood. The dream shows regressive elements and is associated with anxious and miserable feelings. At the same time the dream marks the already accomplished integration process and emotional understanding of the patient. Quinodoz (1999) considers such dreams as "turning over a page" and Winnicott (1949) as a "healing dream."

# References

Beebe B, Lachmann F, Jaffe J. Mother-infant interaction structures and presymbolic self- and object representations. Psychoanal Dialogues. 1997;7(2):133–82. doi:10.1080/10481889709539172.

Bergeret J. La violence fondamentale. Paris: Dunod; 1984.

Blum HP. To what extent do you privilege dream interpretation in relation to other forms of mental representations? Response by Harold P. Blum. Int J Psychoanal. 2011;92(2):275–7. doi:10.1111/j.1745-8315.2011.00419.x.

Bollas C. The Christopher Bollas Reader. Hove and New York: Routledge; 2011.

Brown RE, Basheer R, McKenna JT, Strecker RE, McCarley RW. Control of sleep and wakefulness. Physiol Rev. 2012;92(3):1087–187. doi:10.1152/physrev.00032.2011.

Carta S. J Anal Psychol. 2009;54:85–102. Music in dreams and the emergence of the self. J Anal Psychol. 2009 Feb;54(1):85-102. doi: 10.1111/j.1468-5922.2008.01759.x.

Cavanna AE, Trimble MR. The precuneus: a review of its functional anatomy and behavioural correlates. Brain. 2006;129(Pt 3):564–83.

Christoff K, Gordon AM, Smallwood J, Smith R, Schooler JW. Experience sampling during fMRI reveals default network and executive system contributions to mind wandering. Proc Natl Acad Sci U S A. 2009;106(21):8719–24. doi:10.1073/pnas.0900234106.

Colombi L. The dual aspect of fantasy: flight from reality or imaginative realm? Considerations and hypotheses from clinical psychoanalysis. Int J Psychoanal. 2010;91(5):1073–91. doi:10.1111/j.1745-8315.2010.00327.x.

Crook RE, Hill EC. Working with dreams in psychotherapy: the therapists' perspective. Dreaming. 2003;13(2):83–93.

Da Rocha Barros EM. How do you conceive of the function of dreams? Do you distinguish dreams as a result of trauma from other types of dreams? Response by Elias Mallet da Rocha Barros (São Paulo). Int J Psychoanal. 2011;92(2):270–2. doi:10.1111/j.1745-8315.2011.00426.x.

De Gennaro L, Cipolli C, Cherubini A, Assogna F, Cacciari C, Marzano C, et al. Amygdala and hippocampus volumetry and diffusivity in relation to dreaming. Hum Brain Mapp. 2011;32(9):1458–70. doi:10.1002/hbm.21120.

Ferenczi S. On the revision of the interpretation of dreams. In: Balint M, editor. Final contributions to the problems and methods of psychoanalysis. London: Hogarth Press; 1931. p. 238–43. Reprinted London Karnac Books 1994.

Freud S. The interpretation of dreams (First part), Standard edition, vol. IV. London: The Hogarth Press; 1900.

Freud S. The interpretation of dreams (Second part), Standard edition, vol. V. London: The Hogarth Press; 1900–1901.

Freud S. Creative writers and day-dreaming, Standard edition. London: Hogarth Press; 1908.

Freud S. New introductory lectures on psychoanalysis, Standard edition. London: Hogarth Press; 1933. p. 9.

Giustino G. Memory in dreams. Int J Psychoanal. 2009;90:1057–73.

Goldman-Rakic PS. Topography of cognition: parallel distributed networks in primate association cortex. Annu Rev Neurosci. 1988;11:137–56.

Green A (Ed.). The dead mother. In: On private madness. London: Karnac; 1986. Reprinted 1997, pp. 142–73.

Hartmann E. Meteorite or gemstone? Dreaming as one end of a continuum of functioning: implications for research and for the use of dreams in therapy and self-knowledge. Dreaming. 2010a;20(3):149–68.

Hartmann E. The underlying emotion and the dream: relating dream imaginary to the dreamer's underlying emotion can help elucidate the nature of dreaming. Int Rev Neurobiol. 2010b;92:197–214. doi:10.1016/S0074-7742(10)92010-2. Review.

Hartmann E. The dream is not a series of perceptions to which We respond logically (or Not). the dream is an imaginative creation: a comment on Hobson et al. Dream logic—the inferential reasoning paradigm. Dreaming. 2012;22(1):74–7. doi:10.1037/a0026141.

Hill E, Knox S. The use of dreams in modern psychotherapy. Int Rev Neurobiol. 2010; 92:291–317.

Hobson A, Voss U. A mind to go out of: reflections on primary and secondary consciousness. Conscious Cogn. 2011;20(4):993–7. doi:10.1016/j.concog.2010.09.018.

Ikemoto S, Panksepp J. The role of nucleus accumbens dopamine in motivated behavior: a unifying interpretation with special reference to reward-seeking. Brain Res Brain Res Rev. 1999;31(1):6–41.

Jacob F. The statue within. New York: Basic Books; 1988. ISBN 978-0-465-08223-0.

Jenkins D. The nightmare and the narrative. Dreaming. 2012;22(2):101–14.

Jouvet M. Neurophysiology of the states of sleep. Physiol Rev. 1967;47(2):117–77.

Jus A, Jus K, Villeneuve A, Pires A, Lachance R, Fortier J, et al. Studies on dream recall in chronic schizophrenic patients after prefrontal lobotomy. Biol Psychiatry. 1973;6(3):275–93.

Kahn D, Gover T. Consciousness in dreams. Int Rev Neurobiol. 2010;92:181–95. doi:10.1016/S0074-7742(10)92009-6.

Kaplan-Solms K, Solms M. Clinical studies in neuro-psychoanalysis. London: Karnac Books; 2000.

Kirk GD, Raven JE, Schofield M. Die vorsakratischen Philosophen. Einführung, Texte und Kommentare. Heraklitus, Fragment 93. Stuttgart: J.B. Metzler; 1994.

Köthe M, Pietrowsky R. Behavioral effects of nightmares and their correlations to personality patterns. Dreaming. 2001;11(1):43–52.

LeDoux JE. The emotional brain. New York: Simon & Schuster; 1996.

Levin R, Nielsen TA. Disturbed dreaming, posttraumatic stress disorder, and affect distress: a review and neurocognitive model. Psychol Bull. 2007;133(3):482–528. doi:10.1037/0033-2909.133.3.482, p. 494.

Lin JS. Brain structures and mechanisms involved in the control of cortical activation and wakefulness, with emphasis on the posterior hypothalamus and histaminergic neurons. Sleep Med Rev. 2000;4(5):471–503.

Maggiolini A, Cagnin C, Crippa F, Persico A, Rizzi P. Content analysis of dreams and waking narratives. Dreaming. 2010;20(1):60–76.

Malcolm-Smith S, Koopowitz S, Pantelis E, Solms M. Approach/avoidance in dreams. Conscious Cogn. 2012;21(1):408–12. doi:10.1016/j.concog.2011.11.004.

Martin Cabre LJ. How do you conceive of the function of dreams? Do you distinguish dreams as a result of trauma from other types of dreams? Response by Luis J. Martın Cabre. Int J Psychoanal. 2011;92(2):270–2. doi:10.1111/j.1745-8315.2011.00426.x.

Modell A. Imagination and the meaningful brain. Cambrigde: MIT Press; 2006.

Nielsen TA, McGregor DL, Zadra A, Ilnicki D, Ouellet L. Dream research pain in dreams. American Sleep Disorders Association and Sleep Research Society. Sleep. 1993;16(5):490–8.

Nir Y, Tononi G. Dreaming and the brain: from phenomenology to neurophysiology. Trends Cogn Sci. 2010;14(2):88–100. doi:10.1016/j.tics.2009.12.001.

Ogden TH. What's true and whose idea was it? Int J Psychoanal. 2003;84:593–606.

Ogden TH. This art of psychoanalysis. Dreaming undreamt dreams and interrupted cries. Int J Psychoanal. 2004;85:857–77.

Ohayon MM, Zulley J, Guilleminault C, Smirne S. Prevalence and pathologic associations of sleep paralysis in the general population. Neurology. 1999;52(6):1194–200.

Parsons M. Why did Orpheus look back? EPF Conference. 2007; Bulletin 61, p. 159–66. (162)

Perogamvros L, Schwartz S. The roles of the reward system in sleep and dreaming. Neurosci Biobehav Rev. 2012;36(8):1934–51. doi:10.1016/j.neubiorev.2012.05.010.

Perrin M. Les praticiens du rêve. Un exemple de chamanisme. Paris: Presses Universitaires de France; 1992.

Pitman RK, Rasmusson AM, Koenen KC, Shin LM, Orr SP, Gilbertson MW, et al. Biological studies of post-traumatic stress disorder. Nat Rev Neurosci. 2012;13(11):769–87. doi:10.1038/nrn3339.

Quinodoz JM. Dreams that turn over a page: integration dreams with paradoxical regressive content. Int J Psychoanal. 1999;80:225–38.

Ramaligam V, Chen MC, Saper CB, Lu J. Perspectives on the rapid eye movement sleep switch in rapid eye movement sleep behavior disorder. Sleep Med. 2013;14(8):707–13. doi:10.1016/j.sleep.2013.03.017.

Revonsuo A. The reinterpretation of dreams: an evolutionary hypothesis of the function of dreaming. Behav Brain Sci. 2000;23:877–901.

Sacks O. Hallucinations. London: Picador; 2012.

Sacks O. Musicophilia. Tales of Music and the Brain. Picador 2007; ISBN 1400040817- (280, 281).

Scarfone D. A matter of time: actual time and the production of the past. Psychoanal Q. 2006;75:807–34.

Schredl M. Nightmare frequency and nightmare topics in a representative German sample. Eur Arch Psychiatry Clin Neurosci. 2010;260:565–70.

Schredl M. Frequency and nature of pain in a long dream series. Sleep Hypn. 2011;13:1–2.

Schredl M, Wittmann L. Dreaming: a psychological view. Schweiz Arch Neurol Psychiatr. 2005;156:484–92.

Schredl M, Fricke-Oerkermann L, Mitschke A, Wiater A, Lehmkuhl G. Longitudinal study of nightmares in children: stability and effect of emotional symptoms. Child Psychiatry Hum Dev. 2009;40:439–49.

Shulman RG, Hyder F, Rothman DL. Baseline brain energy supports the state of consciousness. Proc Natl Acad Sci U S A. 2009;106(27):11096–101. doi:10.1073/pnas.0903941106.

Singer JL. Daydreaming, consciousness, and self-representations: empirical approaches to theories of William James and Sigmund Freud. J Appl Psychoanal Studies. 2003;5(4):461–83.

Solms M. Dreaming and REM sleep are controlled by different brain mechanisms. Behav Brain Sci. 2000;23:793–1121.

Solms M. The neuropsychology of dreams: a clinico-anatomical study: March 1, 1997. Mahwah: Lawrence Erlbaum. ISBN-10: 0805815856 | ISBN-13: 978-0805815856

Solms M, Turnbull O. The brain and the inner world. New York: Other Press; 2002.

Stern D. One way to build a clinically relevant baby. Infant Ment Health J. 1994;15(1):9–25.

Terr LC. Children of Chowchilla: a study of psychic trauma. Psychoanal Study Child. 1979;34:547–623.

Terr LC. Life attitudes, dreams, and psychic trauma in a group of "normal" children. J Am Acad Child Psychiatry. 1983;22(3):221–30.

Torda C. Dreams of subjects with bilateral hippocampal lesions. Acta Psychiatr Scand. 1969; 45(3):277–88.

Uga V, Lemut MC, Zampi C, Zilli I, Salzarulo P. Music in dreams. Conscious Cogn. 2006;15: 351–7.

Voss U, Frenzel C, Koppehele-Gossel J, Hobson A. Lucid dreaming: an age-dependent brain dissociation. J Sleep Res. 2012;21(6):634–42. doi:10.1111/j.1365-2869.2012.01022.x.

Vyazovskiy VV, Cirelli C, Pfister-Genskow M, Faraguna U, Tononi G. Molecular and electro-physiological evidence for net synaptic potentiation in wake and depression in sleep. Nat Neurosci. 2008;11(2):200–8. doi:10.1038/nn2035.

Walker A. Music and the unconscious. Br Med J. 1979;2:1641–3.

Winnicott DW. Hate in the countertransference. Int J Psychoanal. 1949;30:69–74.

Winnicott DW. Collected papers: through paediatrics to psycho-analysis. 1st ed. London: Tavistock; 1958.

Winnicott DW. Playing and reality. Publishers, New York: Basic Books; 1971.

Wittmann L, Schredl M, Kramer M. Dreaming in posttraumatic stress disorder: a critical review of phenomenology, psychophysiology and treatment. Psychother Psychosom. 2007;76:25–39.

Yang G, Lai CS, Cichon J, Ma L, Li W, Gan WB. Sleep promotes branch-specific formation of dendritic spines after learning. Science. 2014;344(6188):1173–8. doi:10.1126/science.1249098.

# Part X

# Chapter 16
# Notes to Psychotherapy

## Introduction

In 1895, after years of work on his *Design for a Scientific Psychology*, Freud abandoned his attempt to construct an anatomical–physiological model of the mind and turned to psychoanalysis, predicting however: "We must recollect that all of our provisional ideas in psychology will presumably one day be based on an organic substructure" (Freud 1914: pp. 67–102). "The deficiencies in our description would probably vanish if we were already in a position to replace the psychological terms with physiological or chemical ones . ... We may expect [physiology and chemistry] to give the most surprising information and we cannot guess what answers it will return in a few dozen years of questions we have put to it. They may be of a kind that will blow away the whole of our artificial structure of hypothesis." (Freud 1920: pp. 7–64).

Today with a deeper neurobiological understanding of the brain, the dialogue between psychoanalysis and neuroscience has taken on a new dimension. In particular, using functional MRI, it is possible to demonstrate changes in activation pattern of the brain by psychotherapy. In combining clinical and neuroimaging studies, it is possible to show that transformations induced by psychoanalytical therapy can be assessed in an objective way (Fischmann et al. 2013).

One must be very cautious when trying to explain the underlying neurobiological processes of psychotherapeutic interventions. By its very nature, language represents one of the most powerful tools for communication, impacting on brain connections and leading to secondary internalization in the sphere of the prefrontal cortex. As Solms puts it, the internalization process, taking place during the talking cure, has a "mutative power" (Solms and Turnbull 2002: p. 289).

LeDoux, a neuroscientist studying the mechanisms of emotion, suggests the following interpretation for the beneficial effect of psychotherapy: "Once your emotional system learns something, it seems you never let it go. What therapy does is teach you to control it—it teaches your neocortex how to inhibit your amygdala. The propensity to act is suppressed, while your basic emotion about it remains in a subdued form" (Cited in Goleman 1995: p. 213).

© Springer International Publishing Switzerland 2016

A. Steck, B. Steck, *Brain and Mind*, DOI 10.1007/978-3-319-21287-6_16

## Dialogue between Psychoanalysis and Neuroscience

Psychoanalysis is considered as a scientific method for observing mental processes, especially the unconscious activities of the mind, which become accessible through a therapeutic method, the talking cure. While neuroscience was in the past mainly interested in studying motor or sensory phenomena, recently more complex functions, such as emotions, imagination, and dreams are being studied.

The idea of an unconscious mind goes back to antiquity and was present in various cultures. The term unconscious refers to the unintentional nature of mental processes. In phylogeny and ontogeny, we witness that the unconscious mind precedes consciousness. While neuroscience uses the term nonconscious, unconscious and nonconscious have subtle distinctions depending on the research field of neuroscience and psychoanalysis. For the former nonconscious cognition refers to mental processes such as perceptions from our senses or learning operations, which take place without the subject being aware of it. The unconscious in Freud's theory (1912, 1915) consists of memories, desires, and needs that we are not aware of, but eventually influence our thoughts, feelings, and behavior.

To try to discover neural correlates of subjective phenomena, psychoanalysts looked at models of consciousness such as those proposed by Edelman and Tononi (2000) and Dehaene and Changeux (2011). In these models, the brain is not considered as a computer, but as a complex, self-reflective, and open system, operating and evolving—from conception until death—according to the biological principles of selective-adaptive processes in nature. While we don't yet have a unified theory of consciousness, most current models provide, beyond the core of cognitive processes, room for intersubjectivity, affects, and feelings that all humans share in their embodied mind. What appeals to psychoanalysts such as Modell (1990) and Shields (2006) is the dynamic conception of these neurobiological models, allowing the development of unlimited variables at the root of self-reflective activity characteristic of human fantasy, imagination, and behavior.

Freud's concept of the unconscious mind is still recognized as an important guiding influence in spite of numerous critics. In *The Psychopathology of Everyday Life* Freud demonstrates the unintended behavior of individuals who do not know the cause of their behavior. "In all these cases, the term unconscious referred to the unintentional nature of the behavior or process, and the concomitant lack of awareness was not of the stimuli that provoked the behavior, but of the influence or consequences of those stimuli" (Freud 1901: p. 74).

Flexible and adaptive unconscious functional systems play an important role, especially in times of default behavioral disposition,[1] when our mind drifts away from the present and wanders into fantasies of the past or the future. "It is nice to know that the unconscious is minding the store when the owner is absent" (Bargh and Morsella 2008: p. 78). Unconscious processes are complex, adaptive, and guide us through the

---

[1] The default mode network (DMN), described in the chapter consciousness, is playing a critical role in processes of internal mentation.

living world. In fact, most of the brain activity occurs without conscious awareness, so we can say that the brain maintains stability on an unconscious level.

Affective experiences originating in the visceral brain are the basis for the development of differentiated structures of perceptual and cognitive consciousness within the neocortex. Consciousness relies on affective events, which have survival advantages. "From this perspective, perceptual experiences were initially affective at the primary-process brainstem level, but capable of being elaborated by secondary learning and memory processes into tertiary-cognitive forms of consciousness." (Solms and Panksepp 2012: p. 147).

In psychoanalysis, a particular form of unconscious process is the unconscious communication between analyst and patient. In an analytical situation, the transference relationship facilitates communication of the patient's unconscious formations and permits the search for the meaning of unconscious phenomena in a context of containment (Maldonado 2011). The unconscious includes thoughts, memories, affects, motivations, and dreams; it tends to create meaning and it influences behavior. It is constantly working in sleep as well as in waking state. Conscious and unconscious processes are considered more and more as representations of mental phenomena emerging in a continuous form. Breuer and Freud (1895) already postulated that the unconscious also had a function in sustaining "psychic continuity" when there was discontinuity in consciousness.

While advances in neuroscience have had a significant impact for psychoanalysis with regard to the theoretical concepts of the mind and the way in which psychoanalysts understand their patients, they are still of little relevance for the modus operandi in psychoanalytical therapy with a patient. Thanks to neuroscientific research, a lot has been learned for example about the important differences between various types of memories. Patients undergoing psychoanalytical treatment very often suffered traumatic events in their personal history. The discovery of the different memory encodings has contributed to explaining why some patients are unable to remember traumatic episodes; they were not explicitly encoded and could therefore only appear in dreams, feelings, bodily sensations, and fantasies. Indeed—as therapists know—the (re)construction of these memories is as helpful as the recovery of explicit memories.

What neuroscience cannot yet explain is the individual subjective experience. As Scarfone (2012) states: " 'Mind' … is not secreted by the brain in the way bile is secreted by the liver. It is worth remembering that there are no words' in Broca's area and no 'fear' in the amygdala, although these brain structures are vital for speech and feeling fear respectively" (p. 1288).

One of the goals of psychoanalytical treatment is to understand the inner world of a patient, which unfolds in the significant relationship between patient and therapist. The patient's personal experiences and the meaning he attributes to his experiences are at the core of psychoanalytical investigation, with the aim to favor the patient's specific processes to understand the affective and cognitive contents of his mind. The intention of the therapist is to try to understand the patient's unconscious emotional experiences and to achieve—together with the patient—a careful common understanding of what is "true" for the patient in his unconscious emotional experience (Ogden 2003).

Will neuroscientific research ever be able to demonstrate the variability of symptoms in individual patients, their changes in appearance as well as their disappearance during analytical therapy? Psychodynamic processes are individual, complex, heterogeneous, variable, and inscribed in a unique meaningful relationship with a therapist in the context of a specific and protected setting.

Neuroscience and psychoanalysis—regardless of their multiple differences—deal both with mind and brain and need to interact. The institutionalization of collaborative efforts between psychoanalysts and neuroscientists is already underway (Pulver 2003; Solms 1998). There is a huge gap between the disciplines, rooted in their history and scope, but our capacity to better understand the brain–mind relationship can only come from combining clinical experiences with scientific facts.

## Transference and Intersubjective Relationship

The activation of mental models and states of mind from our relationships with meaningful figures in the past happens all the time in settings both in and outside of the psychotherapeutic relationship (Siegel 2001). Transference is one of Freud's most important contributions and describes a process that takes place in therapeutic interactions and, more generally, in interpersonal interactions. In psychoanalytic theory, "transference" refers to the process in which an analysand's unconscious desires are actualized and projected ("transferred") onto the analyst. "It is a very remarkable thing that the Ucs (Unconscious) of one human being can react upon that of another, without passing through the Cs (Consciousness). This deserves closer investigation … but, descriptively speaking, the fact is incontestable" (Freud 1915: p. 194).

According to Laplanche and Pontalis, transference is the process by which unconscious desires are updated onto certain persons, within a certain type of established relation with them and, particularly, within the analytical relation. The process involves "a repetition of infantile prototypes that are lived out with a deep feeling of reality" (Laplanche and Pontalis 1967). When Freud (1923–1925, 1925–1926) speaks of "transference" or "transference thoughts" in connection with dreams, he is referring to a mode of displacement in which the unconscious wish is expressed in a masked form through the material furnished by the preconscious residues of the day before (Laplanche and Pontalis 1967).

The psychoanalytic process is based on an intersubjective relationship, involving the creation of a relational space in which latent development resources and resilience perspectives of a patient and mutual expectations of the patient and therapist are recorded. New functional possibilities and opportunities for more suitable integrations are explored and a more profound understanding of a commonly shared narrative is elaborated. The aim of the psychoanalytical process is directed towards working out new scope, open space and freedom and creation of alternatives, and more suitable forms of coping with life events (Bürgin and Steck 2013).

For Stern (2004): "The desire for intersubjectivity is one of the major motivations that drives a psychotherapy forward. Patients want to be known and to share what it feels like to be them." (p. 97). Unconscious emotional movements and contents emerge in the patient–therapist relationship, which often follow a latent plan, sometimes like a table of contents, sensitizing the therapist for what is to come. Both intrapsychic fantasies, past relationship patterns and current relationships outside the therapy (especially in the family environment) arise in the transference relationship. These fantasies represent partly conscious, partly unconscious figurative-scenic processes of a relatively fixed nature; they correspond to a sum of different intrapsychic driving forces. Often they are also used as defense configurations against actual drive impulses.

It is the psychotherapist's task to reflect on the changes a patient generates in him and to carefully verbalize his understanding to the patient. The patient—through projective identification[2]—"tells" his therapist on an emotional level what he has painfully experienced. It may be a defense strategy, but above all it is important information for the therapist to understand his patient's emotions to try to help him deal with his painful feelings.

The therapist makes himself available in the intersubjective field to record the patient's information, externalized and projected onto the therapist, then to transform the patient's messages into language (thoughts) and emotion (feelings), and to give them back to the patient in an adequate form. Together with the patient, the therapist further elaborates them to a jointly shared understanding. These transference- and counter-transference movements should—if possible—be accessible for conscious reflection.

Transference contains all the patient's communications in the analytical psychotherapy: his verbal expression such as dreams and narrations, nonverbal communication such as posture, bodily movements, facial expressions, gesticulations, and most importantly his voice, the "musical dimension" of the transference (Mancia 2006). The relationship between patient and analyst represents in part a shared "musical experience," allowing the affective and emotional world to be expressed. This musical dimension is an essential means in the analytical work as it facilitates the affective and emotional, often traumatic experiences, stored in the patient's implicit memory—that cannot consciously be remembered—to be relived in the transferential encounter.

Sometimes, there are mutual and mutative shared experiences called "now-moments" by Stern, "holy-moments" by Winnicott, "implicit relational knowledge" by the Boston Process of Change Study Group (BCPSG 2010). "Implicit relational knowing and meaning" play a key role in the intersubjective field and the reorganization of affective implicit experiences. The mutual implicit relationship, in which patient and therapist share an intersubjective unconscious knowledge and

---

[2] Projective identification is a process, in which—in a close relationship, such as between patient and psychotherapist—an unconscious fantasy of aspects of the self or of an internal relation-representation is attributed to an external person.

understanding, often an experience of surprise, favors emotional changes and (re) organization of the patient's relationship with himself and others (Stern et al. 1998). It lies then in the analyst's ability to record, understand and then verbalize the meaning of the lived emotional expressions in the intersubjective relationship—the primary or primitive emotions that are evoked in the analyst—and finally to connect the symbolic signification to the patient's past.

## Interpretation/Intervention

The therapeutic effect in psychoanalysis is not the result of interpretation but psychic change is carried out by the affective content, the transference being the "key factor in analysis, with interpretation complementing it" (Andrade 2005: p. 682).

Interpretations intend to broaden conscious awareness; they are for example effective when patients can verbalize experiences belonging to explicit memories. But interpretations may also influence unconscious processes such as dreaming, feeling, fantasying, thinking, and behaving. Conscious knowledge helps the patient to examine different procedures for changing his way of feeling, thinking, and behaving. The process of working through comprises unconscious modulations of self-relating and helps the patient to establish better relationships in his real life (Bleichmar 2004).

Often it is not the content of the therapist's verbal intervention the patient listens to, but the sound of the therapist's voice, perceived as emotional expression. A professional musician in analysis tells: "I don't remember what you (her analyst) said to me in the last session, but you appeared in my dream, in which you were a shepherd playing pastoral melodies for me." She experienced the voice of her analyst as soothing and reassuring. According to Freud, "dreams are the royal road to the unconscious" (1900, 1900–1901), and it is true that they are probably the best tools for analytic work with early traumatized patients. The often overwhelming affects and emotions in dreams of experienced events which cannot be remembered, for which no words can be found by the patient, evoke in the intersubjective relationship and in the transference/countertransference emotions, thoughts, and images in the analyst. It is through the shared emotional investment between patient and therapist that these dreams find symbolic representation, meaning, and reconstruction in the analytic process and allow the patient to retrieve lost parts of his self and his livelihood.

Britton (2002) considers the analytical process as effective if:

- The patient's relationship with his self has been enhanced and he has gained a better awareness of his relation to internal and external reality
- The patient is capable of suffering, mourning, and recovering from loss
- His paranoid and depressive anxiety has decreased while his faculty for (self) reflection has increased

## Psychoanalytical Therapy for Patients with Adverse Childhood Experiences

Treatment with adults, adolescents, or children having experienced traumatic events in infancy or early childhood is a demanding task, which has to be executed by a reliable therapist who establishes a secure, protective, and continuous relationship with his patient. Such a therapeutic intervention aims at helping a patient who compulsively repeats his traumatic experiences in actions, somatic states, or emotional distress, by taking in account the unconscious dynamics underlying his reenactments. Patients have to be reassured that expressing the overwhelming feelings associated with the trauma will not bring the trauma back. The goal of working through traumatic experiences is to enable the patient to gradually decrease his highly intense emotional charge and at the same time create meaning of his lived events. It is the responsibility of the therapist to guarantee that re-traumatization does not happen during trauma processing work.

The feelings of (repeated) traumatic experiences need to be extensively expressed, again and again and over a long time to allow the patient—with time—to distinguish the various emotions; therefore, therapists have to be reliable in their emotional attitude and attentive to the nonverbal multiple manifestations of a patient. Some patients may eventually remember traumatic events; others will have no memories at all. What is important for the psychotherapeutic process is the expression of the remembered feelings, as Matte-Blanco stated: "I feel that this repeated expression of most varied feelings connected with the episodes and persons concerned, now made towards a basically respectful and tolerant analyst who tries to understand the meaning of the emotional expression and its connections with the details of early experiences and actual relationships, is the real healing factor"(Matte-Blanco 1988: p. 163, cited in Jiménez 2006). In other words, in psychotherapy the therapist needs to be attentive to the nonverbal expression of emotions emerging in the transference relationship with the patient, as the events of these affects, stored in implicit memory, can neither be recalled nor verbalized. It is the affective resonance of the therapist that the patient needs to hear, in order to feel understood in his infantile demands, wishes, deprivation, and distress. The therapist has to name the affective atmosphere, sensed in the transference. The often very intense and confused emotions of the patient have then to be verbally differentiated in various nuances by the therapist, so that the patient can perceive and consciously experience his feelings and to qualify them with words as for example fear, anger, sadness, pain. Fantasies and images related to the patients' feelings emerge and associations and memories linked to these emotions are then revealed by the patient.

The psychotherapist has to listen carefully to how and what his patient hears from his interventions, interpretations, his voice, or his silence. Often only after "retranscription of memory,"[3] is the therapist able to know what his patient has

---

[3] "Retranscription of memory" according to Modell (1990) or deferred action is a concept that refers to Freud's original term Nachträglichkeit, conceived as early as 1895 in the *Project for a Scientific Psychology* (Freud 1895) "Childhood traumas operate in a deferred fashion as though they were fresh experiences; but they do so unconsciously" (Freud 1896b: p. 167).

recalled and what meaning he has attributed by his own associated reflections (Marion 2012).

In the analytic–psychotherapeutic relationship, implicit emotional and sensory memories have to be transformed into explicit memories, which can then be verbalized and no longer need to be expressed through reenactment. This transformation of unconscious, procedural memories through jointly developed semantic contents into verbal and symbolic representations allows mutual insight of the patient–therapist couple and promotes the psychotherapeutic process.

## Psychotherapy in Children and Adolescents

### *Indication for Psychoanalytical Therapy*

The literature on the evaluation for psychotherapy-indication in children and adolescents is rather sparse. Investigations in the field of psychodynamics are centered on the question of whether and how a child or adolescent patient will be able to use the psychoanalytical approach for better psychic functioning and more favorable development. When assessing the psychopathological difficulties, it is important to evaluate their unconscious symbolic content and the associated developmental aspects.

Anna Freud (1945) already stated that "childhood is a process sui generis, a series of developmental stages in which each manifestation has its importance as a transition, not as a final result". It is essential that "the child's ability to develop does not remain fixated at some stage before the maturation process has been concluded" (p. 136). Integration of heterogeneous psychic functions in children and adolescents depends on the complexities of their development, which is influenced by constitutional, environmental, and maturational factors and their mutual interaction. Indications for psychotherapy are based less on psychopathological manifestations themselves than "on the bearing of these manifestations on the maturation process within the individual child" (pp. 148-149). Emphasis is shifted from purely clinical to developmental aspects.

According to Anna Freud, a neurosis[4] is severe and therapeutic measures have to be taken "if a child shows a faulty knowledge of the outer world, far below the level of his intelligence, if he is seriously estranged from his own emotions, with blank spaces in the remembrance of his own past beyond the usual range of infantile

---

"Deferred action": "It is not lived experience in general that undergoes a deferred revision but, specifically, whatever it has been impossible in the first instance to incorporate fully into a meaningful context" (Laplanche and Pontalis 1973: p. 112).

See also *On Nachträglichkeit: The modernity of an old concept* (Eickhoff 2006).

[4] The term neurosis used by Freud (1896a, b) defines a condition in which unconscious conflicts are expressed as a variety of mental dysfunctions. Neurosis as a diagnostic category has been eliminated from the American DSM. This change reflects the concept to privilege description of behavior and symptoms as opposed to psychological mechanisms, a view that is controversial.

amnesia, with a split of his personality, and with motility out of ego control" (Freud A. 1945: p.148). "Since the decision to seek advice for the child normally lies with the parents, an infantile neurosis is more likely to be brought for treatment when its symptoms are disturbing to the environment. The parents will be guided in their assessment of the seriousness of the situation by the impact of the child's neurosis on themselves." (Freud A. 1945: p. 134). Lebovici (1952) underlined that the difficulty in the psychoanalytical treatment of children lies essentially in the relationship of the therapist with the child's parents.

The assessment of a working alliance with both parents and especially with the child/adolescent has a special meaning. The investigation- and diagnostic procedures should allow the patient to experience how the therapeutic process will evolve. With his functional parts, the patient will work together with the therapist on the dysfunctional structures of his inner world. The overall assessment of the information and the willingness to mental work implies not only the question of whether a psychoanalytic method appears adequate or appropriate, but also includes reflections on the intensity, i.e., the frequency of sessions per week. The indication for a psychoanalytic psychotherapy is the task of professionals (Bürgin and Steck 2013).

When evaluating the indication for psychotherapy, age, gender, developmental features, relational structuring, capacity for communication and expression, as well as the child/adolescent's way of emotional experience and cognitive assimilation must be taken into account. Will the child benefit, take advantage of the therapeutic relationship? On the therapist's side, he or she is always influenced by his or her own education, training, references, and values.

## Psychoanalytical Psychotherapy

In child and adolescent psychotherapy, it is essential to guarantee a safe affective setting for the child so that emotions associated with traumatic events can emerge, be felt, named, and lived as a conscious experience. In the transference relationship, these emotions can be verbalized in symbolic language. Reliving former feelings is very painful. But the grief work is necessary to avoid that the child/adolescent endures secondary traumatization by reenacting traumatic situations. Psychoanalytic psychotherapy has to work with the functional parts of the self, the parts that are not or only mildly disturbed. Some children need repeated recognition of their functional parts before they are ready to deal with dysfunctional or disturbed relationship aspects.

The psychotherapeutic relationship allows an understanding of the sense and meaning of events and to learn—within the therapeutic relationship—to deal with overwhelming emotions, thoughts, representations, and fantasies and to experience that any psychic state can be expressed and contained in the therapeutic relationship. In the working through on a semantic and symbolic level the somatosensory emotional and sensory implicit memories of lived events can be translated into explicit memories, transformed into declarative memory, so that they no longer need to be expressed by the body and/or by acting out.

Within the relationship between therapist and child/adolescent, an exchange characterized by a dialogue and mutual emotional movements, allowing the inner psychic world to appear in the outer world, occurs in the "transitional space"[5] (Winnicott 1971a). Unconscious and conscious emotional fluctuations, fantasies, early relationship patterns, experiences of the past, but also current relationships outside the therapy arise in the intersubjective relationship between patient and psychotherapist.

It is not only the words themselves that are crucial for the analytical process but rather the therapist's accompanying attitude and emotionality, which—through his voice—expresses his self-reflexive emotional commitment. The voice of the therapist may have an important role, for example, a holding or containing function. Brazelton and Nugent (1995), when applying the neonatal behavioral assessment scale with newborn infants, utilized their voice as a holding function.

The communicative exchange between patient and therapist takes place on verbal and preverbal levels. There are always at least two levels to be listened to: what a patient tells or shows both at the infant- or young child age and at the real age of the subject. The self of the infant or young child is the one that presents his suffering in various forms, whereas the self of the real age patient is often present with different contributions and functions such as "helping" or "guiding" the therapist and supporting the therapeutic process. Therefore, the therapist has to continuously adjust his listening according to the different "selves" of his patient: at the infant stage for example, the patient requires a caring and affectionate presence of his therapist.

In the communication units of the present, there are always parts of the past included and usually also of the future. The therapist often functions as an auxiliary ego as well as an independent and separate person. He has to be able to wait, yet never leave a patient—on an emotional level—alone. He has to record any communication (whether nonverbal, enforced by means of projective identification or verbal), preserve, and transform it into language and give it back to the patient. In this way, the therapist documents his "survival"—e.g., against destructive attacks of the patient—and at the same time his separate existence from the patient. For Winnicott (1971a), the trusted therapist, who has registered the patient's (indirect) communication, has to reflect back to his patient the mutual reverberation and resonance. "In these highly specialized conditions the individual can come together and exist as a unit, not as a defense against anxiety but as an expression of I AM, I am alive, I am myself. From this position everything is creative." (Winnicott 1971a: p. 56).

## Play

"It is in playing, and only in playing, that the individual child or adult is able to be creative and to use the whole personality, and it is only in being creative that the individual discovers the self" (Winnicott 1971a: p. 54). Play is different from

---

[5] Transitional space (intermediate area, third area) is that space of experiencing, between the inner and outer worlds, and contributed to by both, in which primary creativity exists and can develop (Winnicott 1971a).

games with established rules.[6] Spontaneous play allows expression of inner psychic processes and may therefore contribute to variations of representations. Without requirements or constraints, it provides an abundance of creativity. "Within the inner life of the child, play is a mental process which takes its stand along with, intermingles with, builds upon and integrates with many other mental processes in the developing child's mind—thinking, imaging, pretending, planning, wondering, doubting, remembering, guessing, hoping, experimenting, revising and working through" (Cohen 2006: p. 137).

Winnicott (1971a) speaks of an area of play, a potential space between an individual and his environment. In this area, two persons can create new representations together, offering different solutions and significant meanings, sometimes out of chaotic and senseless elements. In the mother–child interaction, the mutual play is of essential importance. Already in the second month of life, eye contact and vocal accompaniment are significant interactions between mother and infant.

The child explores in play how things can be accomplished and how roles can be assigned and alternated. He learns to comment with words his play scenes. Playing gives opportunities to distribute attention over longer periods. The play becomes more diverse and meets the growing initiative of the child. The child learns to perform play sequences and to carry out individual movements. With time children participate in interpersonal agreements. Most interactive plays are full of transitions; the adult person introduces something new and gradually the child is able to perform his own ideas in the play.

With repetitive play the child tries to master past experiences. Children explore their relationship with significant persons and show—in their fantasy play—their expectations and wishes, as well as how the meaningful persons should answer their needs and desires (Cohen 2006). The therapeutic and restorative functions of playing have already been discussed by Anna Freud (1965). Later, Winnicott (1971a) considered playing as one of the important features fostering development. Playing allows a child to experiment identifications and solutions of intrapsychic conflict situations and to gain self-understanding and self-awareness. In therapeutic consultations during playing "… the significant moment is that at which the child surprises himself or herself. It is not the moment of my clever interpretation that is significant" (Winnicott 1971a: p. 51). The "just pretend play" facilitates the emergence of unconscious wishes and conflicts; their verbalization in play—that is on a displacement level—may be less anxiety provoking and more acceptable for a child, allowing later a referring of his play-story to himself and his own difficulties.

## Psychoanalytical Therapeutic Group Psychodrama

Human relationships are organized in specific structures, similar to the structure of the myths (Levi-Strauss 1963, 1969). In every civilization, individual or private myths provide a fundamental basis for childhood development, serving the social

---

[6] For a review, see *Play, Playfulness, Creativity and Innovation* (Bateson and Martin 2013).

organization, such as the parent–child relationship. In therapeutic psychodrama, the child has the opportunity to explore—outside the ordinary social order of the family—its individual myths, for example, the Oedipus myth, which Freud used as basis for his concept "oedipal complex."[7]

The dramatic nature of psychodrama can be compared with the classical tragedy: The Greeks have left us poetic and dramatic texts of people and heroes in the struggle with unpredictable gods. The myth in the tragedies is reinterpreted again and again in manifold versions. The therapeutic psychodrama obeys the rule on which the classical tragedy is based, namely the unity of time, place and action. In tragedy, the transgression of the faith-based collective human order and its restitution are presented.

In the psychoanalytical psychodrama, the child experiences the principles of human reality expressed in the myths, such as the difference between generations and gender. The child understands more intuitively than rationally the phenomena of birth, incest, death, love, and hate. He learns to adapt his wishes to the order of human reality. According to Anzieu (1979), the effectiveness of the psychodrama is a symbolic efficiency. The task of the therapists is to represent the private myths in the play and to portray those myths in word and deed. This allows the child to experiment with relationships pattern, to invent new relationship opportunities, and to free himself—due to his increasing awareness—of unconscious conflictual obsessions.

The attraction of the psychodrama is the "realization" of children's phantasms, emotions, and wishes of magic satisfaction. The interindividual relations during the play are in a constant process of development, confront the child with the order of coexistence among persons, which the child over time will no longer deny. The symbolic function of therapeutic psychodrama is situated between looking for an enjoyment and the necessity of recognizing a given and preexisting order. The inner drama of the child is shown in the outside world, in a space that is inhabited by persons who sooner or later symbolize the interindividual situation of the original conflicts. The repetitions of the original emotional disorders lead to symbolic (re)constructions, unknot conflictual situations, and release emotional energy. Inhibitory or pathogenic affects are revived and appear in the transference relationship.

The participation of the therapists is threefold: physical, emotional, and reflective. Between the two poles of body language on one side and verbalized thoughts on the other, the therapists can use opportunities—depending on the situation and moment of the therapeutic process—for therapeutic interventions or interpretations in the hic and nunc. They address their understanding of the child's early psychological trauma, respectively, its consequences, which are actually expressed in the play, without searching for the biographical facts (this information is told by the child' parents in parallel interviews sessions).

---

[7] Already the baby is able to establish triadic exchanges and build triadic relationship structures. Yet the infant has not a clear representation of the sexuality and the relationship between his parents. In the course of development, between about 2 and 5 years, children perceive the sexual differences of their parents. The conflicts associated with this development are called oedipal.

Psychoanalytically oriented psychodrama therapy deals always with the personal history of the child. His story reveals the child's relationships and his interpersonal situation. Children rarely speak directly of themselves. The symbolic interpretation addresses the mythical story. The identity and similarity of the mythical story with the personal drama of the child are at the root of the spontaneous and effective dramatization taking place in the psychoanalytic therapeutic psychodrama (Steck 1998, 1999).

## Psychopharmacological Treatment

The concept of depression or schizophrenia as a brain or neurological disorder is often understood as suggesting that these conditions can be treated with medications only. Yet there is plenty of scientific data showing that this is not the case. While antipsychotic and antidepressive medications are useful, there is so far no evidence that they repair an underlying biological abnormality. Psychiatric diagnostic categories, such as depression or schizophrenia, do not seem to fit biologically distinct diseases, and the goal to define an individual biology of these diseases remains elusive. While genomics research has come up with an array of gene variants associated with mental disorders, these variants are often shared by different conditions such as depression or schizophrenia and confer only minimal risk. Claims that with the help of biomarkers and cognitive tests we may identify groups of patients with better response for pharmacological treatment (Insel 2012) underestimate the underlying tremendous individual variations. It is now increasingly recognized that personal life experiences play a critical role in the development of mental illness. The British Psychological Society on Understanding Psychosis and Schizophrenia (cited by Luhrmann 2015) emphasizes the need for patients with mental illness suffering from distressing symptoms to tell extensively about their lived experiences and to attribute meaning to what they endured. There is ample evidence that adverse or traumatic life events have profound effect on brain development. Treating mental health problems will always require psychosocial interventions and not just a pharmacological approach.

Child and adolescent psychopharmacological treatment is much more than writing prescriptions, even if psychopharmacological interventions in various child and adolescent psychiatric diseases have been helpful to reduce psychological suffering and improve quality of life. Psychopharmacological treatment for children and adolescents requires to consider specific implications: the evaluation and safety profile of various psychoactive drugs indicated for psychiatric disorders is still insufficient; many drugs on the market are not yet legally approved for use in children and adolescents; the long-term effects of a psychopharmacological treatment on child and adolescent development are not sufficiently known; the evaluation of the efficacy of psychopharmacological therapy remains difficult in the child and adolescent age group.

In children and adolescents with serious psychiatric symptomatology, knowledge and application of different treatment methods are mandatory. In most cases of severe psychiatric disorders, psychopharmacological treatment is necessary yet cannot be applied as the only therapeutic intervention. Combination with psychotherapy is indicated. The idea of combining psychotherapy and psychopharmacological therapy is not new. In 1962 Ostow, a neurologist and psychoanalyst already emphasized the benefits of psychotropic drugs during psychoanalytic treatment. He observed that one of the principal effects of psychotropic drugs was on affects and emotions, altering the behavior of the patient to a greater extent than conscious interpretations. Later Sanders (1998) and Stern (1998) confirmed Ostow's findings saying that the changes in unconscious procedural memory are more important for the psychotherapeutic progress than conscious insight.

Today, in serious mental illnesses, combined psychotherapy and psychopharmacological therapy is usually considered the best way to achieve optimal long-term outcomes and reduce disease relapse. In selecting a treatment method, there should never be an either-or decision; but each time the appropriate optimal therapeutic measure must be applied.

The following questions have to be asked: which symptoms or disorders should be treated to improve the child's relationship with his parents and to promote the child's psychological development? The autonomy of the patient and his parent should always be respected. Throughout the therapeutic process, the focus has to be the child's development, not only his symptoms and—besides being a patient—the child has always to be regarded as a person. Listening to the parents' or family's story intensively and over time creates a containment of their anxiety and guilt and helps them to adjust and accept the changes triggered by the therapeutic process (Cohen 2006). It is mandatory to establish a therapeutic concept for the individually ill child and his family.

It is the task of the child and adolescent psychiatrist to integrate knowledge of the advantages of pharmacological treatment and the underlying neurobiological progress to meet the demand of the ill child and his family, and at the same time to offer a significant relationship and a meaningful dialogue. The analytical process is never linear and both patient and therapist undergo unconscious processes; the experience of past events and associated emotions is reactivated in the current relationship. The psychotherapist has always to be aware that it will be the patient who "knows" what he needs in order to be able to change.

Oliver Sacks (1984: p. 164) in *A leg to stand on* states: "Neuropsychology, like classical neurology, aims to be entirely objective, and it's their great power, its advances come from just this. But a living creature, and especially a human being is first and last *active*—a subject, not an object. It is precisely the subject, the living 'I,' which is being excluded" and has to be included by child and adolescent psychiatrists in their discipline. Whatever therapeutic progress is achieved by psychopharmacology, the aim of child and adolescent psychotherapists is to offer— to the suffering individual—a meaningful dialogue and a sustainable relationship, which can sometimes be quite difficult, as Kafka in his story *A Country Doctor* puts it: "To write prescriptions is easy but to come to an understanding with people is hard" (Kafka 1952: p. 152).

# Narratives

## *Introduction*

Narratives belong to the oldest tradition of mankind. This is evidenced, for example, in the epic poems of Greece (Iliad and Odyssey), or the Old and New Testaments of the Bible, the carriers and transmitters of individual and cultural identity and heritage of previous generations to future generations. In all cultures, there is a tendency to create stories about human diversity and to share tradition-based meanings: the soul of the people is reflected in their legends (Murray 1938).

Narratives reveal un- and preconscious representations and phantasms of individual experiences. Telling a story connects—by means of symbolism—memories, images, and scenes with the associated emotions and language (Bucci 1994). The telling of one's own life has a constructive quality; the failure to tell personal narratives or the loss of the ability to bring life experiences into history may represent a personal and familial tragedy that can take a sociocultural historical dimension, as the communicative flow of human experience is interrupted. Narratives may also represent defense mechanisms against unacceptable or painful psychic contents.

The abundant human sciences literature of narratives demonstrates the multiplicity of theories, definitions, and methodologies of personal narratives. According to Bruner and Watson (1983), narratives are embedded in history and culture and arise from these complex influences. A story is a substitute experience, which remains in a domain between the real and the imaginary. The interpretations of narratives need to comply with divergent moral obligations. Human culture contains collectively shared systems of meaning. We learn the everyday psychology of our culture early on, as we acquire language and carry out the interpersonal transactions necessary for living together. The great need for construction of meaning consists of getting things in a proper serial order, marking them with their specific properties and expressing them in the context of a particular point of view. Narrative structures are already inherent in the practice of social interaction before they can be expressed by language. Our innate and primitive predisposition to narrative organization is sustained by our culture with its already developed means of storytelling. It is the sequence of sentences and not the truth or falsity of the meaning of a single sentence that defines the configuration and structure of a story. This unique sequentiality is essential for the meaning of a story and the type of mental organization, according to which it is recorded.

Singer (2004) summarizes the research on narrative identity and meaning attribution across the adult life-span: "Our ability to construct narratives evolves and changes over all phases of the lifespan, as does our capacity for autobiographical reasoning and the ability to make meaning of the stories we tell" (p. 443). New life experiences may change the personal narrative identity, which is related to memory, time, individual factors, and critical circumstances. Personal narratives help a subject to be connected to the past, live in the present and anticipate his future. During developmental phases and transition periods, personal identity may change and the corresponding narrative may present the so-called turning point. According to Riessman (2013), these turning points change the significance of past experiences and have an impact on a subject's identity.

Already infants attempt to grasp courses of action in commonly shared "stories." Damasio (1994) speaks of preverbal narratives. They are established in the earliest relationships with primary caregivers through nonverbal communication and contain perceptions of emotions and bodily sensations. After learning the language, the preverbal narratives are transformed, that is translated into verbal narratives.

A child configures personal events into an historical unity. Significance is expressed in nonverbal (e.g., gestures, facial expressions, tone of voice, body tone and posture) and verbal forms (e.g., narrative representation). Verbal narratives correspond to conscious fantasy formations. At the same time, narratives reveal un- and preconscious ideas and fantasies of individual intrapsychic experiences. The configurations of unconscious or preconscious fantasies often have—at least in verbal "translation"—a narrative character.

The notion of historical "truth" is highly complex as the earliest experiences are not encoded as retrievable memories. "[The analyst's] work of construction, or, if it is preferred, of reconstruction, resembles to a great extent an archaeologist's excavation of some dwelling place that has been destroyed and buried ..." (Freud 1895: p. 259). Where Freud speaks of "the probable historical truth" (p. 261), today the terms "subjective truth" (Frey 2006) or "authenticity" (Collins 2011) are used.

## Narratives in Psychotherapy

The individual history of a person is not a static entity. The mind is composed of more or less integrated areas of lived experiences. Functional parts of thinking and feeling exist besides dysfunctional parts, blocking affects out of fear to feel and to think. In a therapeutic encounter, it is essential that a patient is able to tell the experience of traumatic events with his associated lived emotions and to search for their meaning. The (hi)story of the patient is continually (re)created in the course of an analytical–psychotherapeutic process. The patient attempts to establish a self-continuity, so that his past feels connected—without ruptures—with the self-experience he lives in the present.

### Clinical Vignette Helen

Helen, an Asian girl, arrived in Switzerland at age four-and-a-half years for adoption. Her mother left her when she was 5 months old and her biological father remarried when she was three. Helen lived together with her father and stepmother for one-and-a-half years. At four-and-a-half, she was placed in her prospective adoptive family (parents with two biological sons). After a suicide attempt at age sixteen, Helen left her foster family and lived with her godfather.

One month before her baccalaureate at eighteen-and-a-half, Helen began psychotherapy, which lasted three-and-a-half years. Shortly after passing her baccalaureate and at the beginning of her psychotherapy, Helen left Switzerland for a few weeks—as she had planned for a long time—in search of her biological father who had immigrated to another continent. After the reunion with her father and his family (stepmother and two half-siblings) and her return to Switzerland, Helen suffered from a severe state of depression, multiple somatic symptoms, and consulted various specialists; no organic pathology was diagnosed.

In the next 3 years (19–22), Helen prepared for an admission exam to enter physiotherapist training, which—in spite of considerable efforts—she failed three times. At the same time, she continued to search for her biological mother in her country of origin. Helen described her many very short-lasting heterosexual relationships as disappointing and longed for a stable, continuous relationship. She saw a connection between her emotional relationship difficulties and her inability to start professional training. She believed that if she could succeed in her professional career, she would also be able to engage in a significant emotional relationship.

Helen had her first sexual relationship with her "brother," the biological son of her foster parents, which was the main reason for her suicide attempt at 16 and her desire to leave her family. She had kept the sexual relationship—incestuous in her eyes and against the law—secret from her foster parents. In a few interviews with her family, the secret was revealed, which helped Helen in the elaboration process of her past history in her foster family, promoting greater closeness to all family members.

A few months after these interviews and just before the last opportunity for Helen to pass her entrance exam, Helen—fantasying—said: "If I pass the exam, my success will be related to the death of one of my beloved persons." She knew—she said—that her biological mother was dead because she had been unable to find her, and she was certain that she herself must have caused her death. She thought that it was not her mother who had abandoned her when she was 5 months old, but that she had killed her mother.

One can assume that her fear, a person close to her would die, if she allowed herself to pass successfully the exam, represents the fear of her own breakdown, which Helen had suffered at the moment she lost her biological mother at age five months, a breakdown she has never been able to mourn and integrate in her adult personality.

The fear of breaking down (Winnicott 1974) has its roots in the need to "remember" the original breakdown, which occurred at a development stage, when Helen was dependent on maternal or parental support. Protective forms were missing in Helen's infancy and early childhood. The original experience of "primitive agony" must first be brought into the present experience of an individual and his coping process, before it can belong to the past. To be able to continue emotional development from where it came to a standstill, the patient must return to his early childhood or infancy (Winnicott 1987b). The past is "unknowingly" projected into the future and the recollection can only take place by reliving and mastering the traumatic event in the present. The patient has to return emotionally to the moment when her emotional development was interrupted by the traumatic experience in infancy or early childhood.

Helen endured a very critical time in her psychotherapy, her psychic vulnerability being extreme. In her regressive movements, she was overwhelmed by intense emotions of sadness, pain, rage, and terrorizing fears of annihilation, disintegration, and depersonalization. Finally, she was able to recognize that her fantasies originated from feelings of helplessness and guilt. She learned to distance herself from the upsetting fantasied memories and to tell and envisage different meanings for the traumatic events she had been exposed to in early childhood. By (re)constructing her personal history (narration), she reached a turning point. Helen passed her exams. At this time, she was almost 22 years old, her biological mother's age, when pregnant with her.

According to Guyotat (1980), transmission from parents to children that is from one generation to another is an absolute necessity. If such a legacy cannot be realized, the need for transmission of heritage is replaced by chronology as demonstrated in this vignette, Helen being able to begin a mourning process of her losses at the age when her mother was expecting her. Later, Helen was engaged in a meaningful relationship with a partner.

A mourning process can be considered as engaged if the mourner is able to accept that his love for the new chosen person does not threaten to replace the love for the lost person (Nasio 1996). The image of the lost person must not be wiped out, but has to be maintained up to the moment when the mourning person succeeds to keep the love for the lost person simultaneously with the love for a new chosen person. Pain is alleviated the moment the grieving person finally admits that his love for a new person will never wipe out that for the lost one.

## Narratives of Children with Adverse Childhood Experiences

Storytelling serves to ascribe meaning and significance to life events that interrupted the continuity of one's own personal experience (Riessman 1990). Creating memories of affective experiences helps establish a continuous sense of self. In psychotherapy, narratives are co-constructions by patient and therapist.

Children who have experienced traumatic events try to understand what happened to them by building an imaginary world "explaining" what they endured. A child often tells these fantasies in a story, a form of narrative. The significance a child attributes to the lived event is—in the course of his development—revised again and again. Traumatized children's narratives include the child's desire to shape what happened to him and at the same time meet his basic need to ward off his feelings of despair, helplessness, fear, shame, and guilt. Narratives also represent the child's wishes to repair what he—on a fantasy level—imagines to have destroyed. These fantasies allow narcissistic gratification, which the child desperately needs because of the unbearable injuries he has suffered. The narratives contain elements of reality but mainly represent fantasy—constructions, which the child may tell as if it were a real experience of his past. The stories can also exclude facts of reality that are too painful or too shameful. Children who have suffered physical or sexual violence often deny that they have been abused, even if they bear visible traces of physical abuse. A boy whose scars on his leg showed the shape of an iron explained that the iron *fell* on him. Often children tell weird, seemingly unrelated stories giving the impression not to match to reality. Adults sometimes accuse their child of lying; his narrative cannot be verified. Conversely, the child may highly idealize his past so that his story appears in grotesque contrast to reality. The too painful experience must be warded off or repressed as children are too much afraid to talk about their past, worrying about revealing secrets, which might have catastrophic consequences. Withdrawal into an inner fantasy world is one way to endure the traumatic situation by investing an alternative world and thus expelling the traumatic situation out of consciousness, to repel the memory of the event, or to split off the initial feelings of fear, helplessness, and despair.

According to Wilkinson and Hough (1996), children seek to create memories from affective experiences to control the impacts of such memories and establish a continuous sense of self in relation to others. This allows the child to build a connection—even if of illusory nature—with the past, and thus a way to "neutralize" his experienced traumatic event.

*ALICE*, 8 years old, is severely traumatized: she was hospitalized at age 18 months in a state of grave neglect and marked developmental retardation. She comments on her drawing as follows: "A girl who is 5 years old takes her 18-month-old doll, also named Alice, for a walk in a baby carriage." Alice wishes to be the 5-year-old girl. She draws two hearts as an expression of their mutual love, two flowers, and a watering can, since the two flowers need water. The wish of 8-year-old Alice appears clearly, namely to care for herself in a regressive state (5 years old), to "heal" her inner 18-month-old infant. Children often show or tell in a very transparent way what they "expect" from the psychotherapist, in other words, the help they need.

## Narratives of Children Living with Surrogate Parents (Adoptive or Foster Parents or Caregivers in Institutions)

Storytelling allows children living with surrogate parents to build internal representations of their biological parents. This is an attempt to "repair" the loss of biological parents. Although surrogate parents may replace biological parents in their roles and functions, it is up to the child to build coherent internal parental representations. The older child has to start all over to build up an entirely new relationship with strangers. The construction of a new significant bond with surrogate parents is more difficult for older children because they have not much time to go through earlier developmental stages in a regressive movement and to mourn their often multiple losses before they are confronted with the challenges of adolescence.

Narratives may resemble tales or myths: One theme deals with the fantasy of exposure. According to Moro (1989), the exposed child is faced with an experience of extraordinary danger; he preserves the memory of the threatening situation in the form of interactive fantasies between himself and his environment. These fantasy constructions oscillate between two poles: from extreme psychic vulnerability to the development of extraordinary creative potential. The child grows up in an environment that shares the child's belief of his radical otherness. Exposure and abandonment may have the significance of a hidden potential infanticide. In his fantasies, the child asks the existential question to whom he owes his survival. Has the child survived thanks to a miracle, a good fairy, an angel, a protecting animal, or because of his personal omnipotence? The stories try to give answers to such questions as the following vignette shows.

CHRISTOPHER, a ten-and-a-half-year-old boy from South America, adopted at the age of 3, tells—during the first interview with the child psychiatrist—in the presence of his adoptive mother, the following story: "A whale in the ocean finds a little boy who fell into the water, and brings him to the shore. The whale is caught by fishermen, but they let him go because he had saved a little boy." Asked about the age of the little boy in the story, Christopher answers: "The boy is *three* years old" and he adds:"He lost himself." One does not know, Christopher says, what happened to his parents. This narrative evokes the biblical story of Jonas' rebirth after his stay in the belly of a whale.

The narrative a child tells of his past contains numerous interrogations about guilt and responsibility. Christopher believes to be responsible "the boy lost himself" for having been abandoned. The following vignette shows the frequent phantasm of abandoned children to have been stolen by surrogate or adoptive parents.

RAPHAEL, 6 years old, has lived for 3 years with his surrogate parents. Because of his dangerous auto-aggressive behavior, the school no longer wanted to be responsible for Raphael. In psychoanalytical psychodrama group therapy, Raphael tries repeatedly to hurt himself and has to be almost continually physically contained. He accuses the therapists of being thieves of treasures and children. Finally, he exclaims: "I want to kill myself" and asks:" Why can't I kill myself?" Raphael is overwhelmed by feelings of having been stolen by his surrogate parents. He maintains his emotional bonding to his biological parents and blames his surrogate parents (in the transference the therapists). In the role of a helpless victim of his past traumatic experiences, he expresses his pain and despair in auto-aggressive behavior, driven by the fantasy that only death will relieve him.

Infantile pain occurs when the basic needs of the infant are not fulfilled and is associated with lack of emotional communication at a stage of the infant's absolute dependence. This experience leads to a distorted development process and is accompanied by unimaginable fears of falling, disintegration, and depersonalization. Infantile pain is often warded off by panic and sometimes by suicide (Winnicott 1987a).

Narratives also contain phantasms of narcissistic murderous rage. These phantasms are denied, but expressed in symbolic forms, e.g., in play and drawings or acted out in aggressiveness, representing in most cases the dramatization of an inner reality, too negative to be tolerated. Antisocial tendency arises from loss or deprivation and is an emergency signal. One could say the acting out is an alternative to despair (Winnicott 1965). If a child feels hopeless in terms of repairing the original trauma, he lives in a state of relative depression or dissociation, which conceals the chaotic, constantly threatening state. However, when the child begins to be engaged in a significant relationship, the antisocial tendency often starts to manifest itself as a kind of compulsion to wickedness (e.g., to steal the meaningful person) or—through destructive behavior—to reactivate a severe or even punishing answer, as the following vignette illustrates.

## Clinical Vignette Frederick

Frederick's first child psychiatric examination takes place at age 10 years because of behavioral problems (stealing, lying, and running away) and auto-aggressive acting out (physical injuries). At age five, Frederick was placed in foster care for adoption, but Frederick is not yet legally adopted because of his behavior problems. At the time of his integration into the future adoptive family, Frederick wished to change his name. He named himself after the last name of the foster family and gave himself a new first name.

In the initial contact with the child psychiatrist, Frederick is very cautious, takes great care; he appears suspicious, observing and controlling the relationship with the interviewer. In a squiggle game (Winnicott 1971b),[8] he draws a half fir tree and says it will soon be winter. The fir tree will be a Christmas tree; therefore, the tree is cut and sold, then decorated but finally thrown away.

Frederick seems to tell his own story, namely that of a half-child (deprived of the biological parents), who cherishes the hope to grow into a pretty Christmas tree in the new foster family.

Frederick associates that he has seen a picture of his father in which only half of his father is shown. He knows nothing about his biological parents; he does not want to know since this is linked with too unpleasant thoughts he would rather wipe out.

In the following squiggle, Frederick tells the story of two robbers, whose main concern is to steal. The next squiggle is about a parrot that had flown to America. Frederick adds that he did not have—since age 4—any contact with his biological mother who had left forever to America, and Frederick continues: "Hello, how are you, many greetings from your son." The mother greets him, yet closes the door right away. The parrot flies inside through the window, but the mother has already gone. He tries to reach her by phone, but she pulls the plug from the phone. Frederick (as the parrot) pecks his mother with his beak. He thus demonstrates his anger towards his biological mother rejecting him again.

Frederick has never been able to accomplish a grieving process over the loss of his biological parents and his past history, marked by multiple relationships-ruptures and environmental changes. He is overwhelmed by archaic impulses and feelings that he tries to ward off and control and that he expresses through his physical injuries and in his antisocial and dangerous behavior.

---

[8] The Squiggle Game was described by D. W. Winnicott (1896–1971) pediatrician and psychoanalyst. It corresponds to a modality of diagnostic and therapeutic dialogue and is a way of maintaining contact with the conscious and unconscious personality interests of a patient. Winnicott conceived his game as interactive, as a form of therapeutic communication with children.

Embarrassing, painful memories, especially losses are denied. The subject behaves as if cut off from his memories of the past and lives in a sort of continuous present, where there is neither loss nor death. These children live for the day and are not capable of projecting themselves into the future, or only into all powerful, unrealizable projects.

## Narratives Promote a Grieving Process and the Working Through of Loss and Psychic Trauma

If a child begins, by fantasying, to tell his experienced past to a significant caregiver, it is of little importance whether these narratives actually represent elements of reality or not. Above all it is essential that the child is able to share, in his own way, his inner psychic reality. The adult person whom the child trusts has to be emotionally available and listen to the child's story. He has to identify himself with the child, to empathize with his suffering and pain, without being overwhelmed by such feelings himself. The adult person should neither condemn the child nor the people who took care of or victimized the child. Listening and being emotionally present corresponds simultaneously to bearing the horror and intolerable feelings the child once suffered.

If the child is unable to express in words what happened to him, he may show through symptomatic behavior, what he cannot integrate mentally. By recording the child's narratives during his development, the adult person helps a very important process to take place, namely that unconscious preverbal and emotional contents are symbolized and gain consciousness.

Narratives change, because children perceive and express only gradually their—with unconscious fantasies associated—emotions, according to their development and the ability to tolerate those feelings intrapsychically. Children need an adult person who empathizes with their despair and helps to understand their past experience by ascribing meaning and coherence. This process allows the child to slowly admit his feelings of grief over his painful losses and associated injuries. Mourning allows him to find and build up his identity with respect to the double parental couple (and eventually the double cultures), thus helping to restore his psychic equilibrium.

Thanks to narratives, perception, and expression of fantasies, and emotions of traumatic experiences can take place. The affective history of the child is reactivated with the child's hope that the significant caregivers will be able to help him processing and find meaning of his lived events. Only words make experiences nameable and communicable (Tisseron 1992). If traumatic experiences remain unspoken, i.e., withdrawn from verbal discourse, then secrets of unimaginable or non-pronounceable events emerge. The existence of a secret interferes with any meaningful relationship, also the parent–child relationship. The smooth emotional dialogue between surrogate parents and their child is so important because otherwise unnamed fantasies, desires, fears, and feelings about biological parents and about the origin and the personal history of the child result in additional intra-familial secrets.

The revelation of the fantasied and or real past allows a common shared experience based on the narrated history and strengthens the affective bond of surrogate (foster, adoptive) parents and child. The narratives that children tell to significant caregivers allow integration of split emotional contents, which consist mainly of "translating" un- and preconscious processes into a metaphorical language.

The most difficult and undoubtedly most important task for children is to bring together, in their inner world, their mental representations of biological and other significant caregivers—if any existed—with those of their surrogate (foster, adoptive) parents (Ferrari 1986). Thanks to this fantasied convergence a sense of genetic ancestry and belonging is being built up and with it an authentic parent–child attachment and relationship is created.

# References

Andrade VM. Affect and the therapeutic action of psychoanalysis. Int J Psychoanal. 2005;86: 677–97.

Anzieu D. Le psychodrame analytique chez l'enfant et l'adolescent. Paris: Presses universitaires de France; 1979.

Bargh JA, Morsella E. The unconscious mind. Perspect Psychol Sci. 2008;3(1):73–9, p. 78.

Bateson P, Martin P. Play, playfulness, creativity and innovation. Cambridge: Cambridge University Press; 2013.

Bleichmar H. Making conscious the unconscious in order to modify unconscious processing: Some mechanisms of therapeutic change. Int J Psychoanal. 2004;85:1379–400.

Brazelton TB, Nugent JK. The Neonatal Behavioral Assessment Scale. Cambridge: Mac Keith Press; 1995.

Breuer J, Freud S. Studies on hysteria. 2nd ed. Leipzig: Deuticke; 1895.

Britton R. in: Gabbard GO, Scarfone D. Controversial discussions' the issue of differences in method. Int J Psychoanal. 2002;83:453–456. doi:10.1516/TEJQ-CUY8-FCQ8-85UR.

Bruner J, Watson R. Child's talk: learning to use language. New York: WW. Norton; 1983.

Bucci W. The multiple code theory and the psychoanalytic process: a framework for research. Annu Psychoanal. 1994;22:239–59.

Bürgin D, Steck B. Indikation psychoanalytischer Psychotherapie bei Kindern und Jugendlichen, Diagnostisch-therapeutisches Vorgehen und Fallbeispiele. Stuttgart: Klett-Cotta; 2013. ISBN 978-3-608-94829-5.

Cohen D. Life is with others, Selected writings on child psychiatry. New Haven: Yale University Press; 2006.

Collins S. On authenticity: the question of truth in construction and autobiography. Int J Psychoanal. 2011;92:1391–409. doi:10.1111/j.1745-8315.2011.00455.x.

Damasio AR. Descartes Error. Emotion, reason, and the human brain, A Grosset/Putnam book. New York: G.P. Putnam's Sons; 1994.

Dehaene S, Changeux JP. Experimental and theoretical approaches to conscious processing. Neuron. 2011;70(2):200–27. doi:10.1016/j.neuron.2011.03.018.

Edelman GM, Tononi G. A universe of consciousness: how matter becomes imagination. New York: Basic Books; 2000.

Eickhoff FW. On nachträglichkeit: the modernity of an old concept. Int J Psychoanal. 2006;87: 1453–69.

Ferrari P. La filiation en psychopathologie de l'enfant. Ann Pediatr. 1986;33(8):713–8.

Fischmann T, Russand MO, Leuzinger-Bohleber M. Trauma, dream, and psychic change in psychoanalyses: a dialog between psychoanalysis and the neurosciences. Front Hum Neurosci. 2013;7:877. doi:10.3389/fnhum.2013.00877.

Freud A. Indications for child analysis. The psychoanalytical study of the child, vol. 1. New York: International Universities Press; 1945. p. 127–49.

Freud A. Normality and pathology in childhood. New York: International University Press; 1965.

Freud S. Project for a scientific psychology, vol. I. London: Hogarth Press; 1895. p. 295–391.

Freud S. Heredity and the aetiology of the neuroses, vol. III. London: Hogarth Press; 1896a. p. 143–56.

Freud S. Further remarks on the neuro-psychoses of defence, vol. III. London: Hogarth Press; 1896b. p. 162–85.

Freud S. The interpretation of dreams (First Part), vol. IV. London: Hogarth Press; 1900.

Freud S. The interpretation of dreams (Second Part), vol. V. London: The Hogarth Press; 1900–1901.

Freud S. Psychopathology of everyday life. New York: The Macmillan; 1901. p. 74. A. A. Brill translation; 1914.

Freud S. The dynamics of transference, vol. XII. London: Hogarth Press; 1912. p. 97–108.

Freud S. Remembering, repeating and working-through (Further recommendations on the technique of psycho-analysis, II), vol. XII. London: Hogarth Press; 1914. p. 147–56.

Freud S. The unconscious, vol. XIV. London: Hogarth Press; 1915. p. 159–215.

Freud S. Beyond the pleasure principle, vol. XVIII. London: Hogarth Press; 1920. p. 7–64.

Freud S. The ego and the id and other works, vol. XIX. London: Hogarth Press; 1923–1925.

Freud S. An Autobiographical Study, Inhibitions, Symptoms and Anxiety, The Question of Lay Analysis and Other Works, vol. XX. London: Hogarth Press; 1925-1926.

Frey J (2006): in Collins S. 2011.

Goleman D. Emotional intelligence. New York: Bantam Books; 1995. p. 213.

Guyotat J. Mort/naissance et filiation, Etudes de psychopathologie sur le lien de filiation. Paris: Masson; 1980.

Jiménez JP. After pluralism: towards a new, integrated psychoanalytic paradigm. Int J Psychoanal. 2006;87(Pt 6):1487–507.

Insel TR. Next-generation treatments for mental disorders. Sci Transl Med. 2012;4(155):155ps19. doi:10.1126/scitranslmed.3004873.

Kafka F. A country doctor. In: Selected short stories of Franz Kafka. New York: The Modern Library; 1952. p. 149–56.

Riessman C. Strategic uses of narrative in the presentation of self and illness: a research note. Soc Sci Med. 1990;30:1195–200.

Riessman C. Analysis of personal narratives. In: Fortune AE, Reid WJ, Miller RL, editors. Handbook of interviewing. New York: Columbia University Press; 2013.

Laplanche J, Pontalis JB. Vocabulaire de la psychanalyse. Paris: P.U.F.; 1967.

Laplanche J, Pontalis JB (1973, p 112). The language of psychoanalysis [1967], Nicholson-Smith D, translator. London: Hogarth. 510 p. (International Psycho-analytical Library, No 94.)

Lebovici S. Die Gegenübertragung in der Kinderanalyse. Psyche. 1952;5:680–7.

Levi-Strauss C. Anthropologie structurale (1958, Structural Anthropology, trans. Claire Jacobson and Brooke Grundfest Schoepf, 1963)

Levi-Strauss C. Les Structures élémentaires de la parenté (1949, The Elementary Structures of Kinship, ed. *Rodney Needham, trans. J. H. Bell, J. R. von Sturmer, and Rodney Needham, 1969)

Luhrmann TM. NewYork Times 2015: Jan. 17

Maldonado JL. What is your theory of unconscious processes? What are other theories that you would contrast with your conceptualization? Response by Jorge Luis Maldonado. Int J Psychoanal. 2011;92:280–3. doi:10.1111/j.1745-8315.2011.00425.x.

Mancia M. Implicit memory and early unrepressed unconscious: their role in the therapeutic process (How the neurosciences can contribute to psychoanalysis). Int J Psychoanal. 2006;87(Pt 1):83–103. doi:10.1516/39M7-H9CE-5LQX-YEGY.

Marion P. Some reflections on the unique time of Nachträglichkeit in theory and clinical practice. Int J Psychoanal. 2012;93(2):317–40. doi:10.1111/j.1745-8315.2011.00530.x.

Matte-Blanco I. Thinking, feeling, and being: Clinical reflections on the fundamental antinomy of human beings and world. London: Routledge. 1988; 347 p. New Library of Psychoanalysis, vol. 5. In Jiménez JP; 2006.

Modell AH. Other times, other realities. Toward a theory of psychoanalytic treatment. Cambridge: Harvard University Press; 1990.

Moro MR. L'enfant exposé. Grenoble: Editions La Pensee Sauvage; 1989.

Murray HA. Explorations in personality. New York: Oxford University Press; 1938.

Nasio JD. Le livre de la douleur et de l'amour. Paris: Editions Payot & Rivages; 1996.

Ogden TH. What's true and whose idea was it? Int J Psychoanal. 2003;84:593–606. doi:10.1516/HHJT-H54F-DQB5-422W.

Ostow M. Drugs in psychoanalysis and psychotherapy. New York: Basic Books; 1962.

Pulver SE. On the astonishing clinical irrelevance of neuroscience. J Am Psychoanal Assoc. 2003 Summer; 51(3):755–72

Sacks O. A leg to stand on. London: Duckworth; 1984. p. 164.

Sanders L. Introductory comment. Infant Ment Health J. 1998;19:280–1.

Scarfone D. On: minding our metaphysics. Int J Psychoanal. 2012;93:1286–8. doi:10.1111/j.1745-8315.2012.00639.x.

Shields W. Dream interpretation, affect, and the theory of neuronal group selection: Freud, Winnicott, Bion, and Modell. Int J Psychoanal. 2006;87(Pt 6):1509–27.

Siegel DJ. Memory: an overview, with emphasis on developmental, interpersonal, and neurobiological aspects. J Am Acad Child Adolesc Psychiatry. 2001;40(9):997–1011.

Singer JA. Narrative identity and meaning making across the adult lifespan: an introduction. J Pers. 2004;72(3):438–59.

Solms M. Before and after Freud's Project: neuroscience of the mind—on the centennial of Freud's project for a scientific psychology. Ann N Y Acad Sci. 1998;843:1–10.

Solms M, Turnbull O. The brain and the inner world: an introduction to the neuroscience of subjective experience. New York: Other Press; 2002. p. 289.

Solms M, Panksepp J. The "Id" knows more than the "ego" admits: neuropsychoanalytic and primal consciousness perspectives on the interface between affective and cognitive neuroscience. Brain Sci. 2012;2:147–75. doi:10.3390/brainsci2020147.

Steck B. Die psychoanalytisch-orientierte Psychodrama-Gruppentherapie bei Kindern und Jugendlichen. Teil 1: Kinderanalyse 1998,6, 278–310. Teil 2: Kinderanalyse 1998, 6, 248–77.

Steck B. Die psychoanalytisch-orientierte Psychodrama-Gruppentherapie bei Kindern und Jugendlichen. Teil 3: Kinderanalyse 1999;7:23–52.

Stern DN. The present moment in psychotherapy and everyday life. New York: Norton; 2004.

Stern DN, Sander LW, Nahum JP, Harrison AM, Lyons-Ruth K, Morgan AC, et al. Non-interpretive mechanisms in psychoanalytic therapy. The 'something more' than interpretation. Int J Psychoanal. 1998;79(Pt 5):903–21.

Stern D. The process of therapeutic change involving implicit knowledge: some implications of developmental observations for adult psychotherapy. Infant Ment Health J; 1998;19:300–8.

The Boston Process Change Study Group. Change in psychotherapy: a unifying paradigm, Norton professional books. New York: W.W.Norton; 2010. ISBN 978-0-393-70599-7.

Tisseron S. Tintin et les secrets de famille. Paris: Aubier; 1992.

Wilkinson S, Hough G. Lie as narrative truth in abused adopted adolescents. Psychoanal Study Child. 1996;51:580–97.

Winnicott DW. The maturational processes and the facilitating environment: studies in the theory of emotional development. London: Hogarth; 1965 (International Psycho-analytical Library, No. 64.).

Winnicott DW. Babies and their Mothers. In: Winnicott C, Davis M, Shepherd R, editors. Reading: Addison-Wesley; 1987a.

Winnicott DW. Home is where we start from: Essays by a psychoanalyst. In: Winnicott C, Shepherd R, Davis M, editors. Reading: Addison-Wesley; 1987b.

Winnicott DW. Playing and reality. London: Tavistock; 1971a.

Winnicott DW. Therapeutic consultations in child psychiatry. London: Hogarth; 1971b.

Winnicott DW. Fear of breakdown. Int R Psychoanal. 1974;1:103–7.

# Index

© Springer International Publishing Switzerland 2016
A. Steck, B. Steck, *Brain and Mind*, DOI 10.1007/978-3-319-21287-6

Printed in the United States
By Bookmasters